The Larynx

The Larynx

Harvey M. Tucker, M.D.
Chairman, Department of
Otolaryngology and
Communicative Disorders
The Cleveland Clinic Foundation
Cleveland, Ohio

1987
Thieme Medical Publishers, Inc., New York
Georg Thieme Verlag, Stuttgart · New York

Thieme Medical Publishers, Inc.
381 Park Avenue South
New York, New York 10016

Cover design: Wendy Ann Fredericks

THE LARYNX
Harvey M. Tucker, M.D.

Library of Congress Cataloging in Publication Data
Tucker, Harvey M.
    The larynx.
    Includes bibliographies and index.
    1. Larynx—Diseases. 2. Larynx. I. Title. [DNLM:
1. Laryngeal Diseases. 2. Larynx. WV 500 T892L]
RF510.T83 1987   617′.533   86-30117

Typeset by Maple-Vail Book Mfg. Group, Binghamton,
NY, U.S.A.
Printed and bound by Kingsport Press, Kingsport, TN,
U.S.A.
Printed in the U.S.A.

TMP ISBN 0-86577-241-X
GTV ISBN 3-13-689701-3

5 4 3 2 1

To my wife, Cynthia Ann Tucker, RN,
without whose friendship and love
this book would never have happened.

Preface

I decided to write this book because of my experiences as a student and resident, and later as an educator of students and residents. It became apparent that there was no single text in which the majority of what one might need to know about the larynx could be found. Although such texts exist for otology and for cosmetic and reconstructive surgery, material pertaining to the larynx is scattered through many sources. Textbooks in head and neck surgery may include much of this information and several fine atlases of laryngeal surgery exist, but at this writing there is no single source to which the student can go for a reasonably complete overview of the subject of laryngology. It is my hope and intention that this text will fill this need.

After much thought, I decided to author most of this text myself, rather than to follow the more common format of inviting several recognized experts to write appropriate chapters. This was not done out of belief that I was the best person to write every chapter, but because of the obvious drawbacks inherent in most multiauthor texts: disparity of style and illustrations, lack of continuity, failure to cover some subjects adequately and redundant coverage of others, as well as difficulty in meeting deadlines when failure of only one person to be on time can delay the entire project. In those areas where I was clearly unable to write the chapter myself, I invited recognized experts to participate, but only with their willingness to allow me extensive editorial leeway in order to avoid most of the problems just cited. I am grateful to my contributors for their promptness, adherence to guidelines, and permission to rewrite those portions of their chapters that I deemed necessary.

I have chosen to use extensive margin notes, in the style of the Talmud, for several reasons: I hoped to provide a text that would be useful to beginners in the discipline of laryngology, but also be detailed enough for more advanced individuals, such as residents and practitioners. This format allows the student to read through the basic information presented in continuity, without needing to digress into the detail that might be desirable for the more advanced reader. The reader who wishes to pursue a subject in greater depth can read the margin notes as they appear in the text or go back to them during a second reading of the material, as desired. The bibliography provided with each chapter allows even more detailed study.

Another reason for using margin notes was to permit me to quote specific authors at an appropriate point in the text without interrupting the train of thought. This made it possible to bring in supporting or opposing views in areas of controversy, as well as to emphasize the importance of certain other sources that the student might wish to read later. In a few cases, I have been fortunate enough to obtain comments made by the author specifically for inclusion in this text.

This book proved to be a much greater undertaking than I had first anticipated. I have discovered that the body of knowledge encompassed by laryngology is so great as to defy my efforts to really cover all of it in depth. As a result, this text is probably incomplete in some areas, especially where there is currently great activity and in which changes will have taken place between writing and publication. Nevertheless, it is my hope that it will serve as a starting point for understanding the anatomy, pathophysiology, diagnosis, and management of diseases of the larynx, in much the same way that certain classic texts have for other aspects of otolaryngology and head and neck surgery. If it succeeds in this, the effort will have been worth it.

In closing, a special thank you to the editorial and production staff at Thieme Medical Publishers, whose professional work helped bring my vision for this book to reality.

Harvey M. Tucker, M.D.

Contributors

Melinda Harrison, MA, CCC-Sp
Speech and Language Pathologist
Department of Otolaryngology and
    Communicative Disorders
The Cleveland Clinic Foundation
Cleveland, Ohio

Dennis K. Heffner, MD, CAPT MC USN
Assistant Chairman
Department of Otolaryngic Pathology
Armed Forces Institute of Pathology
Washington, D.C.

Vincent J. Hyams, MD, CAPT MC USN (Ret)
Chairman, Department of Otolaryngic Pathology
Armed Forces Institute of Pathology
Washington, D.C.

Arnold M. Noyek, MD, FRCS(C), FACS
Professor of Otolaryngology
Professor of Radiology
University of Toronto
Toronto, Canada

Harry S. Shulman, MD, FRCP(C)
Associate Professor of Radiology
University of Toronto
Radiologist-in-Chief
Sunnybrook Medical Centre
Toronto, Canada

James T. Suchy, AMI
Medical Illustrator
Cleveland, Ohio

Contents

The Larynx

Chapter 1

Anatomy and Embryology of the Larynx

The larynx is situated at the crossroads of the air and food passages. It must serve not only as a conduit for air and waste gases to and from the lungs but also as a valve to prevent the passage of secretions, of food and of other foreign material into the upper respiratory tract. In many animals it has also come to serve as an organ of communication, the function of which has reached its highest development in the human. This exquisitely balanced and highly developed organ may be an object of wonder to the uninitiated, but even moreso to the sophisticated observer who has a thorough knowledge of its anatomy, development and physiology. This chapter will deal with the adult and developmental anatomy of the larynx with the intention of providing basic information necessary to the student, and to serve as a refresher to the more advanced reader. A thorough mastery of this material is essential to the discipline of laryngology and will permit the reader to better appreciate the pathological conditions and their management dealt with in subsequent chapters.

Adult Anatomy

Structural Support

The skeletal supports of the larynx are provided by the *hyoid bone* and *six cartilages,* of which three are bilaterally symmetrical and paired. These are connected to each other by a series of membranes and ligaments which are usually named for the structures to which they are attached.

The *hyoid bone* (Fig. 1–1) is not strictly considered part of the larynx by some authors, but since it comprises the anterior aspect of the preepiglottic space and is the point of attachment for muscles and ligaments essential to its function, it certainly deserves a place in consideration of laryngeal anatomy. It derives its name from its U shape and is found at the level of the third cervical vertebra in the adult. It is situated just above the thyroid cartilage in the anterior wall of the hypopharynx in relation to the base of the tongue. It is made up of a *body,* bilateral *greater cornua* and bilateral *lesser cornua.* It is a sesamoid bone in that it articulates with no other cartilaginous or bony structure but is suspended between the supra- and infrahyoid musculature and thus is responsible for the concavity be-

Figure 1–1. Hyoid bone and
thyroid cartilage.

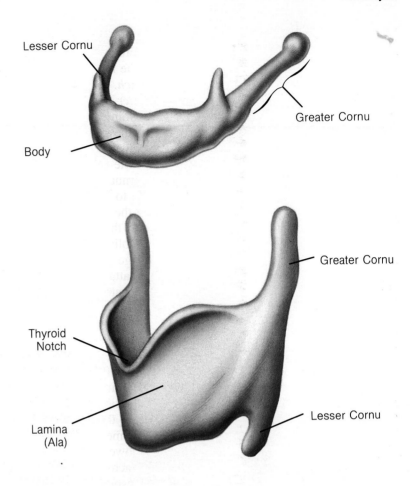

*In performing supraglottic
laryngectomy, the greater cornu of
the hyoid bone can and should be
preserved on the side of noninvolvement. This maneuver
protects the superior laryngeal
nerve, as well as the attachments of
some of the muscles necessary to
coordinated laryngotracheal
movement during swallowing. HMT*

tween the chin and the anterior neck. The *body* is convex forward and from
side to side. It is separated by fat and a bursa from the thyrohyoid membrane, which in turn is separated by fat from the anterior surface of the
epiglottis. At either end of the body on its upper surface is located a small
tubercle called the *lesser cornu.* This is the point of attachment of the medial end of the middle constrictor muscle and of the stylohyoid ligament.
The geniohyoid and genioglossus muscles are attached to the upper surface
and inner surface of the body, while the mylohyoid muscle inserts upon
the anterior surface of the body of the hyoid. The remainder of the middle
constrictor and hyoglossus muscles originate from the *greater cornu,* a
hornlike structure that extends posteriorly and laterally from the body. The
tendon of the digastric muscle is attached to the anterolateral aspect of the
body of the hyoid bone by a retinaculum. The remaining muscles attached
to the hyoid are the infrahyoid group, including the sternohyoid, omohyoid
and, on its inferior surface, the thyrohyoid muscles. The greater cornu of
the hyoid bone is in immediate relationship to the passage of the superior
laryngeal nerve, artery and vein as they traverse the middle and inferior
constrictor muscles to enter the thyrohyoid ligament and thence the larynx
itself.◁

The *cartilages* of the larynx include the *thyroid, cricoid* and *epiglottis*
and the paired *arytenoids, corniculates* and *cuneiforms.* The *thyroid cartilage* (Fig. 1–1), so called because of its shield-like shape when seen *en
face,* is the largest and comprises what the layman refers to as the ''Adam's
apple.'' It is a wedge-shaped structure, the sides of which are called the
laminae. These join each other in the midline at the apex of the wedge,
forming the laryngeal prominence. In the male, these laminae meet at an

angle of approximately 90 degrees, whereas in the female the angle more closely approximates 120 degrees, thus accounting for the more prominent larynx in the male. At their juncture point in the midline is a well-defined *thyroid notch.* Laterally, at the posterior edges of the laminae, are the superior *greater* and the inferior *lesser cornua* of the thyroid cartilage. A more or less prominent oblique line is palpable and visible approximately three-fourths of the way from the anterior commissure to the posterior edge of the lamina, affording attachment for the major muscles and ligaments in this area. The thyroid cartilage articulates with the *cricoid cartilage* at the inferior cornua bilaterally. The inferior border of the thyroid lamina gives attachment to the cricothyroid ligament and along the rest of its inferior margin to the cricothyroideus muscle. The outer surfaces of the laminae give rise to the omohyoid, sternothyroid and inferior constrictor muscles along the oblique line previously mentioned. The upper border of the thyroid cartilage provides attachment for the thyrohyoid membrane and ligament. The attachment of the ventricular bands and the thyroepiglottic ligament is located on the inner surface, at a point approximately halfway between the thyroid notch and the inferior border in males and at approximately the junction of the superior one-third and inferior two-thirds in females.◁ In older specimens there is a palpable tuberosity at this point of attachment. The fibrous attachment of the vocal ligaments penetrates the inner perichondrium and the cartilage and makes contact with the outer perichondrium. This peculiar attachment is referred to as Broyles' ligament.◁ The tips of the greater cornua of the thyroid cartilage are attached to the tips of the greater cornua of the hyoid bone through a dense fibrous band that sometimes contains a small sesamoid cartilage as well (Fig. 1–6). In the lower half of its inner surface, the thyroid cartilage serves as the point of attachment to the thyroarytenoid muscles, which are major adductors and tensors in the vocal cord.

The *cricoid cartilage* (Fig. 1–2) is shaped like an asymmetrical signet ring, the lower border of which is horizontal and the upper border of which constitutes the signet part or *lamina,* which rises above the horizontal between the thyroid laminae posteriorly. The anterior or arch portion is easily palpated immediately below the border of the thyroid cartilage. It is the only complete cartilaginous ring in the upper airway, all the remaining ones being deficient in the posterior aspect.◁ It articulates with the thyroid cartilage through the *cricothyroid joints* bilaterally and with the arytenoids, which rest on the upper surface of its posterior or "signet ring" portion through the *cricoarytenoid joints.* Inferiorly, it is related to the first tracheal ring via ligamentous and musculature attachments only. Anteriorly, along the superior surface of the arch, the cricothyroid ligament and lateral cricoarytenoid muscles are attached, and its inferior rim gives rise to the cricotracheal ligament. The posteriormost aspect of the lamina of the cricoid cartilage gives origin to the posterior cricoarytenoideus muscles on either side of the midline, which are the only abductors of the vocal fold. Laterally, the cricoid cartilage receives the lowermost fibers of the inferior contrictor muscle and the semicircular fibers of the cricopharyngeus muscle, which is the upper sphincter of the esophagus.

The *arytenoid cartilages* (Fig. 1–3) are bilaterally situated and shaped like small, three-sided pyramids, the bases of which are concave, representing the articular facets which glide upon the corresponding facets of the posterosuperior aspect of the cricoid lamina. On their medial surfaces these cartilages are flat and are covered only by mucoperichondrium, very tightly applied to the cartilage. The posterior curved surface receives the fibers of the transverse and oblique arytenoideus muscles (sometimes referred to as interarytenoideus muscles). The thyroarytenoid muscles are at-

The anatomic location of the anterior attachment of the vocal folds may be critical in performance of supraglottic laryngectomy. HMT

Broyles' ligament[4] contains blood vessels and lymphatics within its fibrous tissue. Therefore, if directly invaded by carcinoma, it may serve as an avenue for direct extension of tumor outside the larynx. HMT

If tracheotomy is performed above, through or immediately below the cricoid cartilage, possible chondronecrosis can lead to severe subglottic stenosis. HMT

Figure 1–2. Cricoid cartilage.
a, Anterior view. **b,** Posterior
view. **c,** Right lateral view.

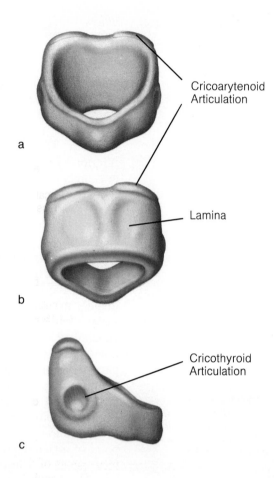

tached to a small tubercle on the posterolateral surface. At the posterolateral corner, a prominent muscular process is found which receives the lateral
and posterior cricoarytenoid muscles. The anteromedial, pointed portion is
referred to as the vocal process. It is the point of attachment of the vocal
ligament, which is connected to the midline of the inner surface of the thyroid cartilage and forms the structural support of the true vocal folds themselves. The upright process or apex of the arytenoid cartilage points pos-
teromedially and serves as the posterior attachment of the aryepiglottic fold.

The *corniculate* and *cuneiform cartilages* (Fig. 1–3) are located within
the substance of the aryepiglottic fold and serve as battens or sesamoid cartilages to support the edges of this membranous structure.

The *epiglottic cartilage* (Fig. 1–4) is composed of elastic cartilage,
unlike the remaining laryngeal cartilages, most of which are hyaline.
Therefore, it does not eventually ossify and remains flexible throughout life.◁
It is leaf shaped and provides the elastic skeleton of the epiglottis. It is
suspended by a series of ligaments and does not articulate directly with any
of the surrounding bony or cartilaginous structures. Its surface is penetrated by multiple small holes that transmit tiny blood vessels and fibrous
tissue attachments from its laryngeal surface to the preepiglottic space. The
laryngeal surface is covered with tightly adherent mucoperichondrium and
provides almost no soft tissue, whereas the anterior or lingual surface is
the posterior wall of the preepiglottic space, which contains loose areolar
tissue and fat. At its inferior end, the epiglottis is attached to the inner
surface of the thyroid cartilage by the strong thyroepiglottic ligament. An-
terosuperiorly, it is attached to the inner surface of the body of the hyoid
bone by the midline hyoepiglottic ligament and laterally to the musculature

*It is this retained flexibility that
permits its use for reconstruction
after near-total laryngectomy. (See
Chapter 13). HMT*

Figure 1–3. Arytenoid cartilages. **a,** Posterior view with cuneiform and corniculate cartilages above. **b,** Inferior view (left), superior view (right). **c,** Anterior view.

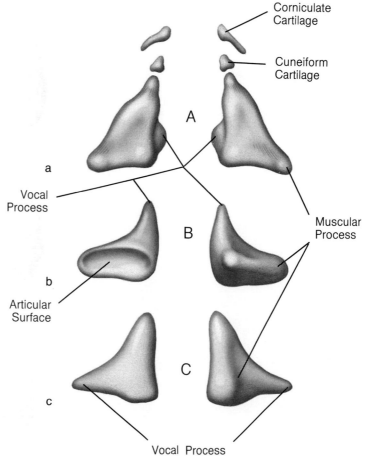

of the base of the tongue by the less prominent glossoepiglottic ligaments. Bilateral pouch-like mucosal reflections between the median hyoepiglottic ligament and these lateral glossoepiglottic ligaments are referred to as the valleculae. The lateral surface of the epiglottis gives rise to the fibers of the oblique and posterior arytenoid muscles, which send slips into the aryepiglottic fold and ligament. Posteriorly, the mucosa of the aryepiglottic fold separates the laryngeal introitus from the opening to the pyriform sinus. The *cuneiform* and *corniculate* cartilages can sometimes be seen as a bulge through the mucosa of the aryepiglottic fold (see Fig. 1–7).

Figure 1–4. Epiglottic cartilage. Note perforations.

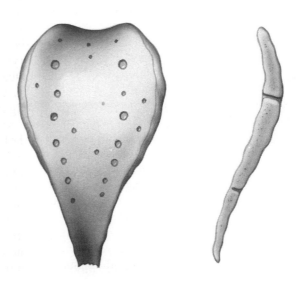

Figure 1–5. Cricothyroid joint,
membrane, and ligament
(above); cricoarytenoid joints,
posterior view (below).

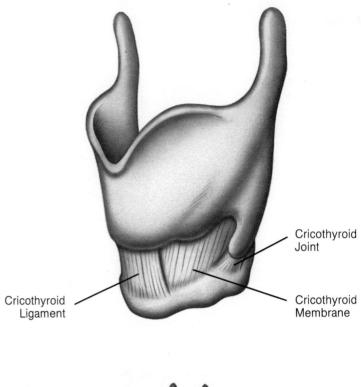

Cricothyroid
Joint

Cricothyroid
Ligament

Cricothyroid
Membrane

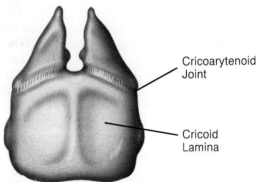

Cricoarytenoid
Joint

Cricoid
Lamina

Joints, Membranes and Ligaments of the Larynx

With the exception of the thyroid, cricoid and arytenoid cartilages, none of the laryngeal cartilages are in direct articulation with any other skeletal structure. The cricoid cartilage may be regarded as the base and support for the entire larynx. It articulates with the other two cartilages mentioned, that is, with the thyroid cartilage via the *cricothyroid joints* and with the arytenoids via the *cricoarytenoid joints* (Fig. 1–5). Both of these are true synovial joints.

The *cricothyroid joint* permits the cricoid cartilage to tilt upward so that the anterior arch will come in closer proximity to the lower border of the thyroid cartilage.[5] In so doing, the distance between the *cricoarytenoid joint* and the inner surface of the thyroid cartilage is lengthened and, assuming that the arytenoids are fixed at this time, increases the tension in the vocal ligaments. The thyroid cartilage is also able to slide in an anterior and posterior direction along the same joint secondary to the pull of the cricothyroideus muscles (see Fig. 1–12).

The *cricoarytenoid joints* are located on the posterosuperior aspect of the cricoid lamina. The articular surfaces on the cricoid lamina are oriented

Figure 1–6. Thyrohyoid
membrane, ligament and
superior laryngeal neurovascular
bundle. Note sesamoid cartilage
between greater cornua of
thyroid cartilage and hyoid
bone.

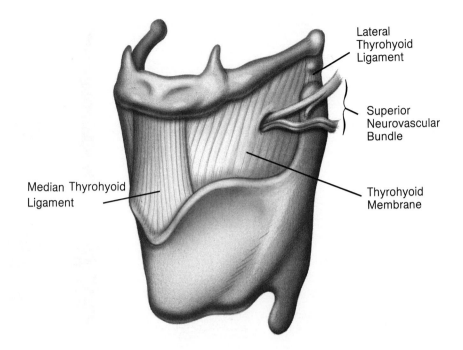

in a slightly posterior direction and are biconcave when seen from above
(Fig. 1–5). The articular surfaces on the under side of the arytenoid cartilages are also biconcave, the concavity being directed medially as well as
inferiorly. When these joints come into contact with each other, the arytenoid will seek the lowest point of the concavity of both joints, unless
there is some muscular pull to the contrary. This accounts for the position
assumed by the vocal cords at rest, which is the intermediate position approximately halfway between the midline and full abduction. The complex
movement of the arytenoids on the cricoarytenoid joints will appear to produce rotary motion. In fact, this apparent rotation is due to the sliding effect both in the anteroposterior direction and in the lateromedial direction
because of the peculiar joint arrangement. Both of these joints, being synovial, are subject to all the disease processes and trauma that afflict any
other joint in the body and can and do become ankylosed under certain
circumstances.

The *thyrohyoid membrane* (Fig. 1–6) is a broad elastic sheet that
stretches from the upper border of the thyroid cartilage, beneath the body
of the hyoid bone to insert on its upper surface. Toward the midline, this
membrane is thicker and can be identified as the *median thyrohyoid ligament* and laterally as the *lateral thyrohyoid ligament*. It is in the lateral-
most aspects of this ligament that a triticeous cartilage is sometimes noted
as a sesamoid structure between the tip of the greater cornu of the hyoid
bone and the greater cornu of the thyroid cartilage. The membrane is penetrated on each side by the superior laryngeal artery, vein and internal laryngeal nerve. The outer surface of this membrane is covered by the infrahyoid muscles. With the hyoid bone, it completes the anterior limits of the
preepiglottic space (Fig. 1–7).

The *cricovocal membrane* or *conus elasticus* (Figs. 1–7, 1–8) arises
from the inner surface of the cricoid arch, passing medially and superiorly
to insert upon the *vocal ligaments* (see Fig. 1–13), which stretch between
the vocal processes of the arytenoid cartilages and the midline inner surface of the thyroid cartilage. The *vocal ligaments* are condensations of the
cricovocal membrane and form the structure of the free margin of the fold.
This *vocal ligament* is surrounded by the medialmost fibers of the lateral

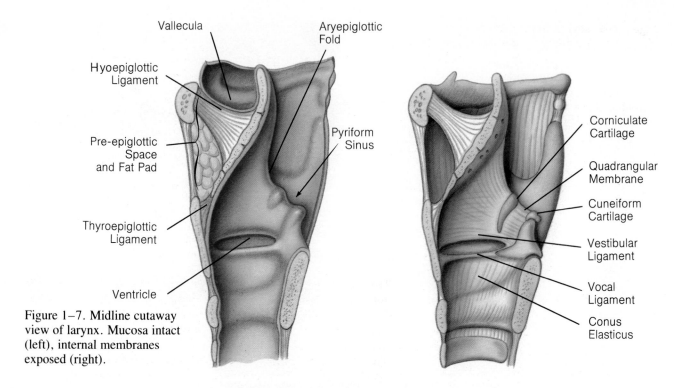

Vallecula

Aryepiglottic
Fold

Hyoepiglottic
Ligament

Pre-epiglottic
Space
and Fat Pad

Pyriform
Sinus

Thyroepiglottic
Ligament

Ventricle

Corniculate
Cartilage

Quadrangular
Membrane

Cuneiform
Cartilage

Vestibular
Ligament

Vocal
Ligament

Conus
Elasticus

Figure 1–7. Midline cutaway
view of larynx. Mucosa intact
(left), internal membranes
exposed (right).

thyroarytenoideus muscles, which are sometimes regarded as a separate muscle called the vocalis.

A less well-defined *quadrangular* membrane (Figs. 1–7, 1–8) arises from the inner aspects of the epiglottis within the aryepiglottic fold and attaches posteriorly to the arytenoid and corniculate cartilages. Inferiorly it attaches to the *vestibular ligament* (false cord) and extends inferiorly around the ventricle to the point of attachment of the upper margin of the true vocal folds.

Figure 1–8. Coronal section of
larynx (semidiagrammatic).

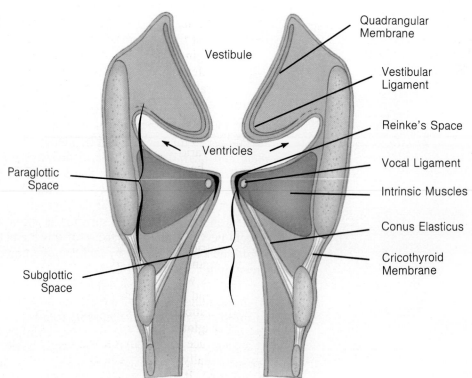

Vestibule

Quadrangular
Membrane

Vestibular
Ligament

Ventricles

Reinke's Space

Vocal Ligament

Paraglottic
Space

Intrinsic Muscles

Conus Elasticus

Cricothyroid
Membrane

Subglottic
Space

Figure 1–9. Larynx from
above. Laryngeal mirror view.

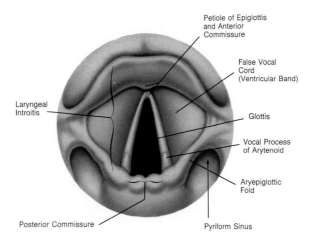

Petiole of Epiglottis
and Anterior
Commissure

False Vocal
Cord
(Ventricular Band)

Laryngeal
Introitis

Glottis

Vocal Process
of Arytenoid

Aryepiglottic
Fold

Posterior Commissure

Pyriform Sinus

*In the great apes, this structure
corresponds to inflatable air sacs
which extend out into the neck.
When distended, the male ape beats
upon them with his fists, thus
producing a booming sound which
can be heard for miles and which
seems to attract females and warn
off other males. HMT*

Cavities and Mucous Membrane

The *laryngeal introitus* (Fig. 1–9) is a roughly triangular-shaped opening in the anterior wall of the pharynx, its base along the free edge of the epiglottis and its apex at the point between the two arytenoid cartilages. The sides are made up of the *aryepiglottic folds* of mucous membrane which stretch between the tips of the arytenoids and the lateral borders of the epiglottis. There are variable aryepiglottic muscle fibers within the aryepiglottic folds. The internal cavity of the larynx may be divided into three parts: the *vestibule,* the *glottis* and the *infraglottic* area. The *vestibule* or *supraglottic area* stretches from the free margin of the epiglottis and aryepiglottic folds inferiorly to the lower margin of the *ventricular bands* (usually referred to as the false cords). The *ventricle* is the laterally directed sac between the undersurface of the ventricular bands and the upper surface of the true vocal folds. At its anterior end is a small blind sac called the *saccule* or *appendix* of the ventricle.◁ Posteriorly the vestibule abuts upon the fold of mucosa between the arytenoids and the interarytenoideus muscles. The *true vocal folds* or *vocal cords* form a *rima glottidis* (glottis, glottic chink) as the space between them. They are approximately 15 mm long in the male and 10 mm in the female. The area within the larynx beginning at the free margin of the vocal folds and extending down to the lower margin of the cricoid cartilage and medial to the cricovocal membrane is referred to as the *subglottic* or *infraglottic* area.

Lateral to the aryepiglottic folds, within the inner surface of the upper portion of the thyroid cartilage and thyrohyoid membrane, is a deep recess which is closed anteriorly but open posteriorly. This is called the *pyriform sinus* (Fig. 1–8; *see also* Figs. 1–9, 1–13).

The various membranes, ligaments and skeletal structures of the larynx have been shown to delineate several potential spaces and compartments. These include the *preepiglottic space,* the *paraglottic space* and the *subglottic space.*

Preepiglottic Space (Fig. 1–7). This is bounded by the hyoepiglottic ligament superiorly (valleculae), by the thyrohyoid membrane and ligament anteriorly and by the anterior surface of the epiglottis and thyroepiglottic ligament posteriorly. It is shaped like an inverted pyramid. It is contiguous with the superior part of the paraglottic space laterally. It contains fat and loose areolar tissue. Carcinoma can spread directly into it via the perforations in the epiglottic cartilage.

Paraglottic Space (Fig. 1–8). This space is bounded laterally by the inner surface of the thyroid cartilage, inferomedially by the conus elasticus, medially by the ventricle, and superomedially by the quadrangular membrane. It communicates superiorly with the space between the thyroid cartilage and hyoid bone, anteriorly with the preepiglottic space near the petiole of the epiglottis and inferiorly with the space between the thyroid and cricoid cartilages. Posteriorly it is closed off by the reflection of pyriform sinus mucosa. At the level of the vocal fold and ventricle, it is effectively divided by muscular and ligamentous attachments into supraglottic and infraglottic parts.

Subglottic Space (Fig. 1–8). This is bounded superiorly by the undersurface of Broyles' ligament at the midline, laterally by the medial surface of the conus elasticus and medially by the subglottic mucosa. Inferiorly, it is continuous with the inner surface of the cricoid cartilage and its mucosa. ◁

With the exception of the vocal folds, virtually all of the larynx is lined by respiratory, pseudostratified, columnar, ciliated epithelium with goblet cells. The vocal folds themselves are covered with stratified squamous, nonkeratinizing epithelium which is glabrous (containing no glands or epithelial appendages). Immediately beneath the mucosa of the vocal folds is a potential space that stretches from the tips of the vocal processes to the anterior commissure and overlies the muscles of the vocal fold and the vocal ligament. This space is referred to as *Reinke's space*. It is essential to the free "flow" of the loose mucosa over the vocal folds during phonation but unfortunately also is prone to the development of edema with the least trauma to the cords. ◁

Studies by Pressman[6] and Tucker[7–9] have demonstrated the ability of these compartments to contain and/or direct the spread of laryngeal cancer within the larynx. Our ability to perform conservation surgery is dependent upon a knowledge of these compartments. HMT

See Chapter 2.

Musculature

Extrinsic Muscles (Fig. 1–10)

The *extrinsic muscles* of the larynx are also sometimes referred to as the *strap muscles*. The *infrahyoid group* includes the *omohyoid, sternothyroid, thyrohyoid* and *sternohyoid* muscles. They are innervated by branches of the descendens hypoglossi portion of the ansa hypoglossi. They are capable of moving the entire laryngotracheal complex as much as one whole vertebral body in going through a full range of two to two and one-half octaves. They are also capable of providing a small degree of increased tension in the vocal folds because when they are very tense, they tend to pull the thyrotracheal complex somewhat forward relative to the cricoid cartilage.

The *suprahyoid group* of muscles, including the *digastric, stylohyoid, geniohyoid, mylohyoid, stylopharyngeus* and *thyrohyoid* muscles, are all elevators of the larynx. The *middle* and *inferior constrictor* muscles are also extrinsic laryngeal muscles but play their most important role in swallowing and have little or no effect on the intrinsic functions of the larynx. The supra- and infrahyoid groups of muscles interdigitate at the hyoid bone and to a lesser extent at the thyroid cartilage. As a result, their synergistic action is capable of fixing the laryngotracheal complex in any position from its most depressed to its most elevated. The depressor (infrahyoid) group of muscles displaces the larynx downward during the inspiratory phase of respiration, while the elevators lift it during most expiratory cycles. The major displacement of the larynx takes place during deglutition, when the elevator muscles move the larynx both forward and superiorly which, associated with the downward movement of the base of the tongue, compresses the epiglottis over the laryngeal introitus as one of the major mechanisms to prevent aspiration. ◁

The *middle* and *inferior constrictor muscles* (Fig. 1–11) are extrinsic muscles of the larynx but play almost their entire role during the act of

See Chapter 2.

Figure 1–10. Strap muscles.

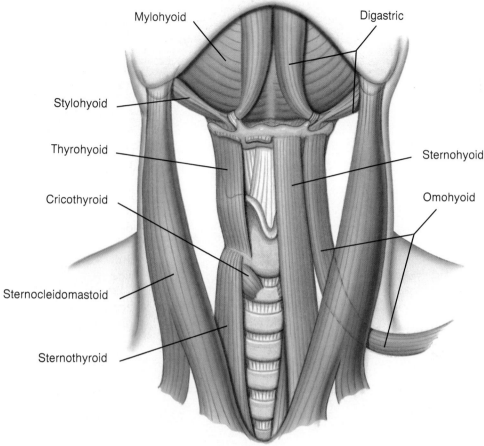

Figure 1–11. Nerve supply of larynx. Also note inferior constrictor muscle.

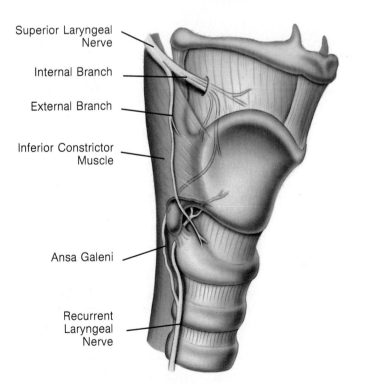

deglutition. The *cricopharyngeus muscle* (Fig. 1–12) may be regarded as an extrinsic muscle of respiration in that if it does not function properly, it favors spilling over of swallowed material directly into the glottis. This becomes extremely important in larynges that are already partially compro-

Figure 1–12. Arterial supply of
larynx. Also note
cricothyroideus muscle.

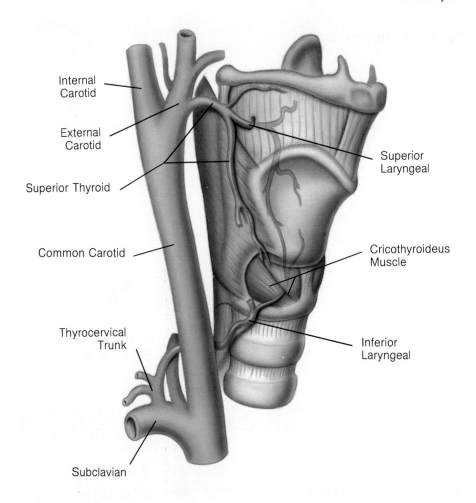

Internal
Carotid

External
Carotid

Superior
Laryngeal

Superior Thyroid

Common Carotid

Cricothyroideus
Muscle

Thyrocervical
Trunk

Inferior
Laryngeal

Subclavian

See Chapters 2 and 11.

mised by vocal cord paralysis or previous surgery. The remaining extrinsic muscle of the larynx is the *cricothyroideus* (Fig. 1–12). This muscle is innervated by the external branch of the superior laryngeal nerve and is ordinarily important during swallowing but also plays a part in increasing tension in the vocal folds, especially at the extreme upper range of pitch or loudness. Its two heads, the *oblique* and the *horizontal,* impart a sliding motion in an anterior-posterior direction, as well as a rocking motion. Recent work[5] has finally resolved the controversy about the movement of this muscle. It has now been shown that it is the thyroid cartilage that is relatively fixed and the cricoid cartilage that moves relative to it. Thus, contraction of the cricothyroideus muscle, which is always bilateral and symmetrical in the healthy state, draws the anteriormost aspect of the cricoid ring upward toward the lowermost aspect of the thyroid ala. This in effect rocks the cricoid lamina posteriorly and applies additional tension to the vocal ligaments, providing that the posterior cricoarytenoid muscle is intact to hold the arytenoids in position. Paralysis of one of the cricothyroideus muscles therefore imparts a rotary motion, because of the intact remaining muscle, so that the posterior commissure is displaced to the side of the paralysis.◁

Intrinsic Muscles (Figs. 1–13, 1–14)

The *intrinsic muscles* of the larynx, all of which are innervated by the recurrent laryngeal nerve, include the *posterior cricoarytenoid* (the only abductor of the vocal cords), *lateral cricoarytenoid, transverse arytenoid, oblique arytenoid, thyroarytenoid* (including the *vocalis*) and the two mi-

Figure 1–13. Horizontal section
of larynx through the ventricles.
Mucosa intact (above), musoca
removed to show intrinsic
muscles of vocal folds (below).

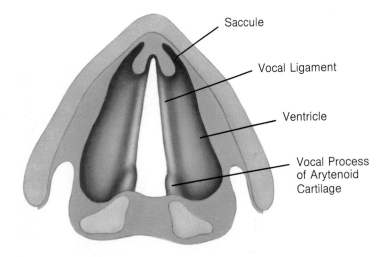

Saccule

Vocal Ligament

Ventricle

Vocal Process
of Arytenoid
Cartilage

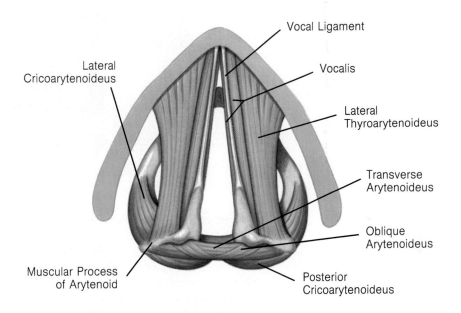

Vocal Ligament

Lateral
Cricoarytenoideus

Vocalis

Lateral
Thyroarytenoideus

Transverse
Arytenoideus

Oblique
Arytenoideus

Muscular Process
of Arytenoid

Posterior
Cricoarytenoideus

See Chapter 2.

nor slips of muscle representing the *aryepiglottic* and *thyroepiglottic* muscles. The *transverse arytenoid* is the only midline, unpaired muscle in the group. The *posterior cricoarytenoid muscle* arises from a midline raphe on the posterior aspect of the cricoid lamina. The fibers run superiorly and laterally, converging to insert on the posterior surface of the muscular process of the arytenoid cartilage. As the only abductor of the vocal cords, it serves to open the glottis by a "rotary" motion imparted to the arytenoid cartilages around an apparent axis of the cricoarytenoid joints. Some of the fibers of the muscle then can draw the arytenoid bodies laterally separating the vocal processes and the vocal folds.◁ During phonation, the posterior cricoarytenoid muscle also serves as a muscle that tenses the vocal fold by acting as an antagonist to the other muscles of the larynx in that the arytenoid is pulled posteriorly or fixed in position, so as to resist the pull of the other tensors. The *lateral cricoarytenoid muscle* has fibers arising from the upper border of the arch of the cricoid cartilage which pass obliquely backward toward the anterior aspect of the muscular process of the arytenoid. Its action is to close the glottis by adducting the vocal folds, which it does by rotating the arytenoid cartilages medially, bringing the vocal processes together. The *transverse arytenoideus* (interarytenoideus) is the

Figure 1–14. Intrinsic muscles
of larynx.

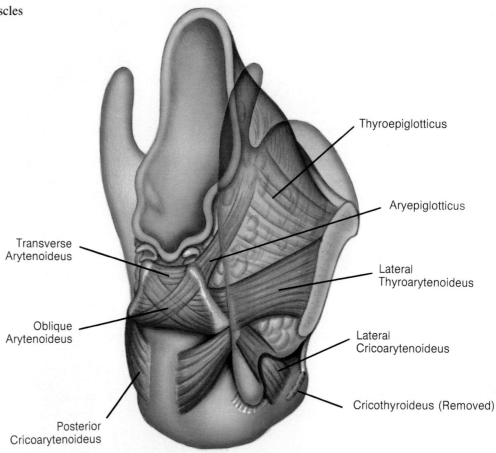

Thyroepiglotticus

Aryepiglotticus

Transverse
Arytenoideus

Lateral
Thyroarytenoideus

Oblique
Arytenoideus

Lateral
Cricoarytenoideus

Cricothyroideus (Removed)

Posterior
Cricoarytenoideus

See Chapter 2.

only unpaired muscle, and its fibers arise from the muscular process and lateral border of the arytenoid on each side, crossing the midline. It makes up most of the posterior commissure of the larynx. Its pull approximates the bodies of the arytenoids, thus closing the posterior aspect of the glottis when the vocal processes have already been brought into apposition. The *oblique arytenoid* muscle is made up of diagonal, transverse fascicles that interdigitate between the upright portions of the arytenoids, in conjunction with the interarytenoid muscles. Its uppermost fibers continue along the aryepiglottic fold, forming the *aryepiglottic muscle.* Combined action of these two muscles has a sphincteric effect on the introitus of the larynx, closing it down like a purse string during the act of swallowing. The *thyroaryten-oideus* is a very broad muscle which arises from the entire inner surface of the inferior half of the thyroid cartilage and also from the conus elasticus. It passes posteriorly and laterally, as well as superiorly, and inserts on the anterolateral surface and vocal process of the arytenoid cartilage. This muscle is usually divided into three parts for anatomic purposes. The first of these are the parallel fibers that arise just lateral to the vocal ligament and sometimes surround it. These are usually referred to as the *thyroarytenoideus internus* or *vocalis* muscle. The muscle is classed as an adductor of the larynx, but once the folds have been brought into close apposition, it is the major tensor of the free edge of the vocal fold. It may also take part in a change in the cross-sectional shape of the free margin, ''thinning'' the vocal fold as higher pitches are approached. ◁ The more lateral and superficial fibers of the *thyroarytenoideus* are referred to as the *externa*. This is the major adductor of the vocal fold. The third part of the muscle is referred to as the *thyroepiglotticus* and is made up of fibers that pass posteriorly and superiorly to insert into the aryepiglottic fold and along the margin of the epiglottis. Contraction of this muscle draws the arytenoid cartilages forward and downward towards the thyroid cartilage, the result of which is shortening of the vocal ligaments and relaxation of the mucous membrane covering them.

Although each of these intrinsic muscles of the larynx can be assigned an apparent function, it is important to note that the function of these muscles changes, depending upon the position of the vocal folds and arytenoids at any given moment. Moreover, as will be discussed in the section

See Chapter 2.

on physiology,◁ the interaction of agonist and antagonist muscles also must be taken into account to understand thoroughly the true function of this exquisitely balanced organ.

Blood Supply

The arterial blood supply of the larynx (Fig. 1–12) is derived from branches of the *superior* and *inferior thyroid* arteries and to a small extent from the *cricothyroid branch* of the *superior thyroid* artery. The *superior thyroid artery* is the first branch of the external carotid artery and, in a few cases, actually arises from the bifurcation of the carotid or even the common carotid. It passes anteriorly in a superiorly directed loop and, usually near the tip of the greater cornu of the hyoid bone, gives off a small *infrahyoid branch*. It then goes on a short distance and bifurcates near the tip of the superior cornu of the thyroid cartilage to give off the *superior laryngeal artery* and continues as the *superior thyroid artery* on the lateral surface of the middle and inferior constrictors. The superior thyroid artery terminates in the upper pole of the thyroid gland, giving off a small branch to the sternocleidomastoid muscle. The *superior laryngeal artery*, in company with the superior laryngeal nerves and veins, enters the larynx by penetrating a hiatus in the thyrohyoid ligament, after which it arborizes to supply the area above the vocal folds. There is, however, extensive interdigitation with the inferior blood supply of the larynx. The *inferior laryngeal artery*, which is a continuation of the *inferior thyroid artery* branch of the thyrocervical trunk, travels superiorly in the groove between the trachea and esophagus in concert with the recurrent laryngeal nerve. It enters the larynx, passing deep to the lowermost fibers of the inferior constrictor muscle with the recurrent laryngeal nerve. It supplies the portion of the larynx inferior to the free margins of the vocal folds, but interdigitates freely with its opposite number and with the branches of the *superior laryngeal artery*. A small *cricothyroid artery*, which is another branch of the superior thyroid artery, may pass across the upper portion of the cricothyroid ligament and anastomose with its opposite number. Small perforators often enter the cricothyroid membrane from this vessel.

Venous Drainage

Venous drainage (Fig. 1–15) is supplied by the *superior* and *inferior laryngeal veins*, which essentially follow the arteries in their course. The superior drainage joins the *superior* and *middle thyroid veins* and thence the internal jugular. The inferior drainage joins the *middle thyroid vein*, which is itself emptied into the jugular vein. There is some venous drainage to the *inferior thyroid vein,* basically a midline structure, and it empties directly into the superior vena cava.

Figure 1–15. Venous drainage
from larynx.

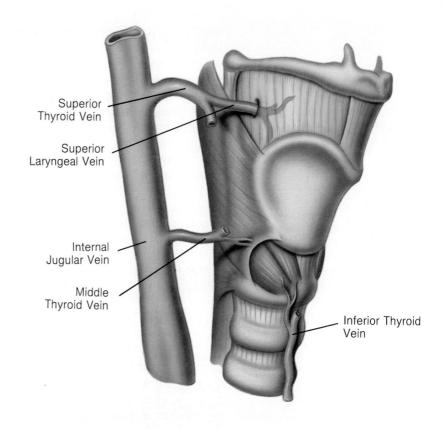

Superior
Thyroid Vein

Superior
Laryngeal Vein

Internal
Jugular Vein

Middle
Thyroid Vein

Inferior Thyroid
Vein

Figure 1–16. Lymphatic
drainage of larynx.

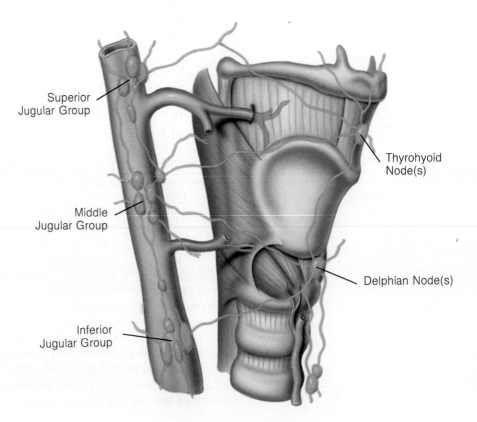

Superior
Jugular Group

Middle
Jugular Group

Inferior
Jugular Group

Thyrohyoid
Node(s)

Delphian Node(s)

Lymphatic Drainage (Fig. 1–16)

The larynx is very well supplied with lymphatics, with the exception of the free margins of the vocal folds themselves. The lymphatics superior to the ventricle cross freely from one side to the other and drain into the *superior* and *middle* group of *jugular nodes*.◁ Drainage from the inferior portion of the larynx, on the other hand, although there is some crossover, tends to be isolated from side to side. The drainage is through the crico-thyroid membrane to the *middle* and *inferior* jugular group and *paratracheal* group of nodes.◁

Supraglottic carcinoma often presents with metastatic nodes because of this rich lymphatic supply. HMT

This phenomenon accounts for the fact that carcinoma of the true vocal fold tends to metastasize to the same side with much higher frequency than to the opposite, although metastasis of any kind from glottic lesions is a relatively late finding in the disease. HMT

Nerve Supply (Fig. 1–11)

The larynx receives its major motor supply and all of the sensory supply below the free margins of the vocal folds via the *recurrent laryngeal branch* of the *vagus nerve*. Sensation above the vocal folds is carried by the *internal* branch of the *superior laryngeal nerve* which also has an *external* motor branch that supplies the cricothyroideus muscle. The larynx likewise receives nerve supply from both the *sympathetic* and *parasympathetic* systems.

The *superior laryngeal nerve* separates from the main trunk of the vagus just outside the jugular foramen. It then travels in close proximity to the main trunk, diverging from it above the greater cornu of the hyoid bone. It passes anteromedially on the thyrohyoid membrane where it is joined by the superior thyroid artery and vein. At approximately this level the *external laryngeal nerve* leaves the main trunk and descends on the surface of the inferior constrictor of the pharynx, deep to the sternothyroid muscles. It sends branches both to the pharyngeal plexus and to the inferior constrictor and finally reaches the cricothyroid muscle, which it supplies.[5] The main *internal laryngeal* nerve continues on the surface of the thyrohyoid membrane in company with and just superior to the superior laryngeal artery and enters the membrane through a hiatus. Immediately within the membrane it divides into three sets of branches: *ascending, transverse* and *descending*. These supply, in the same order, the mucosa of the vallecula and the epiglottis, the pyriform sinus, and the larynx as far down as the vocal fold. On the medial wall of the pyriform fossa, the descending branches give twigs to the transverse arytenoideus muscle via a plexus and then continues behind the cricoid cartilage as a fine filament that communicates with the recurrent laryngeal nerve. This is referred to as the *ansa galeni*.

Parasympathetic fibers destined for the larynx travel with the superior and recurrent laryngeal nerves from their origin within the jugular foramen. *Sympathetic* fibers arrive in the larynx in company with the blood vessels, having arisen from the *superior cervical sympathetic ganglion* near the bifurcation of the carotid.

The *recurrent laryngeal nerve* is derived as a branch of the vagus nerve, on the left side as it passes the arch of the aorta and on the right side as it passes the subclavian artery. In the latter case the nerve passes from anterior to posterior around the subclavian artery and recurs in the tracheo-esophageal groove on the right side. As it travels superiorly, it supplies the trachea and esophagus, especially providing fibers to the cricopharyngeus muscle. The *left recurrent laryngeal nerve* passes lateral to the ligamentum arteriosum behind the arch of the aorta and enters the tracheoesophageal groove. It, too, provides segmental branches to the esophagus and trachea as it ascends. At the lower pole of the thyroid gland it runs between the branches of the inferior thyroid artery and is in intimate proximity to the posterior and medial aspects of the thyroid gland. It reaches the larynx, as does the *right recurrent laryngeal* nerve, by running under the border of the inferior constrictor muscle of the pharynx, which it also supplies. A communication with the *internal laryngeal nerve* (the *ansa galeni*) leaves the recurrent laryngeal nerve some little distance before it reaches the lower margin of the inferior constrictor. The main trunk of the nerve then approaches the larynx at the cricothyroid joint. In the majority of cases the nerve passes behind this joint, but in up to 10 to 15% of adults it passes either anterior to the joint or splits, sending one trunk posterior and one anterior. ◁

It may be that this peculiar arrangement accounts for the small but significant number of uni- or bilateral vocal cord paralyses that are encountered after otherwise atraumatic endotracheal intubation. HMT

Developmental Anatomy

If there is a fifth such apparatus in the human, which is open to question, this is also involved. HMT

The larynx is developed embryologically from ectodermal, endodermal and mesodermal tissues that are derived from the third, fourth, (fifth) and sixth branchial arch and pouch apparatus. ◁ During the fourth week of embryonic life, a ventral and midline diverticulum arises from the foregut, which is referred to as the *respiratory primordium*. As this primordium deepens, it becomes the *laryngotracheal tube*. Examination of the floor of the pharynx of an embryo at this stage shows two midline structures, the more anterior of which arises just behind the mandibular arches and is called the *tuberculum impar,* which eventually develops into the posterior third of the tongue. Immediately behind this is a small diverticulum which is the *primordium* of the *thyroid gland*. Posterior to the thyroid diverticulum is a second raised area lying at the bases of the second and third branchial arches which is called the *copula*. The laryngotracheal groove fuses from caudal to cephalic end, forming a tracheoesophageal septum that separates the laryngotracheal groove from the esophagus. In the fifth to sixth embryologic week, three masses of tissue appear around the primordial glottic slit at the bases of the third and fourth branchial arches. The anteriormost of these, which is immediately posterior to the copula, is the *primordial epiglottis*. Paired bilateral swellings at the bases of the fourth arches are the primordial *arytenoid cartilages*. The resultant T-shaped opening is temporarily closed off by fusion of these epithelial masses, the closure of which persists until the end of the eighth week of embryonic life. During the second month the *thyroid cartilage anlage* begins to be derived from the ventral portion of the cartilages of the fourth branchial arch. The *cricoid* and arytenoid cartilages are likewise derived from the fifth arch (sixth arch) apparatus. During development of the thyroid cartilage, the mucosal anlage of the vocal folds are drawn out between the arytenoids and the inner surface of the thyroid lamina. Simultaneously there is the development of the *vestibular sinus* which will become the *ventricle*. An evagination is present during this stage of development, which ultimately gives rise to the *saccule* of the larynx. The *vocal ligament* forms within the substance of the primitive vocal fold by condensation of mesenchyma.

The primordia of the intrinsic laryngeal muscles are derived from the epicardial ridge and migrate superficially and deeply through the neck to come to rest at the appropriate points within the larynx. The recurrent laryngeal nerves are associated with the sixth branchial arch apparatus. It is understandable, therefore, that these branches would migrate with the muscle masses in a cephalad direction along the anterior neck eventually to rest within the larynx. Because of the persistence of the primordium of the arch of the aorta (ductus arteriosus), the left recurrent laryngeal nerve remains "tethered" in the chest. On the other hand, the right recurrent laryngeal

The derivation of the hyoid bone from both the second and third branchial arch cartilages accounts for the passage of a thyroglossal duct remnant (which is derived from the floor of the primordial foregut anterior to the third arch) through it. This explains the need to remove the body of the hyoid bone during surgery for thyroglossal duct remnant. HMT

nerve can migrate cranially because the fourth and fifth arterial arches on the right side disappear. It, therefore, is "tethered" only by the fourth arch artery (subclavian).

The *hyoid bone* is derived in large part from the second branchial arch cartilage, which gives rise to the styloid process, stylohyoid ligament and, therefore, the lesser cornua of the hyoid bone, as well as most of the anterior portion of the body of the hyoid. The remainder of the body and the greater cornua are derived from the cartilage of the third arch, the two structures fusing in the midline.◁

The Immature Larynx

A study of comparative anatomy shows that the epiglottis extends into the nasopharynx above the level of the soft palate either continuously (whales) or when the head is down in the position for drinking or eating (ungulates, some carnivores). This allows the animal to continue to breathe and to detect warning odors from a predator without interruption. Human infants are obligate nose breathers and therefore benefit from the higher placement of the epiglottis which enables them to breathe while suckling. HMT

The newborn and infant larynx differs in many important ways from that of the adult. In the newborn, the tip of the epiglottis is parallel with the upper portion of the body of the second cervical vertebra. Thus, the tip of the epiglottis may be in direct contact with the soft palate.◁ Also, whereas the narrowest place in the airway of the adult is the glottis itself, in the infant it is the subglottis within the cricoid ring. The epiglottis of the infant is omega or U-shaped and is also much softer than in the adult because of lack of calcification or development of the laryngeal cartilages. This, coupled with the more inferior position of the hyoid bone relative to the thyroid cartilage, allows the base of the tongue to depress the epiglottis to a much more obtuse angle in the infant than in the adult. Indeed, it is possible for the epiglottis to be inverted directly into the laryngeal introitus. This phenomenon, in the presence of the more loose attachment of the mucoperichondrium, may account for the higher incidence of infantile epiglottitis, which is not often seen as a symptomatic condition in the adult. Another important difference between the infantile and adult larynx lies in the fact that more than 50% of the glottic opening is cartilaginous in the infant whereas almost two-thirds of the glottis is made up of soft tissue in the adult. This factor, along with the relative softness of the infantile larynx, may contribute to the condition known as laryngomalacia.

References

1. Lockhart RD, Hamilton GF, Fyfe FW: Anatomy of the Human Body. Philadelphia, JB Lippincott Company, 1960.
2. Hast H: Anatomy of the Larynx. In English, GM (Ed): Otolaryngology. Philadelphia, Harper and Row, 1978.
3. Gray H: The Anatomy of the Human Body. Philadelphia, Lea and Febiger, 1973.
4. Broyles EN: The anterior commissure tendon. Ann Otol Rhinol Laryngol, 52:341, 1943.
5. Abelson TI, Tucker HM: Laryngeal Findings in Superior Laryngeal Nerve Paralysis: A Controversy. Otolaryngol Head Neck Surg, 89:463–470, 1981.
6. Pressman J, Sermon M, Monell C: Anatomi-
cal studies related to the dissemination of cancer of the larynx. Trans Am Ac Ophthalm Otol, 64:628, 1960.
7. Tucker G: A histological method for the study of the spread of carcinoma within the larynx. Ann Otol Rhinol Laryngol, 70:910, 1961.
8. Tucker G: Some clinical inferences from the study of serial laryngeal sections. Laryngoscope, 73:728, 1973.
9. Tucker G: The anatomy of laryngeal cancer. In Alberti PW, and Bryce DP (Eds): Workshops from the Centennial Conference on Laryngeal Cancer. New York, Appleton-Century-Crofts, 1976.

Chapter 2

Physiology of the Larynx

Some 50 different functions have been identified in the literature for the larynx. However, only three of them are of real concern to the clinician. These include provision of an airway, protection of that airway, and phonation. Moreover, these functions have appeared in nature in approximately this same phylogenetic order.

Comparative Anatomy

Provision of Airway

Development of each of the functions of the larynx can be better understood if one examines them as responses to evolutionary needs. Primitive fish, in evolving to permit occasional periods of time on dry land, (such as during droughts or when traveling between discontinuous bodies of water), have developed respiratory diverticula that allow storage of air. Since the walls of these reservoirs are lined with moist mucous membranes and well supplied with blood vessels, a simple but effective form of "air-breathing" can take place.[1]

Upon developing to the point where virtually all respiration is achieved by air breathing, increasing demands for moving larger quantities of air pose new difficulties for the evolving creature. In large, land-dwelling amphibians, such as the axolotl, greater support for the introitus to the air passages is needed than can be provided by the soft tissues alone. Because of the increased demand, air must be moved in and out more rapidly and Bernoulli's effect tends to collapse the walls of the introitus inward. In order to prevent this collapse and to provide support, laterally placed cartilage bars are seen in many salamanders. In the more advanced reptilian forms, these primitive cartilages serve as points of attachment for the valvular muscles and also develop a ringlike structure analogous to the cricoid cartilage in mammals.

Thus, the phylogenetically earliest function of the larynx, provision of the airway, is assured primarily by the skeletal support structures, all of which are incomplete rings except for the cricoid cartilage. Another important anatomic factor that helps to provide a patent airway is the very tight attachment of the mucoperichondrium to the underlying structures, with virtually no submucosal tissue intervening. In this manner, the possibility of edema or other redundancy of tissue that might impinge on the airway is limited.

Protection of Airway

Upon completion of development of an airway mechanism suitable for breathing on land, it became phylogenetically necessary to protect that airway from inadvertent aspiration of food or other foreign material. The next evolutionary step that was required was the development of a valve to control entrance of water or other foreign material into the air reservoir. Such muscular valves are seen in several varieties of lungfish, the more highly developed ones exhibiting fibers capable of opening as well as closing the orifice.

Phonation

Although these primitive animals are able to produce sounds, it is doubtful that there is any significance to them. The somewhat more highly developed salamander larynx, which has identifiable paired *pars arytenoidea* cartilages, is capable of a croaking noise. Since this phonatory behavior is seen mainly during the mating season, it is probably significant, and some of the earliest such activity developed from a phylogenetic viewpoint. Frogs, which may be regarded as the next higher step in laryngeal evolution, become almost totally land dwelling for a large part of their lives. Their larynges demonstrate paired arytenoid cartilages and a cricoid ring to which well-developed sphincter muscles are attached. Frogs use phonatory communication for mating, territorial protection, and to warn of danger. Crocodiles, unlike amphibians, have no capability for transdermal respiration and are thus totally dependent on lung breathing. They are in the first class of animals to employ muscular expansion of the chest to inspire air, as opposed to simply swallowing it. With the development of this highly efficient means of moving air in large quantities, phylogenetic evolution of the upper respiratory apparatus is essentially at the same level as in humans. Thoracic air movement also provides the expiratory control that is necessary for ultimate development of speech.

A fully developed mammalian type larynx, including arytenoid, corniculate, thyroid, cricoid, and epiglottic cartilages, is first seen in small insectivores like the lesser gymnure and the tree shrew. Both of these animals are thought to be derived from ancestors common to man. More advanced structures such as paired true and false vocal folds enclosing a well-developed ventricle appear first in brachiating monkeys like the *rhesus*.◁ Because these animals have to be able to fix the chest wall firmly to permit a stable thorax for the attachment of powerful arm and shoulder muscles, the false vocal folds (ventricular bands) are directed caudally. As subglottic air pressure increases, it is trapped in the ventricle and actually drives the ventricular bands more tightly together, thus preventing air escape (Fig. 2–1).

Most mammals less developed than the great apes and man exhibit some degree of contact between the epiglottis and the soft palate.◁ This relationship becomes particularly pronounced in the head-down position assumed during drinking and eating (Fig. 2–2). It is essential for these animals to drink quickly without aspirating and, at the same time, to maintain the ability to smell approaching danger. Projection of the epiglottis above the level of the soft palate creates an almost continuous tube to divert food or fluids away from the laryngeal introitus, while permitting un-

Besides providing a valve that prevents release of subglottic air pressure, this peculiar arrangement has secondary benefit, at least to certain members of the primate group. In the howler monkey and the orangutan, for instance, the laryngeal saccule is very large and communicates with air sacs that may even extend out over the upper chest wall. These can be expanded at will, providing tremendous vocal resonance and loudness, which permit the monkey vocalizations that can be heard for miles. Gorillas have a similar modification, especially in the male, and can expand these sacs when angry or sexually aroused. He then beats on them with his fists to make a very loud booming noise, with which he can warn off another male or attract a distant female. HMT

In the whales and porpoises, the epiglottis is scrolled to form a continuous tube. This structure extends far above the soft palate to make contact with the "blow-whole" (modified nostrils that have migrated to the top of the head). Since these animals feed while moving rapidly through the water, the tubular epiglottis effectively prevents aspiration, while permitting either breathing at the surface or phonation to continue. HMT

Figure 2–1. Ventricular air trapping combines with increasing supra- and subglottic pressure to seal the glottis.

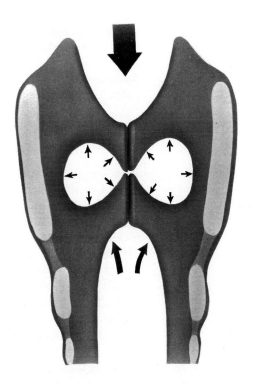

Figure 2–2. Epiglottis is elevated above the posterior edge of the soft palate when in position to drink or graze in most ungulates, thus permitting continuous olfactory sampling to alert the animal to the approach of predators.

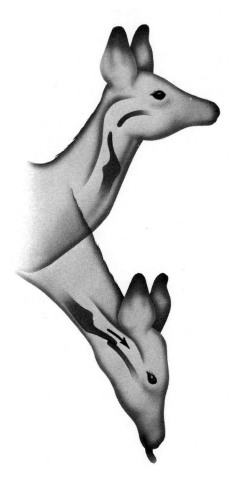

interrupted inspiration and expiration. An analogous arrangement is seen in newborn humans. Infants are obligate nasal breathers, partly to allow them to continue breathing while nursing. The relatively higher position of the infant larynx places the epiglottis in contact with the soft palate and helps to avoid aspiration.

Functional Anatomy

The skeletal structures of the larynx, including the hyoid bone are attached to the mandible by the digastric muscle and hyomandibular ligaments (Fig. 2–3). These structures simultaneously restrict inferior displacement (stylohyoid and hyomandibular ligaments) and coordinate the essential, but exceedingly complex, superior and inferior movements of the larynx that must take place during swallowing. These ligaments may be regarded as "check-reins," that not only passively suspend the laryngeal structures from the skull, but act as antagonists to the infrahyoid muscles, as well. Since some of the movements of the vocal folds during respiration and even phonation may result from muscular pull against this relative fixation, it is important to understand the function of these ligaments (see later).

Strap Muscles

The actions of the strap muscles are outlined in Table 2–1. It is important to remember that these muscles rarely function alone and that for every agonist there is an antagonist. Thus, relative upward or downward displacement of the laryngotracheal structures is a dynamic activity that is the resultant vector of the arithmetic sums of *all* muscles active at any given time.

The suprahyoid muscles are able to move the hyoid bone and the larynx upward or to prevent downward displacement of these structures. The

Figure 2–3. "Check-rein" effect of the suprahyoid muscles and ligaments maintain a fairly constant relationship between the mandible and the larynx, allowing upward movement but preventing downward displacement during swallowing.

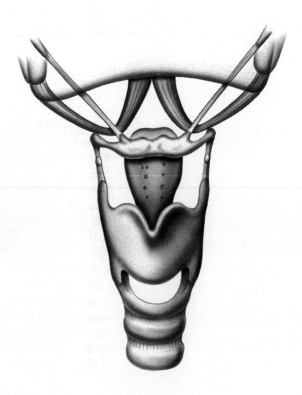

Table 2–1   Movements of the Larynx and Hyoid Bone*

Hyoid bone is moved
  Superiorly and posteriorly by
    1. Stylohyoid
    2. Digastric (posterior belly)
    3. Middle pharyngeal constrictor
  Superiorly and anteriorly by
    1. Geniohyoid
    2. Genioglossus
    3. Mylohyoid
    4. Digastric (anterior belly)
  Inferiorly by
    1. Thyrohyoid
    2. Sternohyoid
    3. Omohyoid
Laryngeal complex is moved
  Superiorly by
    1. Thyrohyoid
  Inferiorly by
    1. Sternothyroid

*Modified from Aronson.[12]

posterior belly of the digastric muscle and, to a lesser extent, the stylo-hyoid muscle also can displace the hyoid bone posteriorly. Since all of the infrahyoid muscles and the laryngotracheal complex are suspended from the hyoid bone, this structure acts as a sesamoid bone, much like the patella, to change the angle of pull of the antagonistic muscles. If, for example, the anterior belly of the digastric and the geniohyoid muscles pull upward and the sternothyroid and sternohyoid muscles pull downward with approximately equal force, the hyoid bone and larynx will move neither superiorly nor inferiorly. Rather, the entire complex will be pulled forward. Such activity is important during swallowing when it may serve to widen the hypopharynx. It may also have some effect on "fine-tuning" tension in the vocal folds, especially near a singer's highest pitch capability.

Intrinsic Muscles

Intrinsic muscles operate the vocal folds and, to some extent, control the movements of the supraglottic structures as well. They include thyroarytenoideus (TA; vocalis), lateral cricoarytenoideus (LCA), cricothyroideus, interarytenoideus, oblique arytenoideus, and posterior cricoarytenoideus (PCA). Of these, all are primarily *adductors* of the true vocal folds except for the PCA muscle, which is the only *abductor*. Although it is customary to designate the medialmost fibers of the thyroarytenoideus (vocalis) muscle as the major tensor of the vocal folds, it is important to recognize that the posterior cricoarytenoideus muscle is also a tensor in that it must oppose the anterior pull of the vocalis muscle for tension to increase. The action of the cricothyroideus muscle is also important in changing tension in the vocal fold during phonation, but it is not, strictly speaking, an intrinsic muscle of the larynx, inasmuch as it is innervated by the superior laryngeal nerve.

In order to understand the complicated activities of the various muscles as they actually occur during phonation and swallowing, it is helpful to consider them first as separate entities. (Fig. 2–4 and 2–5)

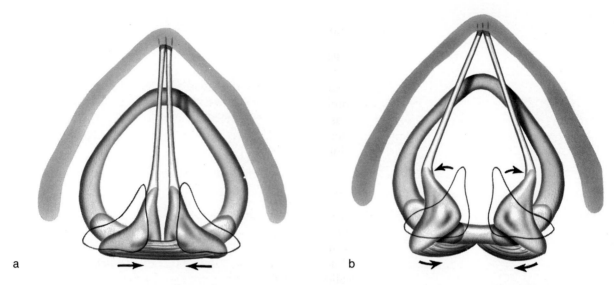

a   b

Figure 2–4. **a,** Action of interarytenoideus and oblique arytenoideus muscles to draw the bodies of the arytenoid cartilages together. **b,** Posterior cricoarytenoid muscles are the only laryngeal abductors.

Posterior Cricoarytenoideus

Because of its insertion near the outer tip of the muscular process of the arytenoid cartilage, contraction of the PCA effectively rotates the tips of the vocal processes away from each other, thus separating the vocal folds. Since all of the other intrinsic muscles are either adductors or tensors of the vocal folds and since they represent a much greater mass of muscle than the PCA, it follows that they must relax during abduction if the PCA is to overcome their pull. If, on the other hand, the vocal folds have been brought into apposition by the adductors, contraction of the PCA serves to prevent anterior displacement of the aryrtenoid and, thus, is essential to normal tensing capability. Therefore, the PCA muscle should be regarded as a primary *abductor* of the vocal fold, but it must also be recognized as a *tensor*.◁

The PCA contains mostly slow contracting motor units,[2] but it is probably the few fast units that are active during its "tensing" function.—HMT

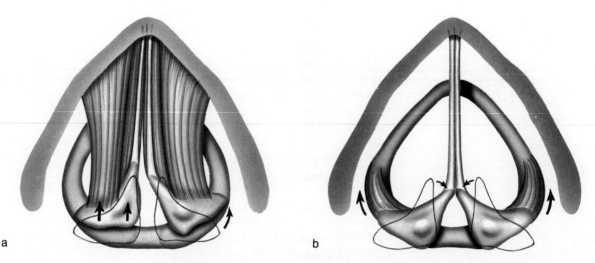

a   b

Figure 2–5. **a,** Vocalis and lateral thyroarytenoideus muscles are adductors and tensors of the vocal folds, depending somewhat on arytenoid position. **b,** Cricoarytenoideus muscles are adductors of the vocal folds. Complete glottic closure requires simultaneous activity of the interarytenoideus muscles.

Interarytenoideus

The interarytenoideus muscle draws the arytenoid cartilages together. It crosses the midline, and is, to some extent, innervated by both recurrent laryngeal nerves. It is important to the integrity of the closure of the posterior commissure, especially during swallowing. Along with the oblique arytenoideus muscles, it must act in concert with the lateral cricoarytenoideus muscles to achieve full adduction of the vocal folds and competence of glottic closure.

Oblique Arytenoideus

These small, diagonally oriented slips of muscle cross the posterior commissure and act in concert with the interarytenoideus muscle. In addition to aiding closure of the posterior glottis, they are important in the "locking" action of the tips of the arytenoid cartilages, which takes place during swallowing and effort closure (see later).

Lateral Cricoarytenoideus

Contraction of this muscle draws the tip of the muscular process of the arytenoid cartilage anteriorly. This displaces the vocal processes toward each other, adducting the vocal folds. Although this activity brings the membranous portions of the vocal folds together, the concomitant adduction of the bodies of the arytenoids provided by the interarytenoideus muscle is necessary to close completely the glottic chink. In addition to its activity as the major adductor of the vocal fold, the LCA can also act as a tensor once the bodies of the arytenoid cartilages have been brought to the midline.

Thyroarytenoideus and Vocalis

It is generally agreed that the vocalis muscle is part of the TA. The lateral fibers of the TA, which make up most of the bulk of the muscle, arise from the anterior body of the arytenoid cartilage, whereas the medial vocalis fibers arise from the vocal process adjacent. The vocalis fibers surround the vocal ligament, so that some of the medialmost fibers are immediately beneath the surface, separated from it only by Reinke's space. These fibers are important in changing the thickness, cross-sectional mass, and, thus, the vibratory characteristics of the vocal fold during phonation (see later). Most of the vocalis muscle functions as a major tensor of the vocal fold, but only after the arytenoid has been brought to the midline by the other adductors. As already noted, this tensing activity requires the opposition of the PCA.

The lateral TA fibers, which make up the bulk of the muscle, act as an adductor when the vocal fold is abducted at or beyond the intermediate position, and as a tensor when the vocal fold is close to the midline.

Cricothyroideus

Although this is not truly an intrinsic muscle of the larynx, its activity is mainly related to phonation and is critical to both adduction and tensing activity of the other laryngeal muscles. Therefore, it can logically be considered in this section. This muscle is innervated by the external branch of the superior laryngeal nerve. Both muscles operate simultaneously under normal circumstances. The resultant motion tends to shorten the distance

Figure 2–6. Action of the
cricothyroideus muscles tends to
tense the vocal folds.

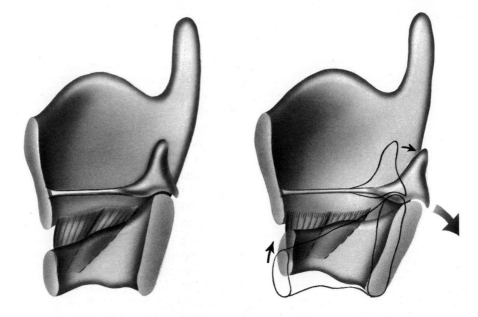

between the two cartilages at the midline anteriorly.[3] In effect, this rotates
the cricoid lamina posteriorly. If the arytenoids are prevented from displacement by the simultaneous balanced pull of the intrinsic muscles, such
posterior rotation will result in increased tension in the vocal folds. (Fig.
2–6) This activity is important in order to increase pitch when singing near
maximum capability and, under certain circumstances, during effort closure.

Respiration

*Fink and Demarest[4] suggest that
both the PCA and LCA are
stabilizers of the arytenoid and that
its abduction results from complex
forces and the peculiar shape of the
cricoarytenoid joint.—HMT*

During quiet breathing, the anatomy of the cricoarytenoid joints would
ordinarily be expected to cause the vocal folds to lie in the intermediate
position (about midway between full abduction and adduction). However,
because of the preponderance of adductor muscle mass, the arytenoids lie
somewhat more toward the midline in the so-called paramedian position.
With quiet inspiration, the vocal folds will abduct slightly, not so much as
a result of activity of the PCA, but because of the combined effect of
downward movement of the entire laryngotracheal complex against the pull
of the abductor muscles.◁ This downward excursion is due partly to the
action of the infrahyoid strap muscles and partly to the expansion of the
thoracic cavity, which also produces a downward pull on the entire tracheobronchial tree. Conversely, during quiet expiration, the vocal folds
adduct slightly. Some of this medial displacement is because of the reversal of the activity previously described above and the medial pull due to
air passage (Bernoulli's effect) between the vocal folds.

*"The short arytenoid vocal
processes in man effectively
increase the relative length of the
membranous vocal cords. . . .
[A]n optimum ratio of arytenoid to
vocal cord length (for efficient
respiration) is found in the gazelle
(7:10), man possessing a 4:10 ratio
instead."—CT Sasaki[5] (p 5)*

As ventilatory demand increases, *all* of the muscles involved in respiration become more active. Increased downward pull on the trachea and
larynx, coupled with more efficient abduction of the arytenoids by the PCA,
results in a wider opening of the glottis. In evolving a larynx suited to
phonation, the relative lengths of the vocal process of the arytenoid and
the membranous portion of the vocal fold have changed.◁ In the human,
the relatively long vibratory segment needed for phonation has decreased
the efficiency with which the glottic area can be increased with each abduction of the arytenoid.

Swallowing

Upward movement of the laryngotracheal complex takes place primarily during deglutition. It is coordinated with simultaneous downward movement of the posterior third of the tongue. Together, these depress the epiglottis posteroinferiorly, effectively inverting it and closing off the laryngeal introitus. In this manner, the bolus of food or liquid is diverted laterally into the pyriform sinus. Simultaneous anterior pull on the thyroid cartilage is provided by the sternothyroid and thyrohyoid muscles, which results in a widened anteroposterior diameter of the hypopharynx just above the esophageal introitus. If the cricopharyngeus muscle relaxes promptly in response to increasing hypopharyngeal pressure, the food bolus can pass the larynx and enter the upper esophagus without aspiration.

A second important protective mechanism intended to prevent aspiration of foreign material during deglutition is firm apposition of the vocal fold. This occurs not only because of the action of the laryngeal adductors, but is also assisted by elevation of subglottic air pressure. As the bolus of food approaches the laryngeal introitus, supraglottic air pressure increases, thus opposing the increase in subglottic pressure. The resultant rise in intraventricular pressure forces the false vocal folds against each other (Fig. 2–1). Because of the overhang of the false cords, expansion of the ventricles increases apposition of the superomedial surfaces of the ventricular bands against each other.◁ In similar fashion, expansion of the ventricles drives the vocal folds against each other. The result is a competent valve at the level of the glottis that is dependent on integrity of the intrinsic adductors only to bring the arytenoids together, after which most of the valvular action is automatic.

Brunton and Cash[6] have shown resistance of the false cords to pressure from below, equaling approximately 30 mmHg. The true cords, on the other hand, will offer relatively little resistance to pressure from below, but can resist up to 140 mmHg pressure from above, when approximated.—HMT

The remaining function that is critical to prompt passage of a food or liquid bolus into the upper esophagus without aspiration is the appropriate and timely relaxation of the cricopharyngeus muscle. If this does not occur quickly enough, the food will tend to spill over into the laryngeal introitus. Timely opening of this sphincter requires normal sensory innervation of the posterior pharyngeal wall so that passage of the bolus toward the larynx can be detected. Esophageal manometric measurements suggest that a critical increase in hypopharyngeal pressure is also necessary to trigger relaxation of the cricopharyngeus, and normal sensory innervation is required to detect this activity as well.[7] Although an otherwise normal upper aerodigestive tract might be able to compensate for failure of any one of these important antiaspiration mechanisms, loss of two or more of them will almost always result in severe derangement of swallowing capability.◁

It is now generally accepted that hypopharyngeal (Zenker's) diverticulum occurs because of delay in timely relaxation of the cricopharyngeus muscle during swallowing.—HMT[8]

Effort Closure

Whereas only the vocal folds are brought into contact during quiet phonation, swallowing and/or straining results in massive, undifferentiated closure of both the true and false vocal folds. The tips of the arytenoids are so forcefully adducted that they may "lock" or interdigitate. The cuneiform and corniculate cartilages are driven against each other, and the distance between the hyoid bone and the upper border of the thyroid cartilage is obliterated, forcing the petiole of the epiglottis down against the tightly apposed aryepiglottic folds. This results in an almost impenetrable "cork" that effectively seals the glottis and permits the needed increase in subglottic and intrathoracic pressure. Such activities as straining at stool, childbirth, and heavy lifting may be difficult or even impossible in the absence of such effort closure.

Functional Neuroanatomy

Function of the larynx is dependent on the complex and timely interaction of all the structures described herein. All of this activity is mediated through the central nervous system and the peripheral neurologic connections of the upper respiratory tract. Although this discussion must be limited primarily to the larynx itself, it is clear that its functions are profoundly affected by and are intimately associated with those of the entire aerodigestive tract.

Afferent System

Sensation from the supraglottic structures reaches the central nervous system via the internal branch of the superior laryngeal nerve on each side. Afferent impulses arising in the glottis and subglottic regions are transmitted via the recurrent laryngeal nerves (Fig. 2–7). Proprioceptive and sensory nerve endings are found most densely situated on the laryngeal surface of the epiglottis and less so on the true vocal folds. More touch receptors are found concentrated toward the posterior commissure than near the anterior, and temperature receptors are almost all found in the supraglottic larynx. Information thus obtained reaches the central nervous system through the nodose ganglion to the tractus solitarius, where further central and integrative connections take place.

Efferent System

Efferent fibers destined for the larynx arise in the nucleus ambiguus of the medulla. All of the intrinsic laryngeal muscles are innervated via the recurrent laryngeal nerves. Only the interarytenoideus muscles are bilaterally innervated. The cricothyroideus muscles, which are not intrinsic to the larynx, are innervated via the external branch of the superior laryngeal

Figure 2–7. Distribution of sensory innervation from the superior and recurrent laryngeal nerves.

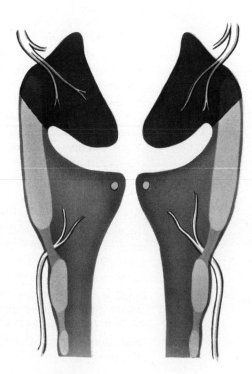

nerves. Parasympathetic fibers travel with the superior and recurrent laryngeal nerves, whereas sympathetic innervation travels with the blood vessels.

Laryngeal Reflexes

The protective, respiratory, and phonatory functions of the larynx are mediated through several polysynaptic reflexes at the level of the brainstem. Whereas the glottic closure reflex, which is essential to protection of the airway, is entirely automatic, the other reflexes can at least be initiated and, to some degree, modified voluntarily.

Glottic Closure Reflex

"This has led [to the suggestion that laryngospasm may be] a form of focal seizure initiated by a local sensory aberration or aura. . . . [I]t consists of prolonged tonic adductor spike activity in [the] recurrent laryngeal nerve that bears no . . . reproducible temporal relationship [or] latency to its initiating stimulus."—CT Sasaki[5] (p 10)

Touch and chemical or thermal stimulation of the supraglottic mucosa subtended by the superior laryngeal nerves results in involuntary forceful closure of the entire larynx. The sequence of events is anatomically the same as that described for effort closure. In man unilateral superior laryngeal nerve stimulation does not result in the contralateral adductor activity seen in most lower animals. This may account, at least in part, for the tendency of unexpected aspiration of saliva associated with unilateral superior nerve palsy.

If the laryngeal closure reflex becomes overly sensitive, laryngospasm may result. It is characterized by electrical activity in the adductor fibers long after the instigating mucosal stimulus has ceased.◁ It can be abolished by heavy sedation, particularly with barbiturates, and also decreases with hypoxia. This may explain why patients are rarely in real danger of asphyxia, since in very severe cases the patient simply faints from hypoxia, at which point the spasm breaks.

Respiratory Reflexes

As far as the larynx itself is concerned, quiet respiration is virtually a passive activity, dependent mostly on chest wall and diaphragmatic activity. However, electromyographic studies demonstrate that there is increased electrical activity in the PCA muscle during each inspiratory effort.[9] Moreover, this activity increases with both rapidity and depth of respiration. The rapid passage of air between the vocal folds tends to draw them together (Bernoulli's effect), and activity in the PCA is necessary to keep them apart. As respiratory effort increases, the PCA separates the vocal folds more and more in reflex response to increasing airway resistance.

"The cross-sectional area of the glottis, . . . modified by expansion of the laryngeal aperture in its anteroposterior dimension, is a direct effect of cricothyroid activity. . . . [T]he greater the rise in subglottic pressure, the larger the laryngeal aperture in expiration."—Sasaki.[5]

A type of ventilatory reflex activity also occurs in the cricothyroideus muscle. Because it is a tensor and, under certain circumstances, an adductor of the vocal folds, this muscle would not be expected to be active during inspiration. Studies show, however, that there *is* activity during inspiration, which apparently results in the lengthening of the vocal folds (and therefore of the glottic chink) in the anteroposterior diameter.[10]

Expiratory resistance and its effect on normal respiratory function is less well understood. It appears, however, that the cricothyroideus muscle also plays a part in adjusting airway resistance during expiration, as well as during inspiration.[5]◁ During expiration, its activity is not modified by concomitant PCA action and, therefore, produces relative narrowing of the airway.

Phonatory Function

The neurochronaxic theory[11] suggested that rhythmic muscular contraction of the vocal folds occurs at the same fundamental frequency as the sound produced.◁ It has been essentially discarded in favor of the myoelastic-aerodynamic theory,[13] which more closely approximates and explains observed phenomena. In simplest fashion, this theory holds that the vocal folds are brought into appropriate position by gross muscular activity, that tension is adjusted, and that sound is produced by puffs of air escaping rhythmically between vocal folds. This rhythmic escape of air takes place because of increasing subglottic air pressure that drives the vocal folds apart, following which Bernoulli's effect immediately begins to draw them together again, only to be driven back apart by subglottic pressure. Changes in tension in the vocal folds is constantly monitored via proprioceptive feedback mechanisms. This monitoring is coupled with auditory feedback to allow adjustment of frequency (pitch) and amplitude (loudness) on an ongoing basis. Loudness is mainly a function of subglottic pressure and is controlled through thoracic and diaphragmatic adjustments. Pitch, on the other hand, is a function not only of vocal fold tension and length, but is also dependent on subglottic air pressure and the relative elevation of the larynx in the neck and the resultant change in pharyngeal dimensions. Although phonation is under voluntary control, the exceedingly complex activities necessary to produce a smooth, clear voice are under reflex control.

References

1. Negus VE: The Comparative Anatomy and Physiology of the Larynx. London, Heinemann, 1949.
2. Edstrom L, Lindquist C, Martensson A: Correlation between functional and histochemical properties of the intrinsic laryngeal muscle units in the cat. In Wycke BD (Ed): Ventilatory and Phonatory Control Systems: An International Symposium. London, Oxford University Press, 1973.
3. Hast M: Anatomy of the larynx. In English GM (Ed): Otolaryngology, vol. III. Philadelphia, Harper & Row, 1978
4. Fink RB, Demarest RJ: Laryngeal Biomechanics. Cambridge, Harvard University Press, 1978.
5. Sasaki CT: Physiology of the larynx. In English GM (Ed): Otolaryngology, vol. III. Philadelphia, Harper & Row, 1984.
6. Brunton TL, Cash T: The valvular action of the larynx. J Anat Physiol, 17:363, 1883.
7. Flores TC, Levine HL, Wood BG, Tucker HM: Factors in successful deglutition fol-

lowing subtotal laryngeal surgery. *Annals Otol Rhinol Laryngol,* 91:579–583, Nov–Dec 1982.
8. Levine HL, Wood BG, Tucker HM: Hypopharyngeal diverticulum and the cricopharyngeus muscle: a posterior surgical approach. *Laryngoscope,* 89:1979 Oct. 1979.
9. Sasaki CT, Fukuda H, Kirchner JA: Laryngeal abductor activity in response to varying ventilatory resistance. Trans Am Acad Ophthalmol Otolaryngol, 77:403, 1973.
10. Suzuki M, Kirchner JA, Murakami Y: The cricothyroid as a respiratory muscle. Ann Otol Rhinol Laryngol, 79:1, 1970.
11. Husson R: Sur la physiologie vocale. Ann Otolaryngol, 69:124–137, 1953.
12. Aronson AE: Clinical Voice Disorders: An Interdisciplinary Approach, 2nd ed. New York, Thieme-Stratton, 1985.
13. Van den Berg JW: Myoelastic-aerodynamic theory of voice production. J Speech Hear Res, 1:227–244, 1958.

Chapter 3

Laryngeal Pathology

Vincent J. Hyams and Dennis K. Heffner

Ideally, the surgical pathologist should be housed physically in the surgical suite, so that immediate consultation is the rule rather than the exception. This type of face-to-face communication is essential not only to the clinician but perhaps even more so to the pathologist. Orientation of specimens, clinical impressions, and description of the gross lesion can be critical to the final diagnosis.—HMT

Following a brief discussion of postmortem examination of the larynx this chapter deals with non-neoplastic laryngeal pathology; neoplasms are considered in the last section. Major emphasis is placed on conditions that can present diagnostic difficulties for the pathologist. It is important for both the clinician and pathologist to be aware of them. Although the pathologist should base his or her diagnosis on the direct examination of tissues, the final interpretation should be one that considers the clinical features as well. In this manner the clinician and pathologist can communicate better, and such communication can perhaps prevent a diagnostic error.◁

Postmortem Examination of the Larynx

If airway obstruction is thought to be involved in a patient's death, postmortem examination of the larynx may be of great importance. There are certain difficulties that can be encountered in the evaluation of the airway at autopsy that both the pathologist and clinician must remember if maximum information is to be obtained.

The pathologist usually examines the internal surfaces of the larynx by splitting and opening the specimen along its posterior midline aspect. Before this is done, the airway should be viewed from above and below to determine if any luminal narrowing is present. Once the larynx is splayed open, it may be impossible to quantify any airway compromise. Attempts to examine the lumen by reclosing the structures after they have been opened are usually unsatisfactory. Formalin fixation makes the situation worse because of tissue distortion caused by the fixation.

Proper laryngeal examination is even more important in the pediatric autopsy. It is virtually impossible to judge the degree of airway compromise in the small larynx of an infant after the larynx is opened. Very slight mucosal swelling can significantly reduce the already small lumen of the pediatric larynx or trachea. It has been estimated that 1 mm of mucosal swelling in the larynx or trachea of a 12-month-old infant reduces the cross-sectional area by 50 percent.[1] In examining the pediatric airway, it may be best not to open the specimen posteriorly. After initial visual inspection from above and below, the laryngotracheal complex can be fixed and sectioned transversely (perpendicular to the airway axis). The effect of the lesion on the airway can then be estimated, after allowing for some fixation shrinkage. The gross sections can be processed for microscopy with the luminal anatomy intact, and this can help preserve anatomic relationships during the microscopic evaluation. An even better result can sometimes be obtained by embedding the larynx whole, without gross sectioning, and then performing serial microscopic sectioning, staining different levels as is appropriate. The infant larynx is easy to process in this fashion because of its small size and lack of calcification of the cartilages.

Radiographs of the specimen might help to define the extent of the lesion, especially in the case of a suspected subglottic lesion. This can be done before fixation and before the shrinkage or distortion of the lesion that may follow fixation.

When airway obstruction may be involved in a particularly important case, it is advantageous that the otolaryngologist join the pathologist during the initial autopsy examination of the larynx. This affords the best opportunity to assess the postmortem airway, and with both the pathologist and clinician present, a mutually satisfactory interpretation is more likely.

Non-Neoplastic Conditions

Some non-neoplastic lesions of the larynx, such as developmental abnormalities or inflammatory conditions in children, can be diagnosed clinically and without biopsy, in which case the surgical pathologist is not involved. When biopsies of reactive or inflammatory lesions are obtained, they are easily misdiagnosed as neoplasm. Clinical correlations can help avoid such errors in diagnosis.

Congenital and Developmental Abnormalities

Laryngomalacia is the most frequent cause of congenital laryngeal stridor. Clinical airway evaluation and exclusion of other causes of stridor is usually sufficient for the diagnosis of this condition. Most patients with this problem improve in time, so that the pathologist is not often involved in their evaluation, although exceptions do occur. If autopsy is performed in such a case, the pathologist can probably add little to the previous clinical assessment other than to exclude other conditions. It has been suggested that there might be alterations of the intercartilagenous supporting tissues in laryngomalacia,[2] but it is difficult to determine or quantify such changes. A rare case in which surgical excision of supraglottic tissues was carried out for a persistent condition suspected of being laryngomalacia in an 18-year-old patient has been reported.[3] The surgical pathologist found it difficult to demonstrate significant histopathologic alterations.

Laryngeal clefts should be diagnosed first by the pathologist only on rare occasions. However, because of physiologic approximation of the cleft between the arytenoids, this condition can be surprisingly difficult to diagnose clinically, even when laryngoscopy and esophagograms in the prone position have been done.[4] Thus, it is occasionally possible for the autopsy pathologist to be dealing with a previously undiagnosed cleft. Examination before the tissues' alteration by posterior incision is important.

Laryngeal webs, atresias, and some *stenoses* may be due to faulty development of the embryologic vestibulotracheal canal. These conditions are most often detected clinically, but in the event of autopsy examination the pathologist may be able to contribute something to the diagnosis, particularly regarding subglottic stenoses. Whether stenosis is congenital or acquired is often not clear and careful autopsy examination may help to determine this. Older literature listed subglottic stenosis as the third most frequently encountered congenital laryngeal anomaly, but it has been less common in the experience of recent investigators.[5] Perhaps some stenoses previously thought to be congenital were in reality of an inflammatory-reactive nature.

Congenital subglottic stenosis can involve only the soft tissues in the region of the conus elasticus, sometimes with an apparent excess of glandular tissue,[6] or it may include cricoid cartilage abnormalities. The cartilaginous stenosis may be circumferential or it may consist of a projecting shelf from only a portion of the cricoid cartilage.[7] An abnormal superior location of the anterior portion of the first tracheal cartilage has been described.[6] In this condition, the anterior portion of the tracheal ring is juxtaposed behind the cricoid arch and there is some loss of luminal diameter. This is a subtle deformity that will probably be demonstrated only by careful autopsy evaluation and suggests a congenital cause for the stenosis. Correlation of embryology with the pathologic findings in developmental anomalies can help explain the lesion. An example of this is a reported instance of subglottic atresia[8] with soft tissue fusion between the vocal cords, but with a narrow, patent tract posteriorly between the arytenoids. This might have resulted from lack of complete development of the vestibulotracheal canal and persistence of the more caudally located pharyngotracheal canal (which normally is obliterated).

Soft tissue stenoses often give the appearance of "subglottic vocal cords,"[7] since there is symmetrical narrowing in the lateral direction. The pathologic examination of these tissues will often show only nonspecific fibrous tissue and the determination of whether the lesion is congenital or acquired may not be possible from the histologic features alone.

Supraglottic cysts may have a developmental basis. *Congenital laryngoceles, large saccules,* and mucin-containing *saccular cysts* may be considered part of a developmental spectrum.[9] The laryngocele is air filled and maintains a communication with the ventricle, but the saccular cyst has lost such a connection. Some congenital cysts in this area are of ductal origin, but examination of the epithelium is seldom helpful in determining the exact origin of the cyst. The location and size of the cyst are probably more important in classification. Saccular cysts tend to be anterolateral and deeply situated; ductal cysts can be located anywhere in the supraglottic area but are usually more superficial.[10] Saccular cysts are usually larger than 1 cm and ductal cysts usually smaller. Congenital subglottic respiratory-lined cysts have only rarely been reported.[11] Small vocal cord cysts might in some instances have a developmental basis.[12]

Cystic lymphangiomas of the supraglottic area have occurred, although rarely.[13] It is important that surgically excised tissue from this type of lesion be correctly identified by the pathologist. A lymphangioma will likely be rather deeply extensive in the tissues and will have poorly defined margins. It will tend to be a more difficult treatment problem with a higher chance of recurrence than a simple cyst. Delineation of the epithelial lining of the cyst as opposed to the endothelial lining of lymphangiomas allows histologic distinction between the two.

Ectopic thyroid gland tissue can occasionally occur within the larynx and may produce a symptomatic airway mass. The condition is a congenital developmental abnormality, but symptoms are usually delayed until adulthood. The lesion is usually in the posterolateral aspect of the subglottic area. There may or may not be an associated defect in the cricothyroid ligament; if there is, the lesion may communicate with the thyroid gland.[14] Because the tissue is likely to be vascular, bleeding may follow biopsy. The surgical pathologist probably will not have difficulty in recognizing that the specimen is thyroid tissue, but it can be difficult to distinguish it from well-differentiated thyroid carcinoma invading the larynx. If both possibilities are kept in mind when the tissue is examined, an error is less likely to occur. *Heterotopic gastric epithelium* within the larynx[15] is even more rare and less readily recognized by the pathologist.

Hamartomas may present as symptomatic, tumorlike masses in the larynx.[16] These lesions are composed of tissues that are normally present in the organ in which the lesion is found, but the amount and organization of the tissues are abnormal. Hamartomas are not true neoplasms and are distinguished from *teratomas* by the greater growth potential and the greater tissue heterogeneity (including tissues foreign to the site of occurrence of the lesion) of the latter.

Whether *subglottic hemangioma* should be considered as malformations, hamartomas, or benign neoplasms is unclear, but it *is* clear that they tend to present in infants, and this suggests congenital origin. The diagnosis is often suggested by the clinical findings, and there is often reluctance to biopsy the lesion because of anticipated bleeding.◁ However, false clinical diagnosis of this lesion can occur, and biopsy may occasionally play a role. Interpretation of the tissue can be difficult if the pathologist is not familiar with the histologic appearance of this lesion. The proliferation can be quite cellular, and the vessels may be minute, collapsed, and histologically inapparent. The lesional tissue can be admixed with the normal glands of the area, and this may be taken for an aggressive invasion (Fig. 3–1). This pattern together with the cellularity of the lesion might cause the hemangioma to be misdiagnosed as some type of sarcoma.[17] Clinical clues, such as associated cutaneous hemangiomas or subglottic location, should be made known to the pathologist. If the possibility of hemangioma is considered while the tissue is being examined, the correct diagnosis can usually be made. Subglottic hemangiomas often extend deeply into the submucosal tissues, even to the perichondrium.[18] Occasionally, they may extend outward between tracheal rings. Perhaps this deep location can contribute to the recurrence of a lesion that has been surgically treated.

It is generally both unnecessary and inadvisable to biopsy a suspected subglottic hemangioma. However, in the event that a biopsy cannot be avoided it is best carried out by laser surgery with partial excision of the lesion. Most of these hemangiomas will be of the mixed capillary and cavernous type and bleeding can be a problem, but usually can be controlled satisfactorily with the laser.—HMT

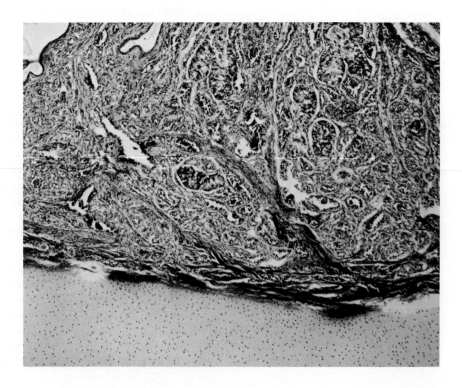

Figure 3–1. Subglottic hemangioma (autopsy specimen with mild autolysis), demonstrating small vessels interspersed among glands. (AFIP #84-5155; H & E, ×60.)

Traumatic Lesions

Accidental Trauma

Fires often cause severe *mucosal burns* in the airway because of in-
haled hot gases. Damage to the laryngotracheal area may be marked even
though pharyngeal injury is slight or inapparent. This may be related to the
more resistant squamous epithelium of the pharynx as opposed to the more
vulnerable respiratory epithelium of the subglottis and trachea.

Fractures of the larynx may stimulate ossification in the soft tissues
near the fracture sites. This can be of some clinical relevance in making
surgical repair more difficult if there has to be a delay in repairing them.

Foreign bodies can cause either acute airway obstruction or a more
chronic problem. If foreign material becomes embedded in the soft tissue,
a marked inflammatory response can eventually occur, especially if there
is secondary infection. If the foreign material is not included in the biopsy,
the cause of the problem may not be determined by histologic evaluation.

Trauma Related to Airway Management

Postintubation granulomas consist of marked proliferation of granulation tissue, usually in the posterior glottis or upper subglottis. If this tissue is biopsied, there will not be anything particularly specific about the
histologic appearance, and the correct interpretation of the condition rests
mainly on the history of recent intubation.

Long-term intubation can result in chronic reactive tissues and *subglottic stenosis*. Occasionally, the posterior glottis develops adhesions between eroded surfaces.[19] In the infant, the posterior subglottic area may be
especially susceptible to intubation injury because of the slightly V-shaped
cross-sectional configuration of the posterior portion of the cricoid cartilage.[20] The resistance of the two flattened sides of the "V" may increase
the pressure on the mucosa trapped between the cartilage and an endotracheal tube.

Injury from long-term airway management may extend into the deeper
laryngeal tissues, occasionally *damaging* the *vocal process* of the arytenoid
or even the *cricoarytenoid joint*.[21] In a case studied by Tucker et al,[22] the
clinical course suggested an acquired subglottic stenosis, but marked changes
were demonstrated in the deep tissues unilaterally. There was fibrosis replacing the vocalis muscle on one side, which extended into the subglottic
area. The cricoid cartilage on the same side was disrupted and there was
ossification in the adjacent tissues. The unilaterality of the changes might
raise the question of a congenital anomaly, but the histologic findings were
unlike congenital anomalies that have been described. This interesting case
illustrates that additional careful examinations of specimens of this type may
be necessary to understand better subglottic stenosis, particularly in determining the contributions of congenital versus acquired causes.

In addition to contributing to most instances of subglottic stenosis,[5]
reactive proliferations from invasive diagnostic or maintenance procedures
on the airway also can cause localized masses that might be mistaken for
neoplasm. Jackson and Jackson[23] indicated as early as 1932 that many lesions of the airway that had been previously diagnosed as neoplasms were
in reality reactive or inflammatory. Even today, the pathologist might mis-
take a cellular, reactive proliferation of this area for a neoplasm. The clinical history of airway procedures should be included in the final interpretation so that the possibility of a reactive lesion is considered.

It may be difficult or impossible for the surgical pathologist to know if fibroblastic tissue obtained from the larynx is reactive or should be considered a tumorlike proliferation such as *aggressive fibromatosis*.[24] Once again, the interpretation must depend, at least in part, on the clinical history.

Lesions Related to Mechanical Function of the Larynx

The vocal cords may develop various lesions related to overly vigorous mechanical action of the glottis. The area of the vocal process is subject to chronic injury by this means, and *contact ulcers* can result. The chronicity of the injury, produced by vocal strain, vocal habits, such as throat clearing, or aggravated by nocturnal gastric reflux,[25] may result in prominent granulation tissue reaction (Fig. 3–2). There also may be reactive squamous epithelial hyperplasia at the edge of such a lesion. If it is biopsied, the tissue will probably appear nonspecific to the pathologist. The clinical findings, such as the posterior glottic location of the lesion, are very important in suggesting the specific diagnosis of contact ulcer.

Other conditions of the posterior glottis, such as *tuberculosis* or *fungal infection,* can be mistaken clinically for a contact ulcer. Usually the pathologist can find some specific histologic clue (such as granulomas or giant cells) to suggest the correct diagnosis in these instances.

The diagnosis of *vocal nodules* and *polyps* can be confusing. This is due in part to somewhat different use of the term ''nodule'' by pathologists from that used by otolaryngologists. Many of the lesions that give the clinical impression of polyp will be composed of reactive tissues that include abundant vessels or moderately sized blood-filled spaces, prominent fibrin exudation, and perhaps some evidence of old hemorrhage (such as hemosiderin) (Fig. 3–3). Lesions of this type have been called ''nodule'' (including laryngeal nodule, singer's nodule, and screamer's nodule) in much of the pathology literature. The otolaryngologist, on the other hand, generally uses the term nodule for tiny, usually bilateral excrescences in the anterior portions of the vocal cords that are smaller than most polyps and that will have a different histologic appearance. Nodules are usually diagnosed clinically and not biopsied or treated surgically,[26] but if they are removed, the histologic composition is essentially a localized excess of otherwise unremarkable fibrous tissue. An awareness of this different terminology can help avoid misunderstandings.

Figure 3–2. Vocal cord contact ulcers, demonstrating the prominent tissue proliferation that occurs in resonse to this condition. (AFIP #85-5454.)

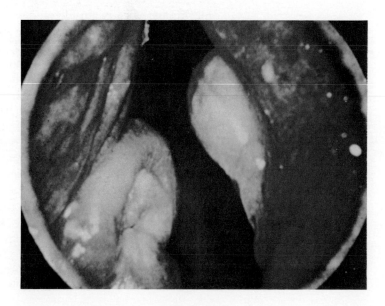

Figure 3–3. Vocal cord polyp with vessels and fibrin exudation; the fibrin can be mistaken for amyloid. (AFIP #85-5762; H & E ×60.)

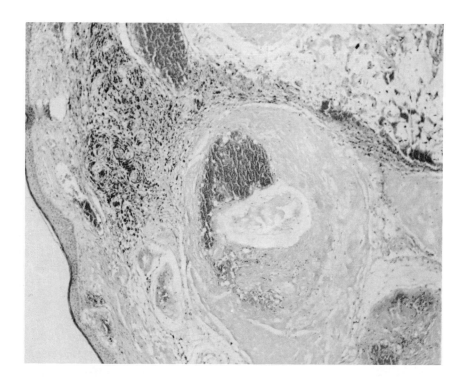

Vocal nodule apparently results from chronic or repeated vocal strain, especially from the generation of higher pitched loud sounds. Many vascular, fibrinous polyps may also result from acute and severe vocal abuse that results in focal hemorrhage or hemorrhagic edema of the cord tissues (Fig. 3–4). These areas can undergo some organizational changes, including neovascularization, and these changes contribute to the histologic appearance when removed surgically. If the lesion is present for a long time, it may become more fibrous and hyalinized (Fig. 3–5).

Figure 3–4. Early hemorrhagic stage in vocal cord polyp formation. (AFIP #85-5456.)

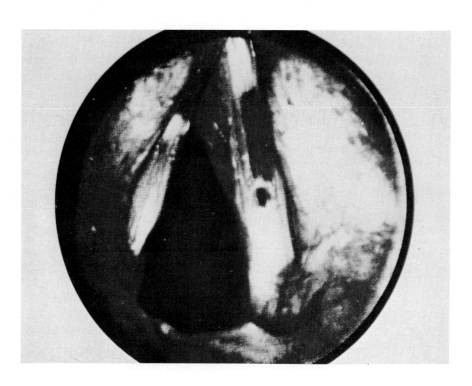

Figure 3–5. Vocal cord polyp that has become fibrous after being present for some time. (AFIP #85-5453.)

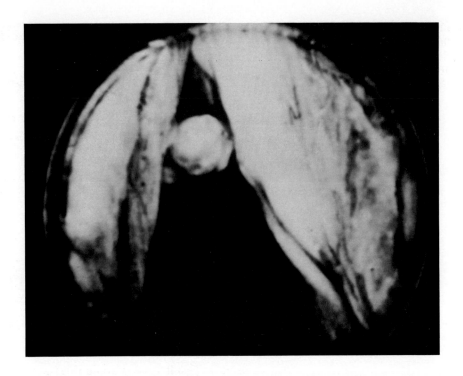

Diffuse fusiform or polypoid change of the vocal folds, especially when it is bilateral and occurs in middle aged and older females, should raise the suspicion of hypothyroidism. Appropriate blood tests should be carried out to rule out low-grade myxedema of the larynx as the cause for such polyps. At biopsy or stripping, they tend to be jellylike and are usually chronic.—HMT

The fibrin deposits in many vocal polyps can suggest *amyloid* to the pathologist (Fig. 3–3), but amyloid deposits in the larynx have clinical and histologic features somewhat different from those of polyps. Amyloid usually will be more sessile or diffusely distributed than would be expected in a polyp. Laryngeal amyloid is often found in more glandular areas of the larynx, and it usually does not have the neovascularity frequently found in polyps. In doubtful cases, special stains for amyloid can be of help.

The vascularity of some polyps can cause them to be mistaken histologically for a *vascular neoplasm* (such as a *hemangioma*). Probably a majority of lesions that have been diagnosed as vascular neoplasms of the glottis are in reality either polyps or contact ulcers (which also tend to have prominent vascularity in the form of granulation tissue). Vascular neoplasms would generally be expected either supra- or subglottically rather than in the glottic area proper.

Some vocal polyps are histologically rather different from the vascular, fibrinous, and fibrous ones just described. They are composed of prominent, uniform myxoid tissue (Figs. 3–6 and 3–7), and they can raise the question of some type of myxoid neoplasm, perhaps a *myxoma*. Myxomas in many parts of the body behave as infiltrative and even locally aggressive neoplasms, but the myxoid polyps of the vocal cords apparently do not have this tendency. Perhaps these polyps are best considered to be the result of some peculiar alteration of the stroma of the vocal cord tissues (especially of Reinke's space), rather than neoplastic. The etiology of the alteration is not clear in most cases but could conceivably be a result of chronic laryngitis from a number of causes. An occasional case may have a relationship to hypothyroidism.◁ These non-neoplastic myxoid polyps should be distinguished from true neoplasms, but since myxoid neoplasms are rare in the larynx, the problem is not a major one. A myxoid rhabdomyosarcoma in the larynx of an adult is very rare. Myxoid nerve sheath tumors can be excluded by using immunohistochemistry for the S-100 protein.

Laryngoceles can occasionally be congenital,[9] but in the adult they

Figure 3–6. Vocal cord polyp
that was histologically myxoid.
See Figure 7. (AFIP #83-
10023.)

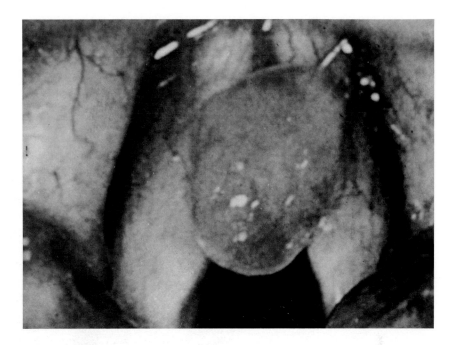

seem to result from chronic dilation of the saccule secondary to increased
airway pressure. The histologic lining of a laryngocele is usually unremarkable respiratory epithelium, perhaps with some slight metaplastic
changes. Distinction of laryngocele from a laryngeal inclusion cyst will,
therefore, depend on the clinical or radiographic finding of an air-filled sac
connected to the ventricle. When there is extralaryngeal extension of lar-

Figure 3–7. Vocal cord polyp
composed of loose, edematous,
myxoid stroma. (AFIP #85-
5764; H & E ×100.)

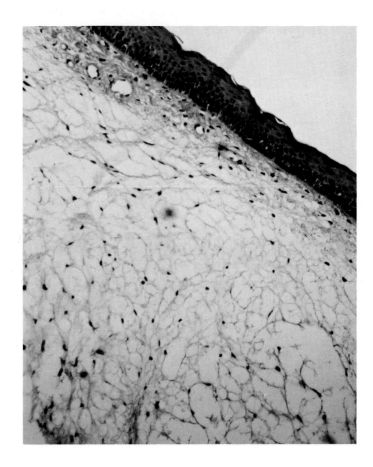

yngocele through the thyrohyoid membrane, this finding can help in diagnosis. A *pharyngocele* will demonstrate a more stratified squamous epithelial lining than in a laryngocele because the clinical site of origin is also different.

Infectious Diseases

Acute Infections

Acute laryngotracheobronchitis is a common infection, probably caused by numerous different viruses,[27] but bacteria are sometimes implicated as well. Generally, the pathologist will not be asked to examine tissue from these cases, but the condition can sometimes be fatal.[27] Cases with bacterial infection are more dangerous.[28] Whether or not bacterial involvement represents secondary infection or a primary viral illness is usually not clear, but, in any event, it is important to recognize the possibility of bacterial infection. Autopsy should include proper examination (cultures, special stains) to determine if such an infection was present.

The inflammation in this kind of infection has a pronounced effect on the subglottic area. The tissues of Pressman's space (in the triangle bounded by the mucosal epithelium, the conus elasticus, and the superior and luminal portion of the cricoid cartilage) become markedly swollen by acute and subacute inflammatory cell infiltrate and especially by edema. There can even be some fibrinous exudate in severe cases.[27] This marked swelling of the subglottic area produces the stridor of croup.

Acute epiglottitis also causes a marked swelling of tissues, but in the supraglottic rather than the subglottic area. The most pronounced edema and inflammatory cell infiltrate occurs in the tissues of the lingual side of the epiglottis. The submucosal tissues here are more loosely areolar and more readily expanded by inflammation than the tissue of the laryngeal side. Marked expansion in this area pushes the epiglottis backward and downward, and this, together with aryepiglottic fold swelling, produces the marked and dangerous supraglottic airway compromise of this disease.

Although acute epiglottitis is most common in children, it can also occur in adults. *Staphylococcus* and *Streptococcus* are probably the most important causative organisms in adults, as opposed to *Hemophilus* being important in children. Epiglottic abscess can be a sequel to acute epiglottitis, and this complication is more common in adults than children.[29] Because of the larger airway of adults, epiglottitis is usually not as dangerous as in children, but if epiglottic abscess occurs, acute airway obstruction and even sudden death can result.[30]

Infection of laryngeal tissues may complicate the tissue reactions that occur after irradiation of the larynx for cancer. When such infection occurs, it tends to extend deeply to the cartilage, and it contributes to *perichondritis* and thence to the egregious chondritis and *cartilage necrosis* that may follow. Cartilage necrosis can be relentless because the perichondrial damage interferes with the sole nutrient support for the cartilage, which has no internal blood supply.

Specific infections, such as *scarlet fever, pertussis, typhoid fever, rubeola, variola,* and *varicella,* may have an associated laryngitis, but the histopathologic reactions of this anatomic area are not especially remarkable in these diseases. *Diphtheria* produces a somewhat specific reaction in the marked degree to which the fibrinopurulent exudate (occurring after surface epithelial erosion) congeals into the well-known "pseudomembrane" of this disease. Diphtheria may initiate subglottic stenosis as a later complication,[31] but this would be a rare cause of stenosis today.

Chronic Infections

Tuberculous infection of the larynx[32] is generally considered secondary to pulmonary infection, but in the instance where the pulmonary infection has not yet been diagnosed, it is important not to misdiagnose the laryngeal infection. Today, there may not be as strong a tendency for a posterior location of the infection as there was in earlier days when therapy of pulmonary tuberculosis usually included bed rest, but involvement of the posterior glottis is still an important finding. This should not be mistaken for contact ulcer. In most cases, the tissues will contain some histologic clues, such as giant cells, that will alert the pathologist to search for a specific granulomatous infection (Fig 3–8).

Once granulomas are found histologically, it is certainly important to rule out infection by all reasonable means before concluding that the granulomas are a manifestation of *sarcoidosis*. If histologic stains are negative for organisms, this does not exclude tuberculous or fungal infection, and other clinical and laboratory methods should be used to search for evidence of infection.

Histoplasmosis, blastomycosis, coccidioidomycosis, actinomycosis, cryptococcosis, sporotrichosis, and *aspergillosis* of the larynx have occurred.[33–38] Histoplasmosis and blastomycosis are probably the most commonly reported. Cryptococcal, aspergillotic, and sporotrichotic infections of the larynx are rare, and the first two would seem to be a problem mostly in persons who are debilitated or immunosuppressed. Except for actinomycosis, most fungal infections are also probably secondary to pulmonary infection. As with tuberculosis, the specific histologic clues of granulomatous infection should not be overlooked by the pathologist. These clues may not be obvious, especially in a small biopsy, and this can be dangerous in the case of some fungal infections (especially histoplasmosis and blastomycosis), since they might be mistaken for carcinoma. The main difficulty is that sometimes these fungal infections stimulate marked pseudocarcinomatous hyperplasia of the overlying squamous epithelium. Such hyper-

Figure 3–8. Multinucleated giant cells within an inflammatory reaction; these giant cells should alert the pathologist to the possibility of a specific granulomatous infection. (AFIP #85-5765; H & E, ×250.)

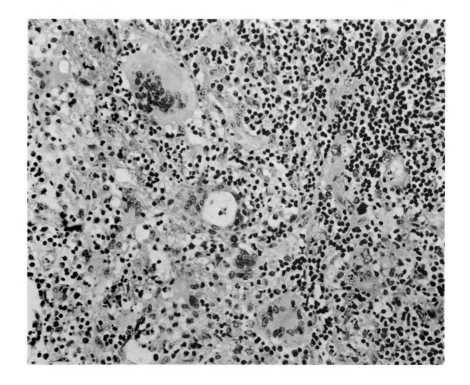

plasia can be mistaken histologically for invasive carcinoma. Histoplasmosis also has been mistaken clinically for carcinoma,[34] and clinical features that are not typical of malignancy should be communicated to the pathologist so that he or she can be especially alert to avoid misdiagnosis. Even a single giant cell would be an important finding to point to the possibility of fungal infection.

Candidiasis can cause superficial mucosal infection of the larynx.[39] This infection is rather easily overlooked, and with relatively superficial and apparently nonspecific inflammation in the laryngeal tissues, the pathologist should scrutinize the surface areas for the fungal hyphae of *Candida*.

Conditions with Metabolic or Genetic Features

Amyloidosis can occur in a localized form in the upper airway, including the larynx. Mass lesions can be produced, particularly in the supraglottic area. A biopsy will reveal deposits of acellular pink material, and special stains, such as the Congo red procedure (with examination under polarized light), can help confirm the diagnosis. If the deposits are prominent, the diagnosis can be strongly suspected by the appearance on routine stains. They often have a somewhat nodular appearance and seem to be replacing glands.[40] Foreign body giant cells are often present, and sometimes calcification can be detected. As previously mentioned, the fibrin deposits that often occur in vocal cord polyps should not be confused with amyloidosis.

Lipoid proteinosis, possibly associated with autosomal recessive inheritance,[41] is a familial disorder that often includes elevated, irregular, somewhat multinodular excrescences in the laryngeal mucosa. Hoarseness is a common sign in infancy. Often there is widespread oral and oropharyngeal involvement, but localized laryngeal involvement may occasionally occur.[42] Airway impingement can be significant, and tracheostomy has occasionally been required.[41] If a mucosal lesion is biopsied, there is a rather diffuse deposition of hyaline, pink material in the subepithelial tissues. Both neutral and acid mucopolysaccharides can be demonstrated by special stains. Lipid material is also supposed to be present, but special stains give variable and unpredictable results. Although amyloid stains would be expected to be negative, the condition might be mistaken histologically for amyloid or some other condition. Clinical features are important in suspecting and supporting the correct diagnosis. Skin lesions are usually present, and small, beady deposits along the eyelid margins can particularly suggest the diagnosis. The usual presentation early in life and the finding of cerebral (hippocampal gyrus) calcification on radiography are other features helpful in diagnosis.

Ligneous conjunctivitis is a rare condition that also involves the deposition of pink material, primarily in the conjunctivae, but airway obstructive symptoms have been described. The diagnosis of this rare disease would rest mostly on examination of the characteristic conjunctival lesions.

Hypothyroidism can cause edema of the vocal cords,[43] and this may occasionally progress to the formation of an edematous or myxoid polyp.

As previously mentioned, *ectopic thyroid tissue* can occur within the endolarynx. Although a congenital condition, this will usually not cause symptoms early in life. Symptoms often first appear only when there are metabolic reasons for enlargement of thyroid tissue. If the person develops an endemic goiter within the normally located thyroid gland, the endolaryngeal tissue can enlarge also. Enlargement and airway symptoms are more common in females and may occur first in connection with pregnancy or in relation to menstruation.

Gouty tophi can involve the larynx, but by the time this occurs there should be definite clinical and laboratory evidence of gout.[44] Therefore, the histologic identification of crystalline deposits with some surrounding reactive tissues as the tophi of gout will probably not be difficult. In persons without gout, there can occasionally be a few tiny crystalline structures within the vocal cord tissues that are discovered incidentally in a biopsy that has been done to evaluate or exclude some condition, such as a neoplasm. They should not be mistaken as indicating gout. These tiny deposits probably represent some type of crystallized protein and most likely are not clinically significant. Perhaps they represent some minor degenerative alteration.

Epidermolysis bullosa,[45,46] *pachyonychia congenita,*[47] and the *blue rubber bleb nevus syndrome*[48] are rare hereditary or congenital skin conditions that have been associated with laryngeal lesions. Epidermolysis bullosa is especially important in this regard, and it can result in significant laryngeal stenosis. The diagnosis will generally be made because of the dermatologic features, and the histopathologic features of the laryngeal lesions will not be critical in this regard.

Miscellaneous Conditions

Wegener's granulomatosis can involve the larynx, usually in the subglottic or upper tracheal area, and this involvement can produce airway symptoms. Biopsy diagnosis of Wegener's disease is often quite difficult, and the specimen may appear to be nonspecific inflammation to the histopathologist. Vasculitis is the pathologic basis if the disease, but histologic proof is often difficult to find in biopsies from the upper respiratory tract (perhaps more so than in biopsies from the lung, kidney, or skin). If inflammation is associated with a vessel, it can be challenging to determine whether that inflammation indicates primary vasculitis or is secondary involvement by diffuse, nonspecific inflammation of the tissues in which the vessel is located.

Wegener's granulomatosis often produces prominent patches of necrosis with fine nuclear "dust" (from karyorrhexis). This "dusty" or "sandy" appearance can be helpful in diagnosis (Fig. 3–9). It is not completely specific, but, if it is prominent, it can be strongly suggestive of Wegener's granulomatosis. A few giant cells are often present, and this is also diagnostically helpful. Although giant cells lend a granulomatous appearance to the histologic features, Wegener's disease generally does not manifest well-defined, dense collections of epithelioid histiocytes to the extent found in many infectious granulomatous diseases. Nevertheless, it may be impossible to exclude mycobacterial or fungal infection by the histologic features alone in a biopsy suspected of representing Wegener's granulomatosis. It is then important to use clinical and laboratory methods to help exclude an infectious process.

Subglottic or upper tracheal involvement by Wegener's granulomatosis usually occurs in females.[49] Involvement of these areas tends to occur only when the disease is already manifested in other areas, and these clinical features are important in determining if the larynx is actually involved when the biopsy interpretation is equivocal.

Sarcoidosis has occurred in the larynx, usually in the supraglottic area.[50] The histologic clue to the diagnosis is finding of noncaseating granulomas, but infection has to be excluded by clinical and additional laboratory means.

Figure 3–9. Wegener's granulomatosis with a patch of necrosis demonstrating the granular or sandy appearance of nuclear debris. (AFIP #85-5763; H & E ×160.)

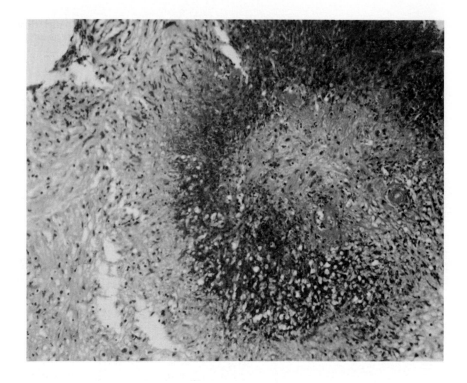

Frequently, the granulomas of laryngeal sarcoidosis are scarce and a small biopsy may miss them and contain only nonspecific lymphoid inflammatory infiltrate. Repeat biopsy might demonstrate granulomas that were not sampled initially.

Vesiculobullous diseases of the skin or mucosal surfaces, such as *pemphigus*[51] or *pemphigoid*, sometimes involve the larynx. Scarring and deformity can occur, particularly with benign mucous membrane pemphigoid.[52] Histologic findings include "splitting" of the mucosal epithelium from the underlying stroma in the basal area, which is the histologic correlate of the clinical blister. Histologic immunologic abnormalities may be demonstrated by immunoflourescence, and this procedure can contribute to diagnosis. However, the histologic diagnostic features can be subtle, and if the biopsy does not include an area where the vesicle is demonstrated, the diagnosis will often be uncertain. The diagnosis can be greatly aided by the total clinical picture; for example, the appearance of other mucosal lesions or of skin lesions in the case of pemphigus and the frequent conjunctival lesions of benign mucous membrane pemphigoid are very helpful.

Rheumatoid arthritis is known to affect the larynx. Histologic evidence of the disease (rheumatoid granulomas with degeneration or "necrobiosis" of tissue with surrounding palisaded histiocytes) can be found in soft tissues of the thyrohyoid and postcricoid regions. Edema and fibrosis associated with these lesions might possibly contribute to airway obstruction,[53] but the most troublesome result of laryngeal involvement is cricothyroid or cricoarytenoid joint involvement that may progress to ankylosis. Histologic changes in these joints are similar to findings in other joints involved with rheumatoid arthritis. Usually, laryngeal involvement occurs in a setting of long-standing disease that is manifested elsewhere in the body, although there are rare exceptions.[54]

Relapsing polychondritis frequently affects the laryngotracheal area,[55] and airway involvement can be a fatal complication of this disease. The histologic changes begin in the outer edges of the cartilage in the perichondrial area, with subsequent inflammatory encroachment on and eventual destruction of the deeper cartilage. In early stages the histologic features can be difficult to distinguish from nonspecific perichondritis. Relapsing polychondritis may be an immunologic disorder involving type II collagen (a component of cartilage) and immunoflourescence studies might demonstrate immune complex deposits at cartilage edges.[56] Again, the clinical findings are important in differential diagnosis and the presence of other cartilage involvement by this systemic disease is helpful. Characteristic auricular and nasal septal cartilage changes are frequent and helpful in diagnosis, as are scleritis (the sclera contains type II collagen) and joint symptoms.

Non-neoplastic lymphoid masses occur rarely in the supraglottic larynx. One interesting case described by Castleman[57] histologically appeared identical to specific lymphoid hyperplasia (or perhaps hamartoma), which usually occurs in the mediastinum. Lymphoid masses of the larynx must be distinguished, if possible, from well-differentiated extranodal lymphomas, a histologic distinction that can be very difficult. It may be necessary to follow the patient to judge the behavior of the lesion before the correct diagnosis becomes clear.

Subglottic stenosis in the adult is usually secondary to inflammation or trauma that can be documented by the clinical history, but occasional idiopathic cases have occurred.[59] Biopsy demonstrates nonspecific fibrous tissue with a few chronic inflammatory cells. Perhaps some of these cases are related to other tumefactive fibroinflammatory masses that occur in the head and neck that are histologically nonspecific but that certainly can be clinically significant.[60] Several cases have been associated with concomitant proptosis and the orbital tissue (which resembled what has been called pseudotumor of the orbit) was histologically similar to the subglottic tissue.[61] A better understanding of these fibrous conditions will require study of more cases.

Laryngeal Neoplasia

Extensive search of the world's literature would probably reveal at least one example of every classifiable human neoplastic entity involving the larynx, but there is neither time nor space for such a complete dissertation. This discussion will be limited to those laryngeal tumors and neoplasms that otolaryngologists might expect to encounter in day-to-day practice. The classification of primary neoplasia of the larynx in Table 3–1 is an adaptation of the World Health Organization Histological Typing of Upper Respiratory Tumors.[62]

Benign Neoplasms

Epithelial

Papilloma is benign, exophytic, epithelial neoplastic proliferation arising from a tissue surface. In the larynx and trachea they account for 10 percent of laryngeal neoplasia recorded in the Armed Forces Institute of Pathology (AFIP) Tumor Registry. Half of the patients have initial involvement before 16 years of age, with the majority of these patients being less than 5 years of age at the onset of the disease. The age range is from 1 month to the eighth decade.[63] There is no apparent sex predilection. Laryngeal papilloma is not generally associated with other papillomas of the upper respiratory tract or other areas of the body. Regardless of the age at onset,

Table 3–1   Classification of Neoplasms of the Larynx

Benign
  Epithelial
    Squamous cell papilloma
    Cyst, epithelial
    Oncocytoma
    Adenoma
      Pleomorphic adenoma (benign mixed tumor)
  Mesodermal, neuroectodermal
    Benign granular cell tumor
    Chondroma
      Osteochondroma
    Hemangioma
      Lymphangioma
    Fibroma
    Fibrohistiocytoma
    Leiomyoma
    Rhabdomyoma
    Lipoma
    Giant cell tumor (? of soft tissue)
    Neurilemmoma (schwannoma, neurinoma)
    Neurofibroma
    Paraganglioma (extra-adrenal)
Premalignant epithelial abnormalities
  Benign squamous hyperplasia (keratosis) with or without epithelial atypia
Malignant
  Epithelial
    Squamous cell carcinoma
    Verrucous carcinoma
    Spindle cell carcinoma
    Undifferentiated small cell (? oat cell) carcinoma
    Adenocarcinoma (carcinoid tumor)
    Adenoid cystic carcinoma
    Mucoepidermoid carcinoma
  Mesodermal, neuroectodermal
    Fibrosarcoma
    Malignant fibrohistiocytoma
    Synovial sarcoma
    Rhabdomyosarcoma
    Angiosarcoma
      Kaposi's sarcoma
    Liposarcoma
    Chondrosarcoma
    Lymphoma
    Plasmacytoma
    Neurofibrosarcoma
    Malignant melanoma
  Teratoid neoplasms (benign and malignant)
    Dermoid cyst
    Teratoma
    Hamartoma
    Choristoma
    Teratocarcinoma
  Metastatic neoplasms involving the larynx

early symptoms include changes in phonation with progressive hoarseness, huskiness, and even aphonia. Chronic involvement may result in personality changes and funnel breast in children. Clinically, papillomas are glistening, elevated, mulberry-like, nodular whitish-gray to reddish-pink masses

Figure 3–10. This specimen represents a larynx removed at the autopsy of a 2-year-old male child with a history of "asthma" for 18 months. The laryngeal luminal masses were benign squamous papillomas, such as demonstrated in Figure 3–11. (AFIP #83-10020.)

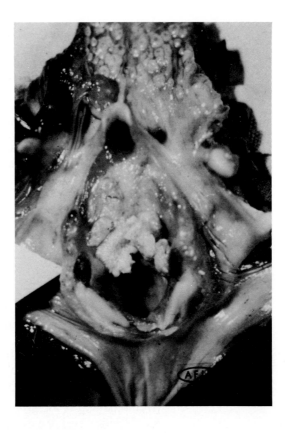

attached to the mucosa by a narrow stalk, although a wide area of continuity with the mucosa can occur (Fig. 3–10). Lesions up to 2 cm may arise anywhere on the laryngeal mucosa but tend to originate from the true vocal cords. Most are friable and bleed easily from slight trauma, which can make complete surgical removal difficult. The micromorphology is nonkeratinizing, uniform squamous epithelium arranged in projecting fronds, with a delicate central vascular connective tissue core (Fig. 3–11). Surface

Figure 3–11. A typical histologic appearance of a laryngeal squamous cell papilloma demonstrating the exophytic uniform squamous cell proliferation with a central fibrovascular core. Surface keratinization is rare. (AFIP #83-10785; H & E ×63.)

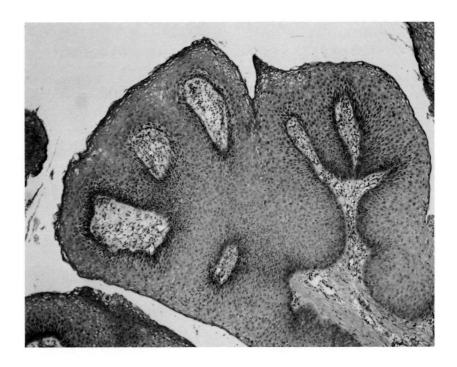

keratosis is rare and, when present, should raise suspicions of other diagnostic possibilities.

Treatment has included removal by techniques such as the carbon dioxide laser, cryotherapy, ultrasound, and microcauterization, all of which are variations of simple surgical removal. Nonsurgical adjuncts such as salves, interferon, and autogenous vaccine have all had their advocates, but at this writing, none has shown superior therapeutic results. Radiotherapy is to be condemned because of the proven relationship of such therapy to carcinomatous degeneration, particularly in those with juvenile onset. Prognosis is guarded, but fatal complications are less than 5 percent in AFIP Otolaryngic Tumor Registry material. Recurrence of laryngeal papilloma is the main complication, particularly in the juvenile-onset group. Holinger et al[63] reported that 80 percent of cases of juvenile-onset papillomas had multiple recurrences, whereas only 36 percent of those with adult-onset recurred. These are found mostly at the initial site, but they may extend to produce massive involvement of pulmonary spaces or infiltration between tracheal and bronchial rings and, on rare occasion, may even have a fatal outcome. Malignant degeneration and metastases are rare.[64] Differential diagnosis of inflammatory and traumatic polyps of the larynx must be considered, but usually cytologic studies indicate the correct diagnosis. In the adult, the possibility of an exophytic squamous cell carcinoma must be ruled out. Any adult laryngeal papilloma with epithelial atypia deserves suspicion and careful clinical follow-up after complete surgical removal.

The cause of laryngeal papillomas seems to be viral. Papova virus and papillomaviral antigen have been demonstrated ultrastructurally within papillomas. Condylomata acuminata involving maternal genitalia at the time of parturition of children who later develop laryngeal papillomas have been reported.[65] Juvenile-onset laryngeal papilloma tends to involve children from the lower socioeconomic levels.

Cysts of the larynx occur at three different age ranges. A congenital cyst may be present at birth as a space-occupying, supraglottic lesion (Fig. 3–12). They are glistening, smooth-walled structures, containing clear fluid. Histologically, the lining is pseudostratified, tall, respiratory ciliated epithelium, which may represent embryologic origin from misplaced laryn-

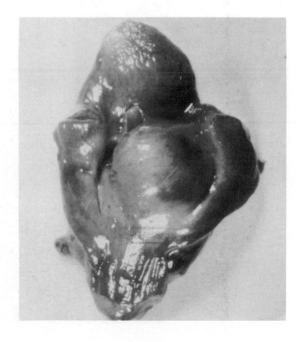

Figure 3–12. A gross larynx removed at autopsy of a full-term male infant who, after a normal birth presentation, failed to breath satisfactorily and died. This large smooth-walled cyst containing clear watery fluid filled the right aryepiglottic fold obstructing the airway. (AFIP #85-6064.)

Figure 3–13. This represents an endoscopic view of the pharynx of a 14-year-old male with several months' complaint of difficulty in breathing and swallowing. At surgery, the paraepiglottic mass proved to be a thin-walled cystic structure filled with a granular gray material. Microscopically, the lining was that of a keratinizing thin band of stratified squamous cell epithelium. (AFIP #85-6063.)

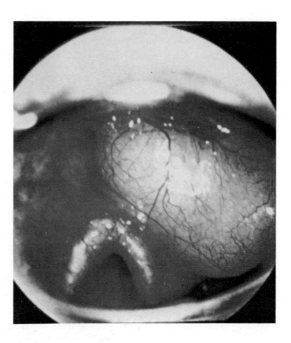

geal epithelium. A second group of laryngeal cysts occurs in the adolescent or young adult in the supraglottic-aryepiglottic fold area (Fig. 3–13). They usually contain a milky-white, puttylike material and are lined microscopically by keratinizing squamous epithelium, possibly derived from a remnant of the upper end of a branchial cleft. The third age group is older adults. These cysts are most frequently located supraglottically and present as mucosal-covered cystic lesions in the laryngeal lumen[66,67] (Fig. 3–14). Histologically, they consist of glandular or cystic epithelial proliferation of oncocytic cells thought to represent degenerative metaplasia of mucoserous epithelium. Difficulty may arise in differentiating between cystic oncocytic metaplasia and an oncocytic neoplasm (oncocytoma, oxyphillic adenoma) (see later). Incomplete surgical removal of the epithelial lining invites recurrence in any of the three types of cysts. Malignant degeneration of these laryngeal cysts has not been reported.

Oncocytoma (oxyphil adenoma) denotes a benign tumor composed of uniform cubiodal to columnar, granular eosinophilic cells arranged in glands

Figure 3–14. A gross larynx removed at autopsy from an 83-year-old female with the stated cause of death being severe arteriosclerotic heart disease. She complained of some shortness of breath and the supraglottic mucosal-covered clear fluid cystic mass was incidentally discovered at autopsy. The histologic features are consistent with that shown in Figure 15. (AFIP #85-6065.)

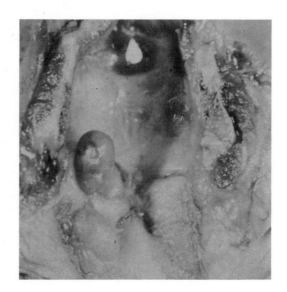

Figure 3–15. A microscopic view of an excisional biopsy of a supraglottic mucosal-covered lesion in a 75-year-old male. Clinically, it resembled the gross lesion depicted in Figure 3–15. The typical tall columnar, sometimes double-layered eosinophilic finely granular cells considered oncocytes are present. They may represent a metaplasia or neoplastic proliferation of local mucoserous glands. (AFIP #83-10709; H & E, ×160.)

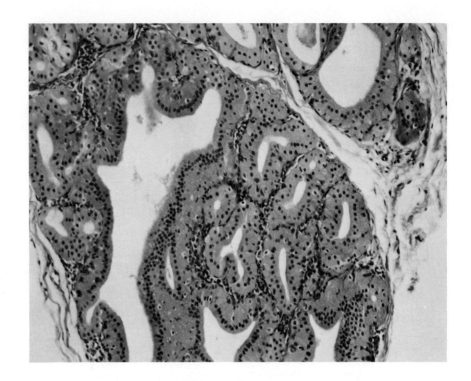

or cords that rarely occur in the larynx. (Fig. 3–15)[66,67] The majority of oncocytic tumors of the larynx represent oncocytic metaplasia of supraglottic mucoserous glands occurring in older patients (see previous section). These have been termed *"prolapse of the ventricle"* due to their gross clinical appearance and supraglottic location. Treatment of laryngeal oncocytoma should be simple complete removal. No malignant oncocytoma has been reported in the AFIP Otolaryngic Tumor Registry material.

Adenoma of the larynx listed in the AFIP Otolaryngic Tumor Registry (1940–1975) includes only *pleomorphic adenoma* (mixed tumor). This well-demarcated usually unencapsulated neoplasm consists of biphasic pattern epithelial cells and mesodermal tissue, the former often arranged in glandular pattern and the latter suggesting myxomatous or chondromatous tissue. In the nine cases recorded in the AFIP Otolaryngic Tumor Registry as arising from the larynx, there was no sex predilection. Ages ranged from 23 to 71 years, with a median of 46 years. Hoarseness was the most common symptom. Eight cases were located supraglottically. Surgical removal or laryngectomy were the main therapeutic modalities, with only one patient dying from the neoplasm secondary to malignant degeneration.

Mesodermal and Neuroectodermal

Benign granular cell tumor is the most common benign laryngeal nonepidermoid neoplasm listed in the AFIP Otolaryngic Tumor Registry (1940–1975). Its classification is somewhat controversial, since it occupies a position between reactive hyperplasia and benign neoplasm.[68,69] Muscle, histocytic, fibroblastic, and neuroectodermal sheath (Schwann) cells have all been blamed as the neoplastic progenitor; thus, the term "benign granular cell tumor," which is noncommital. The larynx is the most common anatomic site in the upper respiratory tract for this tumor, most of which occurs between the ages of 29 and 42 years, with a median of 36 years.[70] There is a slight female preponderance. The tumor presents most often as solitary, mucosal-covered, pink to gray sessile or polypoid nodules located

Figure 3–16. A clinical view of a raised polypoid yellow tumor of the laryngeal posterior commissure area in a 32-year-old female. She had noted hoarseness and some shortness of breath for 2 months. There was no glottic fixation. Excisional biopsy revealed a benign granular cell tumor. (AFIP #83-10612.)

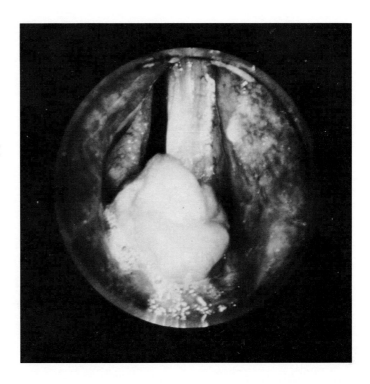

in the posterior vocal cord area, although any part of the larynx may be involved (Fig. 3–16). Mucosal surface ulceration is rare. Since there is no capsule surrounding the neoplasm, there is usually superficial infiltration into surrounding tissues. Microscopically, there are typically large, polygonal cells with eosinophilic granular cytoplasm, occasionally indistinct cellular borders, and central or eccentrically placed, small, hyperchromatic nuclei (Fig. 3–17). Pseudoepitheliomatous hyperplasia of the overlying mucosa is a disturbing histologic finding in more than 50 percent of the laryngeal tumors, because of resemblance to squamous cell carcinoma.[70]

Figure 3–17. A high-power magnification of a portion of the laryngeal tumor shown in Figure 3–16. It shows polygonal cells with intact cell membranes, granular eosinophilic cytoplasm, and small hyperchromatic uniform nuclei. Small spheroidal cytoplasmic diagnostic inclusions (the pustular bodies of Milan, the angular bodies of Bangle) are noted. (AFIP #82-12105; H & E, ×63.)

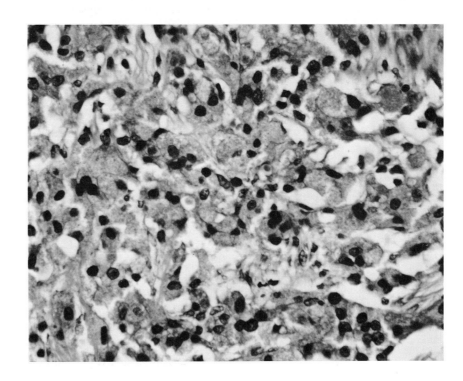

Figure 3–18. This microscopic photograph is from a bony hard spheroidal 1 cm nodule arising from the inner surface of the laryngeal thyroid cartilage. It depicts a chondroma that histologically is identical to normal hyaline cartilage. (AFIP #83-10744; H & E, ×63.)

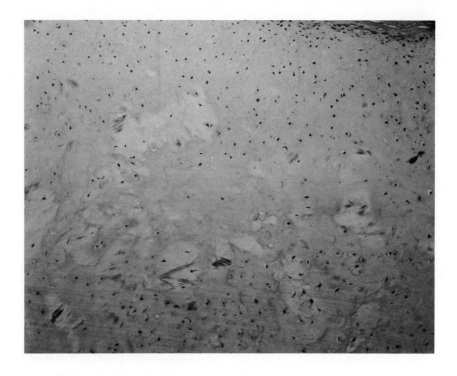

The malignant alveolar soft part sarcoma is occasionally referred to as malignant granular cell tumor, but there is no apparent relationship to benign granular cell tumor. Alveolar soft part sarcoma is not recorded as involving the larynx in our experience. There was only one case among more than 50 patients in the Armed Forces Institute of Pathology Otolaryngic Tumor Registry that required laryngectomy for a locally aggressive granular cell tumor.— Hyams and Heffner

According to the laryngeal cartilage of origin: elastic-epiglottic, true vocal cord; hyaline-thyroid, cricoid, arytenoid.— Hyams and Heffner

Granular cell tumor is benign, with no report of malignant behavior in any of the cases in the AFIP Otolaryngic Tumor Registry.◁ Complete surgical removal of the tumor with minimal sacrifice of laryngeal function is recommended.

There are 36 *chondromas* and two osteochondromas among the 1000 benign neoplasms of the larynx listed in the AFIP Otolaryngic Tumor Registry (1940–1975), occurring from the second through the eighth decade with no sex predilection. They can involve the epiglottic, thyroid, arytenoid, or cricoid cartilages and may also arise from the soft tissue of the vocal ligament (Reinke's space).[71] Clinically, the symptoms include hoarseness, shortness of breath, and wheezing. Laryngeal chondromas or osteochondromas seldom exceed 1 cm in diameter at the time of diagnosis. Microscopically (Fig. 3–18), chondromas are composed of histologically normal cartilage that can either be hyaline or elastic in type.◁ Osteochondroma has an outer layer of histologically benign cartilage with an underlying core of benign osteoid tissue. Simple surgical removal with minimal functional loss usually suffices. AFIP Registry experience demonstrates rare recurrence and no instances of malignant degeneration in laryngeal chondromas. (Chondrosarcoma of the larynx is discussed under malignant mesodermal neoplasms of the larynx.)

Hemangioma of the larynx is encountered in two distinct clinical varieties, *infantile* and *adult*.[72,73] The infantile type presents in the early months of life twice as frequently in females as males and most often consists of a sessile, diffuse subglottic lesion. Rapid growth is possible, and 50 percent of patients have hemangiomas elsewhere.[74] Grossly, it presents as a distinctive reddish-blue lesion localized to one side of the subglottic area, usually in the posterolateral portion. Microscopically, either capillary or cavernous forms may be present, with the former presenting as a firm, noncompressible tumor, whereas the latter is more likely to have a soft, compressible consistency. Treatment methods have included radiotherapy (least desirable), systemic steroids, chemical injection, cyrosurgery, laser removal, and observation for spontaneous regression. In the adult, laryngeal hemangioma may be present with minimal symptoms for years. Males are involved almost exclusively. The tumors are rounded, purplish growths arising on or above the true vocal cords. Hoarseness is the most common symptom, and serious airway obstruction is unusual. Spontaneous hemorrhage can occur but is most often a complication of operative interference. If at all possible, adult hemangioma should be left alone or managed conservatively.

Lymphangioma is a rare neoplasm of the larynx, most often occurring as an extension of lesions in adjacent tissues. A form of vallecular or pre-epiglottic cyst has been attributed to angiomatous malformation (blood or lymph vessels).[75]

Fibroma may be defined as a localized proliferation of histologically benign fibrocytes. It is difficult to be sure whether such a tumor is a true neoplasm or represents reactive proliferation of fibrous tissue in response to inflammation, infection, or trauma.[76] There are 29 cases of laryngeal fibroma among 935 benign laryngeal neoplasms contained in the AFIP Otolaryngic Tumor Registry (1940–1975). They most often present as soft, polypoid, mucosa-covered tumors within the larynx. Local, nonmutilating surgery is usually sufficient for cure. Rarely, *fibromatosis* may involve the larynx either alone or with systemic lesions. This lesion shows gross and microscopic infiltration of histologically benign fibrous tissue and could cause obstructive symptoms of the larynx.

Myxoma (fibromyxoma) is a benign but often infiltrating neoplasm of uncertain mesenchymal cell origin, characterized by irregular round, spindle, or stellate cells within a matrix containing abundant mucoid material, scant vascularity, and a variable meshwork of reticulum and collagen (Fig. 3–19). This entity is much more commonly seen in the sinonasal tract and bones of the jaws, but several laryngeal cases are reported in AFIP Otolaryngic Tumor Registry material. All cases presented as a soft polypoid mucosal mass and occasionally recurred after local removal but did not metastasize. When the true vocal cords are involved, a diagnosis of inflammatory myxomatous polyp cannot be ruled out. Recurrence, especially when

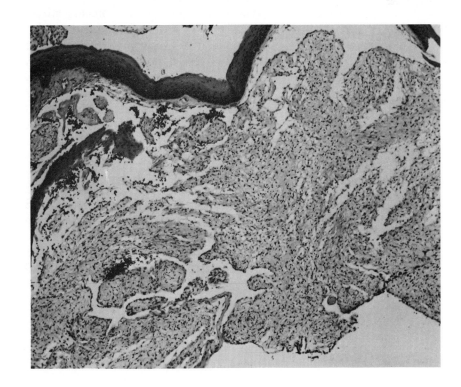

Figure 3–19. This histologic specimen represents a portion of a large recurring translucent pink polyp (2 cm in diameter) arising from the ventricular surface of the right true vocal cord. A similar polyp had been previously removed 3 months before at the identical anatomic location. The tumefaction shows myxomatous proliferation that could be supported cytologically either as an edematous Rienke's glottic space or a true neoplastic myxoma. (AFIP #83-10372; H & E, ×63.)

Figure 3–20. This microscopic view of a rare subglottic fibrohistiocytoma supports the typical proliferation of benign histiocytes along with the multinucleated giant cell (Touton cells). (AFIP #83-10566; H & E, × 160.)

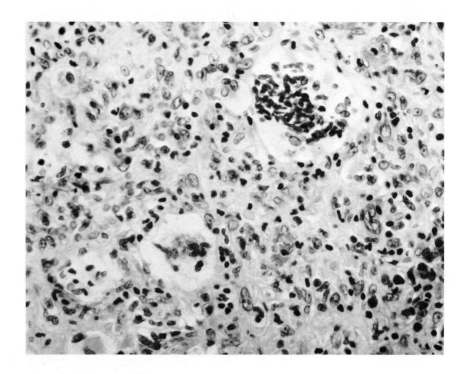

associated with extraglottic sites, supports the diagnosis of myxoma (fibromyxoma) of the larynx.

Fibrous histiocytoma (xanthoma, fibroxanthoma) is a generic term applying to tumors composed of cells differentiating into fibroblasts and histiocytes. The histologic interplay of the histiocyte and fibroblast yields a heterogenous and often bewildering spectrum of lesions, some neoplastic and others apparently of a reactive nature. Certain of these facultative fibroblastic tumors (such as *nodular fasciitis*) have not been reported in the larynx. There are 12 cases of laryngeal fibrohistiocytoma listed in the AFIP Otolaryngic Tumor Registry (1940–1975). There is male preponderence, with ages ranging form the first to ninth decades but occurring mostly in the third to sixth decades. They are usually polypoid, firm, mucosa-covered, and yellow or orange in color. Micromorphology can vary from cells that are large, polygonal, and histiocytic in appearance to mixtures with elongated spindle shapes resembling fibrocytes. (Fig. 3–20). Multinucleated cells with foamy cytoplasm (Touton cells) can be seen. All cells retain a benign appearance and may form a pattern that is described as cartwheel, pinwheel, or storiform. The tumors are rarely encapsulated. Local surgical removal is adequate, since complications are generally related to recurrence or rare metastasis.

Leiomyoma[77] is a benign neoplasm of smooth muscle, which is the least frequent of all nonepithelial lesions of the head and neck. This may be due to the paucity of smooth muscle in the anatomic area other than that occurring in blood vessels. Association with vascular structures is reflected in the prominent blood vessel component usually seen in leiomyoma of the head and neck, leading to the suggestion that the lesion be called angioleiomyoma. Fifteen acceptable examples of laryngeal leiomyoma are discussed in the literature. Five cases are listed in the AFIP Otolaryngic Tumor Registry (1940–1975). Although reported in children, they occur most often in the adult with a 2:1 male preponderance. The typical leiomyoma usually arises in the vestibular folds. It is a slowly enlarging, relatively discrete, solitary, submucosal mass, either sessile or polypoid with a small pedicle. They vary from a few milimeters to several centimeters in diam-

Figure 3–21. The surgical laryngectomy specimen of a 17-year-old male. This obvious airway obstructing neoplasm reveals good demarcation. The histologic findings are noted in Figure 3–22. (AFIP #83-10616.)

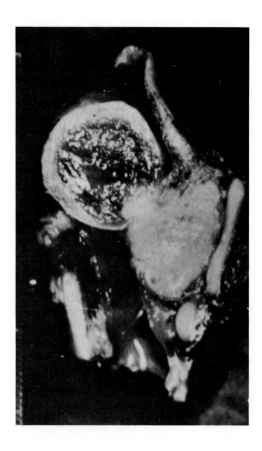

eter with a gray-pink to red surface, due to the vascularity of the neoplasm. Microscopically, these vascular leiomyomas demonstrate blood vessels with thick walls consisting of leiomyocytes, with nodular and whorllike cellular patterns in addition to spongelike structures rich in fibers but containing few nuclei. Surgical removal leads to a good prognosis.

Rhabdomyoma of the larynx is a benign neoplasm usually presenting as a solitary, lobulated and well-circumscribed fleshy yellow to red-brown appearance (Fig. 3–21). They are reported up to 10 cm in size. Histologically, the cells are most often polygonal, frequently vacuolated, and have granular, deeply acidophilic cytoplasm with intracellular cross-striations (Fig. 3–22). Of the two types of head and neck rhabdomyoma, adult and fetal, only the former is found in the larynx. Most such patients are older than 35 years of age. The tumors may arise in any portion of the larynx, but with a slightly higher incidence in the vocal cord.[78] These tumors have never been associated with malignant transformation and simple surgical removal will provide an excellent prognosis.

Lipoma is infrequent in the larynx.[79] There were four cases in the AFIP Otolaryngic Tumor Registry (1940–1975). They occur mostly in adults and present as a soft, yellow polypoid lesion projecting into the upper respiratory tract (Fig. 3–23). Suffocation has resulted from the large size of some of these tumors. The possibility of multiple lipomas must be investigated. The histologic configuration is simply normal adult fat arranged in lobules delineated by thin fibrous septa (Fig. 3–24). Simple surgical removal is the treatment of choice.

There were eight cases of *giant cell tumor* arising in the larynx listed in the AFIP Otolaryngic Tumor Registry (1940–1975). Whether these neoplasms arose from ossified cartilage or from laryngeal soft tissue is difficult to determine. They do not metastasize; however, their size occasionally

Figure 3–22. A high-power histologic view of the laryngeal neoplasm seen in Figure 3–21 confirms a relatively uniform proliferation of striated muscle cells. Under the microscope the characteristic cross-striations are evident. (AFIP #83-10399; H & E, ×160.)

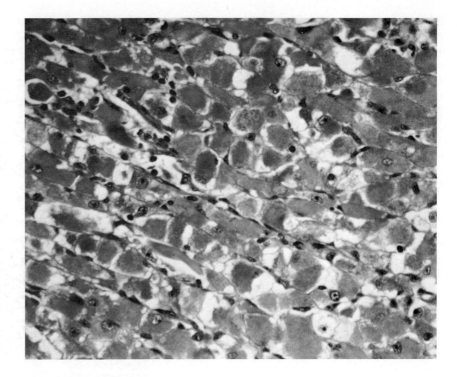

causes airway obstruction. There was no sex predilection, and age incidence was the second through seventh decades. Histologic structure resembled that of central giant cell granuloma of the bones of the skull with focal collections of small multinucleated giant cells and intervening fibrous tissue stroma. There is some question as to whether these laryngeal giant cell neoplasms might represent fibrohistiocytoma, but the large size does not seem to support this diagnosis. Two of the cases reported prominent vascularity, suggesting an aneurysmal bone cyst type of micromorphology. Several required total laryngectomy because of the large size of the lesion and the obstructive laryngeal symptoms.

   Neurilemmoma (schwannoma, neurinoma) is a benign neoplasm arising from the Schwann cell of peripheral and some cranial nerves. There are 13 cases reported to involve the larynx in the AFIP Otolaryngic Tumor Registry (1940–1975). The *neurofibroma* is a neoplasm that also arises from

Figure 3–23. A gross autopsy laryngeal specimen of a 62-year-old female who was found dead in her sleep. This yellow soft fatty polypoid mass arising from the posterior cricoid cartilage area was found wedged into the glottic inlet. (AFIP #10622.)

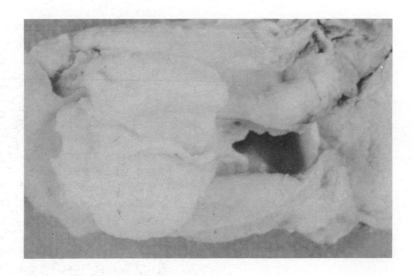

Figure 3–24. A histologic examination of the laryngeal tumor seen in Figure 3–23 reveals essentially normal fat tissue consistent with the diagnosis of lipoma. (AFIP #83-10565; H & E, ×63.)

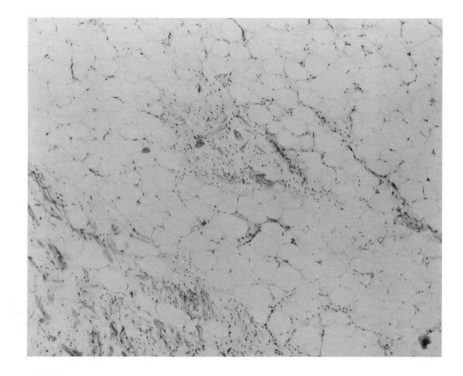

peripheral nerve sheaths and eight cases of this lesion are noted to involve the larynx in the AFIP material. Usually neurofibroma tends to be multiple (as opposed to neurilemmoma), nonencapsulated, and sometimes demonstrates local infiltrative behavior. Both neoplasms occur from 3 months to 75 years of age, with most of them in the third decade.[80] The majority involve the aryepiglottic fold or the false cords. The larynx, like the rest of the upper airway, is infrequently involved in patients with multiple neurofibromatosis *(von Recklinghausen's disease).* Therapeutically, the usual tumor demarcation with overlying intact mucosa leads to complete surgical removal and an optimistic outlook, except where multiple systemic neurofibromatosis complicates matters.

The larynx is relatively well-supplied with paraganglia. There are four normal paraganglia, one each at the point of entrance of the superior and inferior laryngeal vessels and nerves into the larynx proper.[81] The literature reports 27 cases of primary laryngeal *paraganglioma,*[82] and there are six cases contained in the AFIP Otolaryngic Tumor Registry (1940–1975). The patients ranged from 14 to 86 years of age, and 75 percent were male. Origin was usually from the supraglottic area. Hoarseness, dysphagia, neck mass, and pain were the presenting symptoms listed in order of frequency. Clinically, the tumor presents as a smooth, cystic-to-fleshy mucosal covered swelling of the supraglottic larynx, varying from 0.5 to 6 cm in diameter, with the larger masses extending unilaterally from the aryepiglottic fold into the ventricle. The histologic findings are those that of the typical ''cell nest'' pattern of the temporal bone and carotid body paraganglioma. Clinical behavior of laryngeal paraganglioma has been generally localized to the organ, and treatment is best directed toward complete surgical removal. Metastases have been reported in the literature, but in our experience, the possibility of misdiagnosing an aggressive adenocarcinoma of the larynx as a paraganglioma is a real one, and perhaps this accounts for the reported metastases of ''laryngeal paraganglioma.'' None of the AFIP Otolaryngic Tumor Registry cases exhibited metastasis.

Malignant

Premalignant epithelial abnormalities include those neoplastic changes of the laryngeal mucosa originating mainly in the glottis. They are usually due to the "wear and tear" on the anatomical area secondary to environment, personal habits (smoking), or other noxious stimuli. Metaplasia of normally ciliated respiratory columnar pseudostratified epithelium or hyperplastic or dyplastic change of the normal nonkeratinizing squamous cell mucosa (particularly of the glottic area) may occur. These changes have been considered premalignant, but less than 25 percent of cases develop into squamous cell carcinoma, especially when the condition is recognized and steps taken to relieve predisposing factors.[83] We have generally recognized two grades or stages of premalignant change. The first and the less likely to develop serious complications is *benign squamous cell hyperplasia (acanthosis, keratosis)* (Fig. 3–25). This is actually an increase in the mucosal epithelial cell mass due to an increase in the *number* of squamous cells. If the process is diffuse and related to a healing reaction, such as following a biopsy, it may be termed *"pseudoepitheliomatous hyperplasia,"* which seldom leads to malignant degeneration, especially when recognized and treated. *Pachydermia laryngis* is a condition that may present particularly in the older male with long-term histologic evidence of laryngeal abuse. This entity presents with a history of prolonged hoarseness. The appearance of diffusely irregular mucosal thickening involving the immediate glottic area is typical. Microscopic examination reveals only irregular, histologically benign hyperplasia involving the mucosa. It is unusual for this condition to develop into frank invasive squamous cell carcinoma.

The second grade or stage of premalignant changes is *dysplasia (epithelial atypia).* The clinical appearance of dysplasia and benign hyperplasia may be very similar. Histologically, however, dysplasia exhibits squamous cells, particularly in the basilar zones of the mucosa, whose micromorphology suggests malignant appearance. Mucosal hyperplasia may be minor, and the basement membrane is intact. There is a higher inci-

Figure 3–25. This biopsy of a roughened area of the vocal cord reveals an irregular hyperplasia of uniform stratified squamous epithelial mucosa. No dysplasia is noted (AFIP #83-10329; H & E, ×63.)

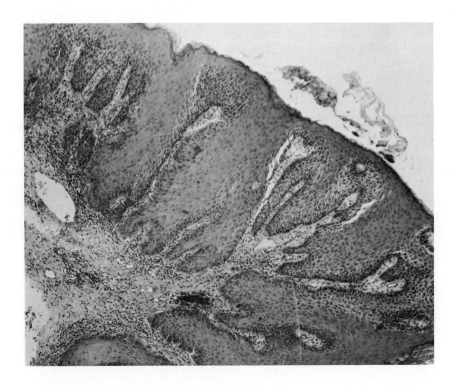

Figure 3–26. This focal squamous cell carcinoma-in-situ from a biopsy of a clinically suspicious glottic surface is characterized micro-morphologically by a zone of epithelial dysplasia (atypia) extending from the mucosal surface to the basement membrane, but not beyond. Adjacent is a normal area of mucosa. (AFIP #83-10321; H & E, ×63.)

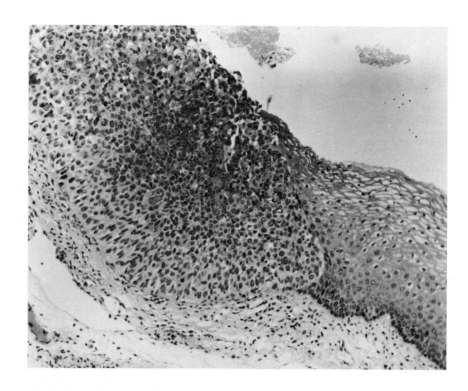

dence of malignant degeneration in dysplasia than in benign hyperplasia.[84] Some investigators[83] have graded dysplasia as mild, moderate, or marked and found squamous cell carcinoma developing later in 2, 12, and 25 percent of such cases, respectively.

Occasionally, terminology such as *hyperkeratosis, keratosis, parakeratosis,* and *dyskeratosis* is utilized to signify a premalignant diagnosis; however, we consider these terms histologic descriptions rather than specific diagnoses. Any of these findings may be seen in either benign or malignant squamous cell mucosal proliferation. *Leukoplakia* is to be discouraged as a microscopic diagnosis, since it has been interpreted by different authorities as meaning so many different pathologic conditions. We prefer to define leukoplakia as a descriptive term meaning a white patch seen on a mucosal surface. Premalignant changes, if properly managed, offer a good prognosis when originating in the glottis. Those originating in extraglottic areas (supra- and subglottic sites) are, in our experience, more likely to develop invasive carcinoma eventually, even with prompt therapy.

Squamous cell carcinoma in situ (intraepithelial carcinoma, Bowen's disease) is defined as cellular dysplasia involving the entire thickness of mucosa from the basement membrane to the outer surface, but without microscopic evidence of invasion beyond the basement membrane (Fig. 3–26). It is most often detected on the anterior vocal cord and clinically may present circumscribed or diffuse involvement with a grayish-white or red, smooth to granular appearance. Therapeutically, radiation, mucosal stripping, and local surgical removal (laryngofissure) have all been advocated. The relation of this lesion to invasive squamous cell carcinoma is not clear; however, those patients who do develop invasive carcinoma may well have had concomitant invasive disease that was overlooked at the time of the original diagnosis.[85]

Squamous cell carcinoma (epidermoid carcinoma) accounts for 99 percent of mucosal malignancy of the larynx. Ninety percent of patients are men, and the age incidence is from the fourth through the ninth decades, with the mean age in the fifth decade. Etiology of laryngeal carci-

Figure 3–27. A postsurgical laryngectomy specimen revealing the typical exophytic gross appearance of squamous cell carcinoma. (AFIP #10025.)

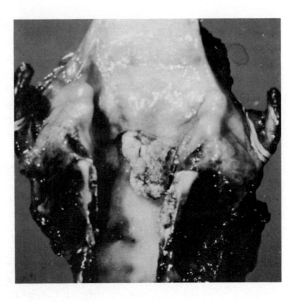

noma has long been linked to tobacco and alcohol, but socioeconomic, geographic and racial factors, vocal stress, and asbestos and nickel exposure have all been less definitely incriminated. Hoarseness is the presenting symptom in more than 90 percent of cases; less frequent symptoms, such as airway obstruction, throat pain, dysphagia, or hemoptysis suggest more advanced involvement. The majority (40 to 75 percent) of these carcinomas arise from the glottis with 20 percent occurring in the supraglottic area and less than 5 percent subglottic (Fig. 3–27). Laryngeal carcinomas will generally vary from 1 to 4 cm in largest diameter, with a fungating pink to gray appearance, often with central ulceration. The TNM system of the American Joint Committee for Cancer Staging and End Results Reporting[86] is the best available prognostic index. Histologic staging is difficult because of the inability to obtain diffuse sampling of the morphology throughout the entire neoplasm at diagnostic biopsy (Fig. 3–28).

Figure 3–28. Micromorphologic aspects of an invasive squamous cell carcinoma of the larynx. The typical squamous cell histologic features consisting of intercellular bridges and focal collections of keratin can be imagined. (AFIP #83-10787; H & E, ×63.)

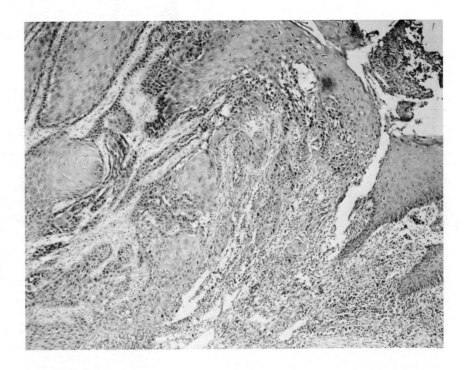

Small or *oat cell carcinoma* is a controversial neoplasm.[87] It represents the most undifferentiated of the laryngeal carcinomas and carries the poorest prognosis, only about 20 percent of cases surviving beyond 1 year. There is some evidence to suggest that it is an undifferentiated form of squamous cell carcinoma. However, because of electron microscopic findings of intracellular neurosecretory granules in the neoplastic cells similar to those found in oat cell carcinoma in the lung, the assumption has been made that they arise from Kulchitsky-like cells apparently present in the larynx.

Therapy for laryngeal squamous cell carcinoma is discussed in detail in Chapter 13. There is a direct and linear relationship between clinical staging and 5-year survival.

Verrucous squamous cell carcinoma (verrucous carcinoma, Ackerman's tumor) is a malignant neoplasm usually defined as verrucoid, highly differentiated squamous cell carcinoma of mucosal or skin surfaces. It tends to produce prominent surface keratin and, even though capable of local tissue destruction and invasion, does not usually metastasize. Clinical and histologic differentiation from conventional squamous cell carcinoma is of prime importance in diagnosis.

Verrucous squamous cell carcinoma occurs most often in the oral cavity, but the next most common area of involvement is the larynx. They constitute 0.7 percent of the 6500 cases of squamous cell carcinoma contained in the AFIP Otolaryngic Tumor Registry (1939–1976). Ages may range from the fourth to eighth decades, with a mean age of 60 years. Four of five patients are male. Probably the same etiologies that are responsible for squamous cell carcinoma are also involved in verrucous carcinoma. The typical lesion is a pale, warty, fungating, locally aggressive, ulcerated tumor attached by a broad base (Fig. 3–29). Ninety percent of laryngeal involvement is in the glottis. The symptoms are the same as those of laryngeal squamous cell carcinoma.

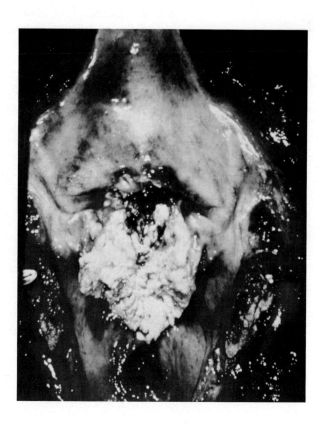

Figure 3–29. A postsurgical total laryngectomy specimen of a 68-year-old male who had several previous removals at yearly intervals of what was diagnosed as a keratin papilloma of the larynx. Eventually, the diagnosis of verrucous carcinoma was entertained because of the local destruction of the adjacent thyroid cartilage by the tumor mass. (AFIP #83-10029.)

Figure 3–30. A low-power microscopic view of the previous gross specimen emphasizing the so-called church spire surface hyperkeratosis, the irregular hyperplasia of benign-appearing squamous epithelium forming the broad bands that push rather than infiltrate in the submucosal fibrous tissue. The prominent chronic lymphocytic infiltrate in the latter is another regular finding. (AFIP #83-10312; H & E, ×25.)

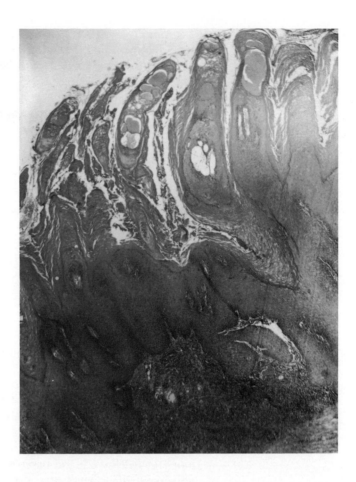

Probably in no other neoplasm of the larynx is there more need for cooperation between surgeon and pathologist than in the diagnosis of verrucous squamous cell carcinoma. Because of the uniform micromorphology of the prolilferating squamous cell elements of verrucous squamous cell carcinoma, differentiation from benign squamous cell proliferation and squamous cell papilloma may only be achieved through the clinician's gross observation and information (Fig. 3–30). There is an entity described as a *keratotic "wart"* or *verruca vulgaris* of the larynx[88] that is difficult to differentiate either clinically or histologically from verrucous squamous cell carcinoma, but complete surgical removal of such a lesion is in the best interest of the patient. The other important differential diagnostic problem is with well-differentiated squamous cell carcinoma. Identification of dysplastic epithelium and infiltration of irregular cords of dysplastic squamous cells into adjacent stroma rather than the broad, pushing bands of uniform squamous cells of verrucous squamous cell carcinoma should help clear up the difficulty.[89]

Treatment of choice for laryngeal verrucous squamous cell carcinoma appears to be surgical removal. One must remember that in this nonmetastasizing neoplasm, incomplete excision is not necessarily disastrous. Although this may lead to later recurrence, it is not life-threatening, and perhaps more radical approaches may then be selected. There are those who advocate radiation therapy alone, but others have reported anaplastic transformation of verrucous squamous cell carcinoma after radiotherapy. Certainly the well-differentiated keratin surfaced verrucous squamous cell carcinoma would not seem to be very susceptible to radiation cure. In our experience, those cases that were represented as radiation-cured verrucous squamous cell carcinoma were in reality well-differentiated squamous cell

Figure 3–31. A postsurgical laryngectomy specimen from a 65-year-old male with the complaint of increasing difficulty in breathing for several months. The microscopic diagnosis was spindle cell carcinoma and the gross polypoid clinical appearance is typical of the particular spindle cell carcinoma of the larynx. (AFIP #85-6006.)

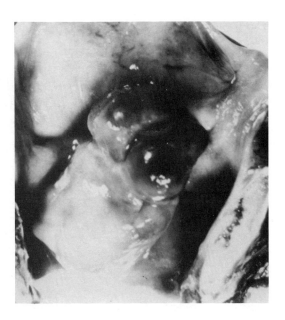

carcinoma. The prognosis of verrucous squamous cell carcinoma is excellent. There was actually no patient listed in the AFIP Otolaryngic Tumor Registry with treated verrucous squamous cell carcinoma of the larynx who succumbed to the neoplasm. One patient who had refused treatment died of airway obstruction.

Spindle cell carcinoma (sarcomatoid squamous cell carcinoma) usually presents in the larynx as a polypoid mass with infiltrating and metastasizing capabilities and is characterized histologically by foci of squamous cell carcinoma contained in a volume of pleomorphic cells.[90,91] This entity accounts for 1.5 percent of the laryngeal squamous cell carcinomas contained in the AFIP Otolaryngic Tumor Registry (1940–1975). Ninety percent of patients are males between the fifth and ninth decades, with a median age of 68 years. There appears to be a relationship to laryngeal irritants (smoking, alcohol); moreover, a significant number of patients have had previous irradiation therapy for previous laryngeal squamous cell carcinoma. The true nature and histogenesis of this neoplasm has been questioned. The most commonly accepted interpretation is that it represents squamous cell carcinoma that has undergone metaplasia into a spindle cell morphology. Some theories suggest that the spindle cell element is a nonneoplastic reactive component; others believe that it is a collision or dual growth of carcinoma and sarcoma (collision tumor, carcinosarcoma). The concept that this lesion represents squamous cell carcinoma undergoing neoplastic spindle cell metaplasia is best supported by electron microscopic and other laboratory studies. Clinically, laryngeal spindle cell carcinoma presents almost exclusively as a polypoid tumor varying from 1 to 6 cm in diameter (Fig. 3–31). The base of attachment may be narrow or wide. The surface presents a glistening gray-pink appearance, although histologic examination usually demonstrates marked denuding of the mucous membrane. Three quarters of our series[90] arose from the true vocal cord, with the remaining cases originating from supraglottic, subglottic, and pyriform sites.

Microscopic examination should contain an area of histologically conventional squamous cell carcinoma; however, in some cases this characteristic is difficult to detect (Fig. 3–32). The bulk of the neoplasm will usually contain the spindle cell element, which may be represented by cellular fibromatosis or moderately anaplastic fibrosarcoma-like morphology. In about

Figure 3–32. The histologic section of the spindle cell carcinoma shown in Figure 3–31 emphasizes the conventional squamous cell carcinoma and the adjacent malignant-looking spindle cell portion that seems to be a transformation from the regular squamous cell carcinoma. (AFIP #83-10302; H & E, ×63.)

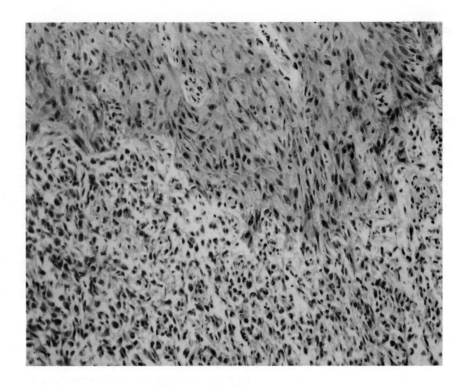

5 percent of cases, dystrophic bony or occasionally cartilagenous foci may be seen. This finding usually follows previous irradiation to the anatomic area. Transition of squamous cell carcinoma into the spindle cell variety is a helpful diagnostic criterion (Fig. 3–32), but occasionally the only epidermoid element will be a surface of squamous epithelium with only the basal areas revealing dysplastic cells that seem to "drop off" into the underlying atypical spindle cell neoplasm. Electron microscopic and immunoperoxidase studies confirm that the spindle cell element is actually undifferentiated squamous cell carcinoma. Distal and regional metastases may contain the squamous cell carcinoma or the spindle cell malignancy or both. Differential diagnosis will include fibrosarcoma (a rare laryngeal malignant neoplasm) and atypical inflammatory polyp.

The treatment[90,91] is essentially surgical, with the therapeutic goal of complete removal of the neoplasm. This may entail a local surgical procedure or a partial or total laryngectomy. Radiation therapy alone has not provided a cure in the AFIP Otolaryngic Pathology Registry material (1940–1975). Follow-up of 20 cases from the Registry revealed a 60 percent five-year survival.

Adenocarcinoma (carcinoid tumor) is represented in the AFIP Otolaryngic Tumor Registry (1945–1975) by 26 cases of primary laryngeal origin (0.4 percent of all laryngeal neoplasia). Ages ranged from 19 to 75 years (median age, 59 years), and 22 were male. Symptoms averaged 4 months previous to diagnosis and consisted of hoarseness, dysphagia, pain, hemoptysis, and dyspnea. Most of these lesions arose supraglottically and had a gross clinical appearance varying from a mucosal-covered small nodule to a large ulcerated mass. The histologic picture was variable, quite often revealing sheets of cells and occasionally a "cell nest" pattern suggesting paraganglioma. In all cases at least a focus of glandular pattern could be identified, varying from small tubular structures to cystadenomatous patterns. The individual tumor cell is a moderately well-differentiated cuboidal to columnar type, with rare mitoses and no surface cilia. Cell mucin content could occasionally be demonstrated, but not usually. Positive

Figure 3–33. A post surgical total laryngectomy specimen from a 37-year-old female with signs and symptoms of supraglottic laryngeal mass, which proved histologically to represent an adenoid cystic carcinoma. The neoplasm had infiltrated the lower surgical margin of the laryngectomy specimen, although grossly the margin seemed clear. (AFIP #83-10604.)

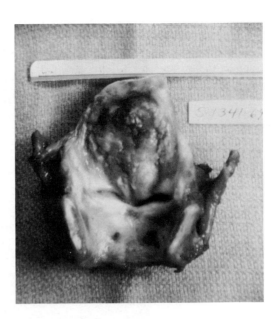

immunoreactivity against calcitonin, somatostatin, and adrenocorticotropic hormone has been demonstrated.[92] Electron microscopic and special histochemical studies demonstrate cellular inclusions resembling neurosecretory-type granules. This latter finding has suggested that laryngeal adenocarcinoma is a carcinoid tumor,[92] although no systemic hormonal activity has been described. Surgical removal has been the treatment of choice. After local removal by partial laryngectomy, there was recurrence or metastasis in approximately 50 percent of cases; after total laryngectomy, there was no recurrence or metastasis. Only two cases were treated by radiation alone, and both succumbed to the laryngeal neoplasm.

Adenoid cystic carcinoma is a nonepidermoid laryngeal carcinoma that behaves in a similar manner to its counterpart in other areas of the upper respiratory tract and salivary glands. It is an aggressive neoplastic process with poor prognosis regardless of therapeutic approach. It constituted 0.26 percent of the malignant laryngeal neoplasms in the AFIP Otolaryngic Tumor Registry (1945–1975). Ages ranged from 32 to 83 years, with a median of 57 years. Males predominated 3:1. Symptoms of hoarseness, pain, dyspnea, and cough preceded diagnosis by an average of 1½ months. The primary site of the neoplasm was distributed evenly between the supraglottic and subglottic anatomic areas. Adenoid cystic carcinoma has no typical appearance (Fig. 3–33). Our experience is that quite often the extension of the neoplasm is underestimated clinically, and when laryngectomies or local attempts at complete surgical removal are done, there is often an unsuspected microscopic extension of neoplasm through the surgical margin. Histologic examination shows a cribriform pattern of small hyperchromatic cells lacking distinct glandular pattern orientation (Fig. 3–34). A tubular and a solid form has been noted in the larynx but does not appear to relate to any difference in prognosis among the different histologic types. Perineural space invasion is common and is a finding that assists in microscopic identification of adenoid cystic carcinoma. This neoplasm rarely metastasizes to the regional lymph nodes. Distal spread is most often blood borne. Recommended therapy has been radical surgery. The addition of radiation may not be curative, but is certainly worthwhile in this overwhelmingly fatal disease.[93] Follow-up of the AFIP Otolaryngic Tumor Registry cases revealed that all patients had residual disease or died of the neoplasm regardless of the therapeutic approach.

Figure 3–34. The histologic
view of the adenoid cystic
carcinoma of the specimen
pictured in Figure 3–33. This
micromorphologic pattern
represents in part the tubular
and cribriform architecture of
neoplastic entity. Regardless of
histologic pattern of the adenoid
cystic carcinoma of the larynx,
the outcome is dismal. (AFIP
#83-10558; H & E, ×25.)

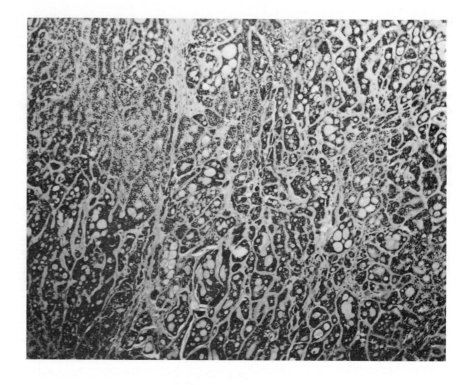

Mucoepidermoid carcinoma (adenosquamous cell carcinoma) comprises 0.3 percent of malignant laryngeal neoplasms in the AFIP Otolaryngic Tumor Registry (1940–1975). Age incidence is from 25 to 76 years,
with a median of 57 years. The male to female ratio was 6:1. Practically
all of these neoplasms arose in the supraglottic larynx with symptomatology similar to laryngeal squamous cell carcinoma. Clinical gross appearance is indistinguishable from squamous cell carcinoma (Fig. 3–35). Histologically, there is an admixture of squamous cell carcinoma and mucus-
producing carcinoma (Fig. 3–36). Degree of anaplasia should help determine classification into well-differentiated versus poorly differentiated mucoepidermoid carcinoma, inasmuch as such qualification seems to bear directly on treatment and prognosis.[94]

Because of histologic support for the origin of these neoplasms from
laryngeal mucosa, the term "adenosquamous carcinoma" has been sug-

Figure 3–35. A postsurgical
laryngectomy specimen from a
56-year-old male with signs and
symptoms of a destructive
supraglottic laryngeal mass. The
biopsy results supported
mucoepidermoid carcinoma.
(AFIP #85-06067.)

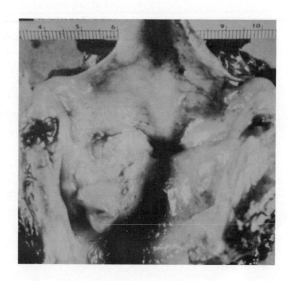

Figure 3–36. A histologic view of the specimen in Figure 3–35 where the epidermoid and mucus carcinomatous elements support the diagnosis of mucoepidermoid carcinoma. Also, the micromorphologic findings tend to lend support to the origin of the neoplasm directly from the overlying laryngeal respiratory mucosa. (AFIP #83-10701; H & E, ×63.)

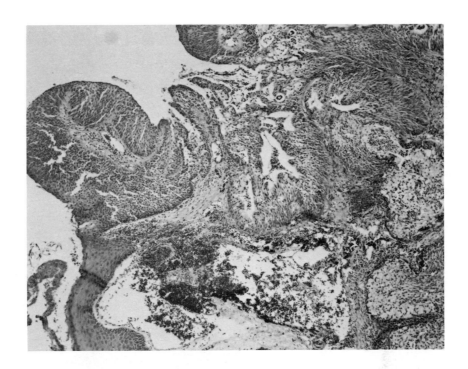

gested to distinguish it from the mucoepidermoid carcinoma of salivary gland origin; however, this distinction only causes additional confusion and the name seems better left as mucoepidermoid carcinoma. Experience gained from the AFIP Registry material suggests that an approach similar to that which is employed for squamous cell carcinoma is appropriate. Small lesions and those of low-grade malignancy showed 100 percent 5-year survival, whereas those of high-grade micromorphology or extensive lesions, or both, had only a 50 percent 5-year survival.

Mesodermal, Neuroectodermal

There were 33 laryngeal fibrosarcomas in the AFIP Otolaryngic Tumor Registry (1940–1975) and 32 additional acceptable cases have been reported in the English medical literature.[74] The majority were more than 50 years of age at diagnosis and males predominated over females 4:1. Most of these lesions arise from the anterior vocal cords or commissure. Rarely, they present as fungating or ulcerating masses, the majority appearing as nodular or pedunculated lesions. Prognosis appears to depend largely on whether the micromorphology is well or poorly differentiated. Regardless of degree of differentiation, laryngeal fibrosarcoma rarely metastasizes. It spreads most often by infiltration along fascial planes or muscles in the environs of the larynx. Distal spread is usually through blood vessels. Most patients with poorly differentiated firbosarcoma of the larynx are dead within 3 years after diagnosis. The main microscopic diagnostic problem is differentiation from spindle cell carcinoma.

Malignant fibrous histiocytoma (malignant xanthoma, malignant histiocytoma) has not been listed for the larynx in the AFIP Otolaryngic Tumor Registry (1940–1975); however, some investigators believe that it is a common laryngeal mesenchymal malignancy. The benign counterpart was discussed previously. Anaplasia of stromal cells, extensive cellular pleomorphism, atypical mitoses, diffuse and often intense neutrophilic infiltration not associated with necrosis, or a large neoplasm all support a malignant diagnosis. The registry does contain eight cases of giant cell tumors

Figure 3–37. Microscopic appearance of a synovial sarcoma demonstrating the spindle cell fascicular arrangement with epithelial-lined glandlike spaces, which together make up the biphasic histologic characteristics of this aggressive neoplasm. (AFIP #83-10725; H & E, ×63.)

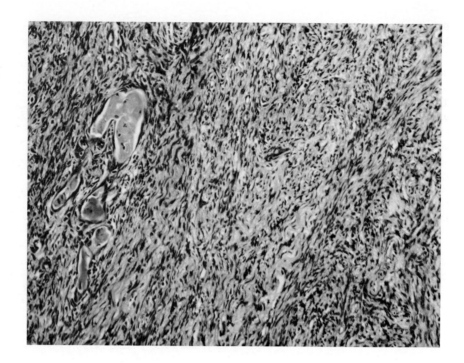

of the larynx, and their histologic features could fit into a category of fibrous histiocytoma, but even though they were quite often large (necessitating laryngectomy), they did not demonstrate regional or distal metastasis.

Synovial sarcoma (synovioma) is represented among the laryngeal malignant neoplasms of the AFIP Otolaryngic Tumor Registry (1940–1975) by eight cases. This neoplasm is believed to evolve from synovial membranes that normally consist of an inner epithelioid-like layer and an outer connective tissue layer. This might explain the common dysplastic histologic characteristics of the neoplasm. Origin of synovial sarcoma of the larynx may be from synovial membranes within the joints of the organ or from connective tissue with the ability for synovioblastic differentiation. The exact anatomic area has been difficult to determine because of the large size and infiltrative nature of these neoplasms at diagnosis. It occurs in young adults, mostly between the ages of 20 and 40 years and with a slight preponderance in females. Patients usually present with gradual onset of hoarseness, dyspnea, and dysphagia. Gross clinical appearance is an ill-defined, deep-seated, mucosal-covered mass in the larynx, although sometimes they are pedunculated. A soft, rubbery consistency is common and on sectioning there is a yellow to gray surface that may be well circumscribed and often pseudoencapsulated. The histologic findings (Fig. 3–37) are mostly biphasic, consisting of a stroma of spindle cells resembling fibrosarcoma that may include spaces, clefts, or cysts lined by epithelial cuboidal cells. Occasionally, a uniphasic pattern presents with the micromorphology of a fibrosarcoma. Correct diagnosis requires a search for epithelioid cells to prove synovioblastic origin. Prognosis for laryngeal synovial sarcoma appears better than is reported for those arising in the extremities. An approximately 50 percent 5-year survival is reported in head and neck synovial sarcomas.[95] Metastasis to the lungs is the usual cause of death, with less frequent involvement of the lymph nodes and bones. Best therapeutic results seem to follow complete surgical removal of the neoplasm, usually total laryngectomy, followed by radiation.

Rhabdomyosarcoma is the most common soft tissue malignancy in the

Figure 3–38. A biopsy of an infiltrating laryngeal mass in a 17-year-old male that was diagnosed as being an embryonal rhabdomyosarcoma. The main tumor mass is made up of spindlelike fetal muscle resembling cells, and the outer edge is formed of compact more rounded neoplastic cells comprising the ''Cambrian'' layer. No cross-striations are identified in this microphotograph. (AFIP #83-10475; H & E, ×63.)

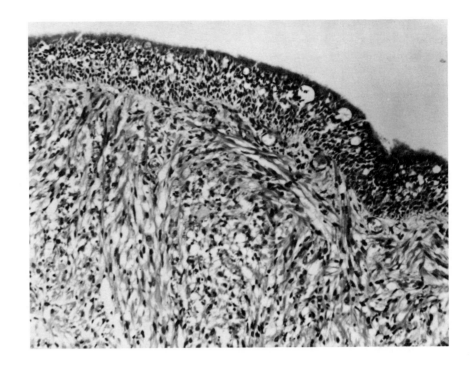

head and neck area in patients less than 16 years of age but is rare in the larynx (only six cases reported in the AFIP Otolaryngic Tumor Registry (1940–1982). The literature reports approximately a dozen cases ranging in age from 1 to 72 years[96] with a preponderance in the first three decades. Males are affected as often as females. Symptoms are usually vague, with hoarseness and dyspnea related to a bulky, sessile, or pedunculated mass arising mainly in the glottic area, often covered by ulcerated mucosa. Histologic findings of rhabdomyosarcoma encompasses the so-called embryonal, alveolar, and botryoidal types, all of which can also occur in the adult (Fig. 3–38). Micromorphology resembles developing muscles as seen in the 7- to 10-week-old fetus. It is characterized by round and spindle cells in a background of myxomatous stroma. The cells may reveal cross-striations, but these are not essential for diagnosis. Alveolar arrangement of rounded cells may occur. In addition to the juvenile type, there is the so-called pleomorphic or adult type wherein the neoplastic cell is more mature and resembles adult muscle. This type is rare in the head and neck regardless of the age of the patient. The prognosis was almost universally dismal in the past, but with the advent of combination therapy (radiation, surgery, and chemotherapy), there is now hope for cure. The size of the lesion and the occurrence of metastases at the time of diagnosis are important to prognosis.

Angiosarcoma is a malignant vascular neoplasm that is rare in the larynx, with only four substantiated cases in the AFIP Otolaryngic Tumor Registry (1940–1975). The patient will most likely be male, in the fourth to seventh decades of life. The tumor is usually supraglottic, presenting either as an ulcerating nodule or diffusely spreading bluish or purple tumefaction, often demonstrating intralesional hemorrhage. There is no capsule. The neoplasm tends to spread throughout adjacent soft tissues for considerable distances. The histologic examination may show low- or high-grade differentiation; the former will resemble granuloma pyogenicum, but the vascular spaces are lined by large, plump, and atypical endothelial cells; the vascular spaces penetrate stroma, and there are papillary fronds of endothelial cells. Undifferentiated or high-grade angiosarcoma is composed

Figure 3–39. The typical histologic findings of a Kaposi's sarcoma from the larynx of an elderly male with the so-called classic Kaposi's disease. The laryngeal dark blue hemorrhagic 1.5 cm mass occurred after a mass had developed on the ankle. The micromorphologic findings are those of spindle fibrosarcomatous-looking cells with numerous intercellular vascular slits filled with red blood cells (AFIP #83-10526; H & E, ×63.)

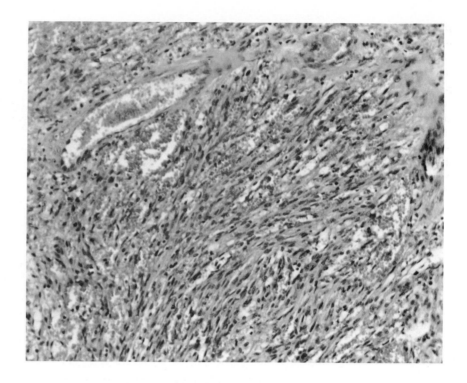

of anaplastic spindle cells forming vascular channels with cells suggesting pleomorphic endothelial cells. Mitotic activity is plentiful, and necrosis is usually prominent. Angiosarcomas are resistant to therapy, requiring total surgical removal for any hope of survival. Those angiosarcomas in the upper respiratory tract seem to have a better prognosis (50 percent survival) than that of the overall head and neck area, perhaps because of earlier diagnosis and the usually younger age of the patient.[74]

Kaposi's sarcoma rarely involves the larynx and those that do are of the "classic" Kaposi's disease, occurring in older men without the acquired immune deficiency syndrome. The majority of laryngeal cases are associated with previous skin lesions;[98] however, there has been occasional primary origin of the neoplasm in the larynx, where it is usually supraglottic (epiglottic). It presents as a reddish-purple, nodular, or pedunculated tumor, covered with intact or ulcerated mucosa. The classic histologic feature is that of spindle cell fibrosarcomatous neoplasia, but with the addition of slitlike, nonendothelial lined vascular channels (Fig. 3–39). Irradiation and chemotherapy have been utilized with success. Approximately 25 percent of the classic Kaposi's sarcoma patients succumb to the disease, usually due to gastrointestinal involvement.

Hemangiopericytoma is a rare laryngeal vascular neoplasm not listed in the AFIP Otolaryngic Tumor Registry (1940–1975). There is only one published case of malignant laryngeal hamangiopericytoma that has come to our attention.[97]

Liposarcoma (myxoid liposarcoma, myxoliposarcoma) of the larynx is represented by five cases in the AFIP Otolaryngic Tumor Registry (1940–1983). Five more are listed in the English medical literature,[99] all of which occurred in middle and older aged males. A lobular, fleshy yellow gray mass is seen most often in the aryepiglottic fold. Histologic examination will reflect a malignant neoplastic variation of fat cells (round, pleomorphic, or well differentiated) accompanying a myxoid tissue stroma. Follow-up after laryngectomy and postoperative radiation therapy has been generally encouraging.

Figure 3–40. The histologic view of a low-grade chondrosarcoma arising from the anterior surface of the posterior lamina of the cricoid cartilage. The increase in tumor cell number as well as the increased anaplasia present supports the malignant diagnosis. (AFIP #83-10747; H & E, ×63.)

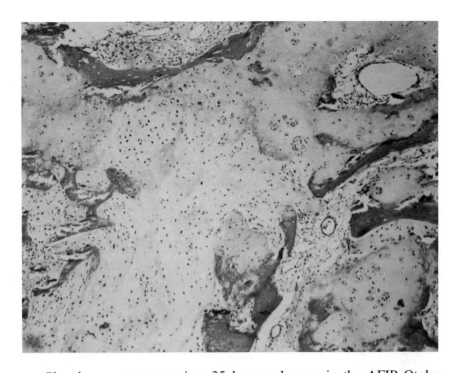

Chondrosarcoma comprises 35 laryngeal cases in the AFIP Otolaryngic Tumor Registry (1940–1975), or 0.4 percent of all malignant laryngeal neoplasms listed during this period. The patients are in the fifth to eighth decades of life and the male to female ratio is 3:1. The most common anatomic area of origin is the anterior surface of the posterior lamina of the cricoid cartilage, with the thyroid cartilage much less frequent and none primary in the epiglottis. Common involvement of the luminal surface of the cricoid cartilage leads to early airway obstruction. Gross appearance of a mucosal covered mass, 2 cm or larger, involving the posterior lamina of the cricoid cartilage is typical. The overwhelming majority of these lesions are classified as low grade, and quite often because of the minimal increase in cellularity and slight anaplasia of tumor cells, the diagnosis of benign chondroma is made initially (Fig. 3–40). The diagnosis of chondrosarcoma is justified by a definite increase in cellularity and anaplasia of neoplastic cells when compared with the histologic configuration of normal cartilage.[71] Approximately 10 percent of the AFIP cases reveal higher grade and anaplastic micromorphology. Prognosis of laryngeal chondrosarcoma is definitely better than when the tumor occurs in other areas of the head and neck, perhaps due to the low-grade histologic appearance of most of the laryngeal cartilaginous neoplasms. Only 3 of 16 cases reported from the AFIP material exhibited regional or distal metastasis, and these were of high-grade histologic changes. The most effective treatment appears to be complete surgical removal of the neoplasm, especially if this can be accomplished without sacrificing the entire larynx; however, in most cases studied the neoplasm was of a size that required total laryngectomy. There are cases we know of wherein local removal or laser destruction of low-grade chondrosarcoma was carried out for comfortable survival of many years. The low incidence of metastasis seems to support a conservative therapeutic approach.

Although there are three cases of laryngeal *osteosarcoma* reported in the AFIP Otolaryngic Tumor Registry (1940–1945), we doubt that this neoplastic entity exists in "pure" form. All cases studied with the diagnosis of laryngeal osteosarcoma seem to represent part of some other malignant neoplastic process, such as osteoid metaplasia of laryngeal spindle cell carcinoma or osteoid differentiation in a chondrosarcoma of the larynx.

Primary lymphoma of the larynx is rare. Most of the literature suggests that only non-Hodgkin's lymphoma involves the larynx. There was a 0.2 percent incidence of laryngeal non-Hodgkin's lymphoma listed in the AFIP Otolaryngic Tumor Registry (1940–1975). Although there were four cases of Hodgkin's disease involving the larynx during this same period, such cases probably represent either misdiagnosis or secondary involvement from another anatomic site. There is no sex predilection; the ages of involvement are usually the fifth through the eighth decades, although a patient at any age is susceptible. Non-Hodgkin's lymphoma is most likely to occur in the supraglottic area (epiglottic and aryepiglottic fold), appearing grossly as a mass covered by intact mucosa. The histologic examination will show monotonous profusion of atypical lymphocytes. Space does not permit a discussion of the confusing state of non-Hodgkin's lymphoma classification; it is sufficient to say that the prognosis is generally related directly to differentiation of the neoplastic lymphocyte, with the better differentiated neoplasms having a better outlook. We still utilize the Rappaport classification as the one best suited to relate differentiation of the neoplasm to prognosis. In a recent review, 18 cases of non-Hodgkin's lymphoma, varying from well to poorly differentiated, were present as primary neoplasms in the larynx, but none of these patients died from the disease, even though follow-up was for 10 years or longer.[100] Radiotherapy was the treatment of choice. Lymphocytic leukemic infiltrate can produce a tumor in the larynx. The histologic features may be identical to the primary non-Hodgkin's lymphoma; however, identification of leukemic cells in the marrow and peripheral blood will help make the correct diagnosis.

Malignant midline reticulosis (Lethal midline granuloma) is accepted as representing a mixed type non-Hodgkin's lymphoma of the sinonasal tract, and involvement of the larynx by this entity is not likely unless by secondary spread of lymphoma.

Plasmacytoma (extramedullary) of the larynx is represented by 13 cases in the AFIP Otolaryngic Tumor Registry (1940–1975). It is a circumscribed mass of infiltrate involving the soft tissues of the larynx composed of recognizable plasma cells. The fifth to seventh decades is the usual age at presentation, with the male preponderance of 3:1. The patient has symptoms of a slow-growing laryngeal mass, such as dyspnea, hoarseness, and dysphagia. The clinical appearance may be a soft, polypoid mass, but more often it presents as a submucosal, infiltrating, reddish rubbery tumor. Histologically, there is a monotonous infiltrate of plasma cells in varying degrees of maturation. Differentiation from a plasma cell granulomatous process is essential. This latter condition exhibits mature plasma cell cytologic features that are mixed with other inflammatory cell elements and may show Russell bodies (microscopic spheroidal collections of eosinophilic gamma globulins) (Fig. 3–41). Radiation therapy of localized extramedullary laryngeal plasmacytoma has yielded good results in our cases. Secondary laryngeal involvement accompanying plasma cell neoplasia of other anatomic areas generally does poorly, occasionally proving to be *multiple myeloma.*

Neurofibrosarcoma (malignant schwannoma) occurred in the larynx on only one occasion according to the AFIP Otolaryngic Tumor Registry (1940–1975).

Malignant melanoma of the larynx was noted five times in the AFIP Otolaryngic Tumor Registry (1940–1975). It was difficult to ascertain whether these were primary or metastatic from elsewhere, since pigmented melanocytes have been noted in the normal larynx. The medical literature[101] supports the primary origin of malignant melanoma in the larynx but indicates that it is an infrequent occurrence. The treatment, behavior, and

Figure 3–41. A histologic example of an inflammatory cell granuloma of the larynx secondary to a chewing gum sensitivity in an 18-year-old male. The obvious plasma cell infiltrate consists of mature cells, mixed with lymphocytes and numerous round cell Russell bodies, all of which are against the diagnosis of a plasma cell malignancy. (AFIP #83-10498; H & E, ×63.)

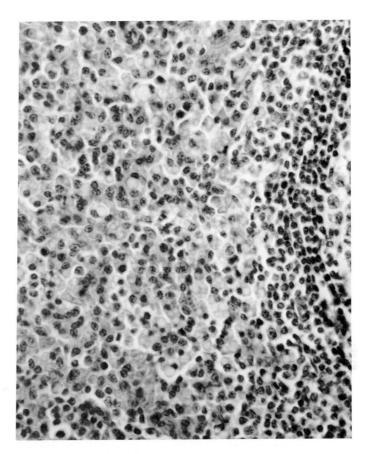

prognosis of laryngeal malignant malanoma parallels that of the same neoplasm in other sites, and survival depends on the size of the primary lesion and its metastatic behavior at the time of diagnosis.

Miscellaneous

Teratoid Neoplasms are composed of tissue derivatives of one or more germinal layers, sometimes foreign to the area of occurrence. They may be benign or malignant. They are a rarity in the larynx.

Hamartoma is simply a benign congenital malformation composed of tissue indigenous to the anatomic area of occurrence. We have seen two cases involving the larynx, and they presented as slowly growing masses that, when surgically removed, offered a good prognosis. *Choristoma*, on the other hand, is a benign congenital malformation formed of tissue derivatives not indigenous to the anatomic area. We have encountered thyroid tissue in the larynx, but whether this qualifies as a choristoma or represents congenital ectopia is debatable.

Histologically, keratinizing squamous cell cystic structures are not usually found in the larynx, particularly in the aryepiglottic fold, but adnexal tissue is absent in the cyst wall so that they should not qualify as dermoid cysts.—Hyams and Heffner

Dermoid cysts are benign teratoid neoplasms containing ectodermal tissue derivatives only (squamous cell epithelium, skin adnexa).◁

Teratoma is a benign neoplasm composed of two or more germinal layer derivatives. A rare case is reported in the larynx. There is no evidence in the literature or in our experience to support a malignant teratoma arising in the larynx.

Metastatic Neoplasia

In any diagnosis of malignant neoplasm of the larynx (particularly adenocarcinoma), the laryngologist should consider the possibility that the neoplasm represents metastasis from an undetected regional or distant primary site. Certainly, clinical evaluation is in order to rule out such possibility. Malignant melanoma metastatic to the larynx is the most common neoplasm in this category,[102] followed in decreasing frequency by renal cell, breast, lung, gastrointestinal, and prostatic carcinoma.

References

1. Blahova O, Brezovsky P: Stenosing processes due to endotracheal intubation and tracheostomy in children. Int J Pediatr Otorhinolaryngol, 3:199–203, 1981.

2. Kelemen G: Congenital laryngeal stridor. AMA Arch Otolaryngol, 58:245–268, 1953.

3. Templer J, Hast M, Thomas JR, Davis WE: Congenital laryngeal stridor secondary to flaccid epiglottis, anomalous accessory cartilages and redundant aryepiglottic folds. Laryngoscope, 91:394–397, 1981.

4. Jahrsdoerfer RA, Kirchner JA, Thaler SU: Cleft larynx. Arch Otolaryngol, 86:108–113, 1967.

5. Cotton RT, Richardson MA: Congenital laryngeal anomalies. Otolaryngol Clin North Am, 14:203–218, 1981.

6. Tucker GF, Ossoff RH, Newman AN, Holinger LD: Histopathology of congenital subglottic stenosis. Laryngoscope, 89:866–877, 1977.

7. McMillan WG, Duvall AJ III: Congenital subglottic stenosis. Arch Otolaryngol, 87:272–278, 1968.

8. Puveendran A: Congenital subglottic atresia—a case report. J Laryngol Otol, 86:847–852, 1972.

9. DeSanto LW: Laryngocele, laryngeal mucocele, large saccules, and laryngeal saccular cysts: A developmental spectrum. Laryngoscope, 84:1291–1296, 1974.

10. DeSanto LW, Devine KD, Weiland LH: Cysts of the larynx—classification. Laryngoscope, 80:145–176, 1970.

11. Chamberlain D: Congenital subglottic cyst of the larynx: A case report. Laryngoscope, 80:245–259, 1970.

12. Monday LA, Cornut G, Bouchayer M, Roch JB: Epidermoid cysts of the vocal cords. Ann Otol Rhinol Laryngol, 92:124–127, 1983.

13. Ruben RJ, Kucinski SA, Greenstein N: Case report: Cystic lymphangioma of the vallecula. Can J Otolaryngol, 4:180–184, 1975.

14. Bone RC, Biller HF, Irwin TM: Intralaryngotracheal thyroid. Ann Otol Rhinol Laryngol, 81:424–428, 1972.

15. Wolff M, Rankow RM: Heterotopic gastric epithelium in the head and neck region, Ann Plast Surg, 4:53–64, 1980.

16. Zapf B, Lehmann WB, Snyder GG III: Hamartoma of the larynx: An unusual cause for stridor in an infant. Otolaryngol Head Neck Surg, 89:797–799, 1981.

17. Jaffe BF: Unusual laryngeal problems in children. Ann Otol Rhinol Laryngol, 82:637–642, 1973.

18. Brodsky L, Yoshpe N, Ruben RJ: Clinical-pathological correlates of congenital subglottic hemangiomas. Ann Otol Rhinol Laryngol, 92 (Suppl 105):4–18, 1983.

19. Hawkins DB, Luxford WM: Laryngeal stenosis from endotracheal intubation: A review of 58 cases. Ann Otol Rhinol Laryngol, 89:454–458, 1980.

20. Tucker GF, Tucker JA, Vidic B: Anatomy and development of the cricoid: Serial-section whole organ study of perinatal larynges. Ann Otol Rhinol Laryngol, 86:766–769, 1977.

21. Morrison MD, Maber BR: Cricoarytenoid joint obliteration following longterm intubation in the premature infant. J Otolaryngol, 6:277–283, 1977.

22. Tucker GF Jr, Newton L, Ruben RJ: Histopathology of acquired subglottic stenosis: A documented case report. Ann Otol Rhinol Laryngol, 90:335–338, 1981.

23. Jackson C, Jackson CL: Benign tumors of the trachea and bronchi with especial reference to tumor-like formation of inflammatory origin. JAMA, 99:1747–1754, 1932.

24. Rosenberg HS, Vogler C, Close LG, Warshaw HE: Laryngeal fibromatosis in the neonate. Arch Otolaryngol, 107:513–517, 1981.

25. Ward PH, Zwitman D, Hanson D, Berci G: Contact ulcers and granulomas of the larynx. Otolaryngol Head Neck Surg, 88:262–269, 1980.

26. Strong MS, Vaughn CW: Vocal cord nodules and polyps—the role of surgical treatment. Laryngoscope, 81:911–922, 1971.

27. Szpunar J, Glowacki J, Laskowski A, Miszke A: Fibrinous laryngotracheobronchitis in children. Arch Otolaryngol, 93:173–178, 1971.

28. Liston SL, Gerhz RC, Jarvis CW: Bacterial tracheitis. Arch Otolaryngol, 107:561–564, 1981.

29. Heeneman H, Ward KM: Epiglottic abscess: Its occurrence and management. J Otolaryngol, 6:31–36, 1977.

30. Sopher IM, Fisher RS: Epiglottic abscess: Fatal acute airway obstruction in an adult. Arch Otolaryngol, 93:533–535, 1971.

31. Robin PE, Dalton GA: Subglottic stenosis in infants: Eight cases and their surgical and

conservative management. J Laryngol Otol, 88:233–247, 1974.

32. Travis LW, Hybels RL, Newman MH: Tuberculosis of the larynx. Laryngoscope, 86:549–558, 1976.

33. Lyons GD: Mycotic disease of the larynx. Ann Otol Rhinol Laryngol, 75:162–175, 1966.

34. Donegan JO and Wood MD: Histoplasmosis of the larynx. Laryngoscope, 94:206–209, 1984.

35. Feder RJ and Acquarelli, MJ: Blastomycosis of the larynx. Ann Otol Rhinol Laryngol, 74:1091–1101, 1965.

36. Benitz WE, Bradley JS, Fee WE Jr and Loomis JC: Upper airway obstruction due to laryngeal coccidioidomycosis in a 5-year-old child. Am J Otolaryngol, 4:367–370, 1983.

37. Reese MC and Colclasure JB: Cryptococcosis of the larynx. Arch Otolaryngol, 101:698–701, 1975.

38. Ferlito A: Primary aspergillosis of the larynx. J Laryngol Otol, 88:1257–1263, 1974.

39. Yonkers AJ: Candidiasis of the larynx, Ann Otol Rhinol Laryngol, 82:812–815, 1973.

40. Michaels L and Hyams VJ: Amyloid in localized deposits and plasmacytomas of the respiratory tract, J Pathol, 128:29–38, 1979.

41. Richards SH and Bull PD: Lipoid proteinosis of the larynx, J Laryngol Otol, 187–190, 1973.

42. MacKinnon DM: Hyalinosis cutis et mucosae (lipoid proteinosis), Acta Otolaryngol, 65:403–412, 1968.

43. Bicknell PG: Mild hypothyroidism and its effects on the larynx. J Laryngol Otol, 87:123–127, 1973.

44. Marion RB, Alperin JE and Maloney WH: Gouty tophus of the true vocal cord. Arch Otolaryngol, 96:161–162, 1972.

45. Cohen SR, Landing BH, Issacs H: Epidermolysis bullosa associated with laryngeal stenosis. Ann Otol Rhinol Laryngol, 97(Suppl 52):25–28, 1978.

46. Thompson JW, Ahmed AR, Dudley JP: Epidermolysis dystrophica of the larynx and trachea: Acute airway obstruction. Ann Otol Rhinol Laryngol, 89:428–429, 1980.

47. Cohn AM, McFarlane JR, Knox J: Pachyonychia congenita with involvement of the larynx. Arch Otolaryngol, 102:233–235, 1976.

48. Crepeau J, Poliquin J: The blue rubber bleb nevus syndrome. J Otolaryngol 10:387–390, 1981.

49. McDonald TJ, Neel HB III, De Remee RA: Wegener's granulomatosis of the subglottis and the upper portion of the trachea. Ann Otol Rhinol Laryngol, 91:588–592, 1982.

50. Neel HB III, Mcdonald TJ: Laryngeal sarcoidosis: Report of 13 patients. Ann Otol Rhinol Laryngol, 91:359–362, 1982.

51. Charow A, Pass F, Ruben R: Phemphigus of

the respiratory tract. Arch Otolaryngol, 93:209–210, 1971.

52. Weinstein S, Sachs AR: Pemphigus of the oropharynx and larynx: Report of a case. Arch Otolaryngol, 62:214–217, 1955.

53. Bridger MWM, Jahn AF and van Nostrand AWP: Laryngeal rheumatoid arthritis. Laryngoscope, 90:296–303, 1980.

54. Friedman BA and Rice DH: Rheumatoid nodules of the larynx. Arch Otolaryngol, 101:361–363, 1975.

55. Daly JF: Relapsing polychondritis of the larynx and trachea. Arch Otolaryngol, 84:570–573, 1966.

56. Foidart JM and Katz SI: Subtle clues to diagnosis by immunopathology. Am J Dermatopathol, 1:257–260, 1979.

57. Climie ARW, Waggoner LG and Krabbenhoft KL: Lymphoid hamartoma of the larynx. Laryngoscope, 74:1381–1388, 1964.

58. Pellettiere EV 2d, Holinger LD and Schild JA: Lymphoid hyperplasia of larynx simulating neoplasia. Ann Otol Rhinol Laryngol, 89:65–68, 1980.

59. Mikaelian DO: Idiopathic subglottic laryngeal stenosis in an adult. J Laryngol Otol, 88:467–472, 1974.

60. Wold, LE and Weiland LH: Tumefactive fibro-inflammatory lesions of the head and neck. Am J Surg Pathol, 7:477–482, 1983.

61. Brandenburg JH: Idiopathic subglottic stenosis. Trans Am Acad Ophthalmol Otolaryngol, 76:1402–1406, 1972.

62. Shanmugaratnam K: Histological Typing of Upper Respiratory Tract Tumors. International Histological Classification of Tumours, No. 19, Geneva, World Health Organization, 1978.

63. Holinger PH, Johnston KC, Anison GC: Papilloma of the larynx: A review of 109 cases with a preliminary report of Aureomycin therapy. Ann Otol, 59:547–564, 1950.

64. Bewtra C, Krisnman R, Lee SS: Malignant changes in nonirradiated juvenile laryngotracheal papillomatosis. Arch Otolaryngol, 108:114–116, 1982.

65. Quick CA, Watts SL, Krzysek RA, Faras AJ: Relationship between condylomata and laryngeal papillomata. Ann Otol, 89:467–471, 1980.

66. Gallagher JC, Puzon BQ: Oncocytic lesions of the larynx. Ann Otol, 78:307–315, 1969.

67. Holms-Jensen S, Jacobsen M, Tommesen N, Ferreira O: Oncocytic cysts of the larynx. Arch Otolaryngol, 83:366–371, 1977.

68. Sobel HJ, Marquet E: Granular cells and granular cell lesions. Pathol Ann, 4:43–79, 1974.

69. Frable MA, Fischer RA: Granular cell myoblatstomas. Laryngoscope, 86:36–42, 1976.

70. Compagno J, Hyams VJ, Ste-Marie P: Benign granular cell tumors of the larynx: A re-

view of 36 cases with clinicopathologic data. Ann Otol, 84:308–314, 1975.

71. Hyams VJ, Rabuzzi DD: Carcilaginous tumors of the larynx. Laryngoscope, 80:755–767, 1970.

72. Bridger GP, Nassar VH, Skinner HG: Hemangioma in the adult larynx. Arch Otolaryngol, 92:493–498, 1970.

73. Ferguson GB: Hemangioma of the adult and the infant larynx. Arch Otolaryngol, 40:189–195, 1944.

74. Batsakis JG, Rice DH: The pathology of head and neck tumors: Vasoformative tumors. Part 9a. Head Neck Surg, 3:231–239, 1981.

75. Ruben RJ, Kucinski SA, Greenstein N: Cystic lympangioma of the vallecula. Can J Otolaryngol, 4:180–184, 1975.

76. FU Y-S, Oerzom KH: Nonepithelial tumors of the nasal cavity, paranasal sinuses and nasopharynx. A clinicopathologic study. VI. Fibrous tissue tumors (fibroma, fibromatosis, fibrosarcoma), Cancer, 37:2912–2928, 1976.

77. Kleinsasser O, Glanz HL: Myogenic tumours of the larynx. Arch Otolaryngol, 225:107–119, 1979.

78. Ferlito A, Grugoni P: Rhabdomyoma purum of the larynx. J Laryngol, 99:1131–1141, 1975.

79. Mansson I, Wilske J, Kindblom L-G: Lipoma of the hypopharynx. A case report and a review of the literature. J Laryngol Otol, 92:1037–1043, 1978.

80. Batsakis JG, Fox JE: Supporting tissue neoplasms of the larynx. Surg Gynecol Obstet, 131:989–997, 1970.

81. Lawson W, Zak FG: The glomus bodies (paraganglia) of the human larynx. Laryngoscope, 84:98–111, 1974.

82. Hordyk GJ, Reuter DJ, Bosman FT, Mauw BJ: Chemodectoma (paraganglioma) of the larynx. Clin Otolaryngol, 6:249–254, 1981.

83. Hellquist H, Lundren J, Olagsson V: Hyperplasia, keratosis, dysplasia, and carcinoma-in-situ of the vocal cords. A follow-up study. Clin Otolaryngol, 7:11–27, 1982.

84. McGavran MH, Bauer WC, Ogura JH: Isolated laryngeal keratosis. It's relation to carcinoma of the larynx based on clinicopathologic study of 87 consecutive cases with long term follow-up. Laryngoscope, 70:932–951, 1960.

85. Bauer WC, McGavran MH: Carcinoma in situ and evaluation of epithelial changes in laryngopharyngeal biopsies. JAMA, 221: 72–75, 1972.

86. American Joint Committee for Cancer Staging and End Results Reporting. Staging of Cancer of Head and neck Sites and of Melanoma. Chicago, 1980.

87. Gnepp DR, Ferlito A, Hyams VJ: Primary anaplastic small cell (oat cell) carcinoma of the larynx. Preview of the literature and report of 18 cases. Cancer, 51:1731–1745, 1983.

88. Fechner RE, Mills SE: Verruca vulgaris of the larynx. Am J Surg Pathol, 6:357–362, 1982.

89. Ferlito A, Recher G: Ackerman's tumor (verrucous carcinoma) of the larynx. A clinicopathologic study of 77 cases. Cancer, 46:1617–1630, 1980.

90. Hyams VJ: Spindle cell carcinoma of the larynx. Can J Otolaryngol, 4:307–313, 1975.

91. Leventon GS, Evans HL: Sarcomatoid squamous cell carcinoma of the mucous membranes of the head and neck. A clinicopathologic study of 20 cases. Cancer, 48:944–1003, 1981.

92. Paladugu RR, Nathwani BN, Goodstein J, Dirde LE, Memoli VE, Gould VE: Carcinoma of the larynx with mucosubstance production and neuroendocrine differentiation: An ultrastructural and immunohistochemical study. Cancer, 49:343–349, 1982.

93. Spiro RH, Huvas AG, Strong EW: Adenoid cystic carcinoma: Factors influencing survival. Am J Surg, 138:579–583, 1979.

94. Damiani JM, Damiani KK, Hauck K, Hyams VJ: Mucoepidermoidadenosquamous carcinoma of the larynx and hypopharynx: A report of 21 cases and a review of the literature. Otolaryngol Head Neck Surg, 89:235–243, 1981.

95. Roth JA, Enzinger FM, Tannenbaum M: Synovial sarcoma of the neck: A follow-up study of 24 cases. Cancer, 35:1243–1253, 1975.

96. Duhn KW, Hyams VJ, Harris AE: Rhabdomyosarcoma of the larynx: A case report and review of the literature. Laryngoscope, 94:210–212, 1984.

97. Ferlito A: Primary malignant haemangiopericytoma of the larynx. J Laryngol Otol, 92:511–519, 1978.

98. Abramson AL, Simons RL: Kaposi's sarcoma of the head and neck. Arch Otolaryngol, 92:505–507, 1970.

99. Gaynor EB, Ragkausan J, Weisbrot IM: Primary myxoid liposarcoma of the larynx. Otolaryngol Head Neck Surg, 92:476–479, 1984.

100. Swerdlow JB, Merl SA, Davey FR, Gacek, RR, Gotlieb AJ: NonHodgkin's lymphoma limited to the larynx. Cancer, 53:2546–2550, 1984.

101. Shanon E, Covo J, Loeventhal M: Melanoma of the epiglottis: A case treatment by supraglottic laryngectomy. Arch Otolaryngol, 91:305–306, 1970.

102. Whicher JH, Carder GA, Device KD: Metastasis to the larynx. Report of a case and review of literature. Arch Otolaryngol, 96:182–184, 1972.

Chapter 4

Diagnostic Imaging
of the Larynx

Arnold M. Noyek and Harry S. Shulman

This chapter explores concepts of laryngeal imaging, its applications, potentials, and the limitations of contemporary "radiologic" evaluation. Effective diagnostic imaging of the larynx requires rational, cost-effective, and innovative use of a variety of radiologic modalities. Diagnostic radiologic examinations (both reoentgenographic[1] [dependent on a primary x-ray beam] and nonroetgenographic,[2] such as ultrasound, radionuclide scans, and magnetic resonance imaging [MRI]) can provide selective and critical perspectives on the patient and his laryngeal disorder. Effective imaging of the larynx helps to establish a realistic provisional diagnosis and an appropriate treatment plan.

Need for Laryngeal Imaging

As with other structures in the upper airway, the framework or skeletal supports of the larynx remain largely inaccessible to clinical assessment. Even with improved optics, only surface elements of the mucous membrane, which are readily seen from above, can be evaluated effectively by the clinician. Even so, many of the surface structures of the larynx remain hidden (the ventricles, the subglottic region). Laryngeal radiology can permit morphologic and functional assessment of the airway, as well as evaluation of the laryngeal soft tissues and supporting cartilaginous skeleton. Thus, laryngeal diagnostic imaging has the potential to improve accuracy of diagnosis greatly when combined with history, conventional mirror examination, telescopic examination, and direct endoscopic examination.

Radiology as an Allied Specialty

A functional approach to laryngeal diagnosis is necessary if imaging studies are to be requested and used in a meaningful way. High technology does not by itself guarantee instant answers; there is a human being at either end of the piece of diagnostic equipment. The clinician need not understand all of the details of the physics of radiologic (or nonradiologic) evaluation of the larynx; however, he *does* need to understand technologic applications as well as indications, contraindications, and kinds of information that the various studies can provide.

Radiology should be viewed as an "allied" specialty, rather than a provider of technical support. The radiologist must be brought into the management of the patient as a *consultant,* since the images that he creates may be pivotal in determining, for example, whether a patient needs to have his larynx removed or not. When the radiologist understands the impact his studies may have on the patient's welfare, he becomes an integral component in the diagnostic process. It is therefore imperative that the clinician help the radiologist to understand the specific clinical problems facing the patient. The radiologist can then recommend those studies most likely to provide the information needed.◁

Factors related to technologic availability, geography, economics, and, not least of all, qualified and interested laryngeal radiologists, determine what kind of diagnostic service will be rendered to patients.

Functional Approach to Imaging

Radiologic evaluation of the larynx should be based on certain principals. The studies requested should provide:

1. Maximal *anatomic* information concerning the entire larynx, viewed regionally
2. Maximal *functional* information (i.e., vocal cord mobility)
3. Adequate *evaluation of the airway* from a structural point of view (i.e., the level of airway obstruction, its precise localization, and dimension)
4. Assessment of *occult* or hidden *areas* of the larynx, such as the ventricles or the subglottic region

"Major league" disease requires "major league" imaging. For example, if carcinoma of the larynx is already advanced on clinical presentation (some T2, all T3, all T4), a valid treatment approach cannot be planned without the best imaging technology available. Here computed tomography (CT) has its widest application, not only in improved T staging, but in the possibility of improved N staging. Laryngeal trauma also deserves CT diagnosis.

Axial CT exactly matches our surgical approaches to the larynx. It should therefore be utilized freely when major interventions are considered. In addition, CT constructions allow a full, three-dimensional assessment of laryngeal pathologic conditions. As a result, few exploratory operations should be needed. MRI may help us deal with these problems even more effectively.

Functional approach suggests that the larynx be viewed as a dynamic organ with the supraglottis, glottis, and subglottis all available for detailed study by a variety of radiologic modalities. The adjacent framework and the extralaryngeal structures of concern (thyroid gland, major vessels, lymph nodes, hypopharynx, and esophagus) are all increasingly subject to accurate anatomic, physiologic, and pathologic assessment. Each modality should be considered in turn as a possible means of study, considering the specific clinical problem at hand. Key clinical problems must be formulated as each radiologic consultation is requested. Is the laryngeal cartilage involved? Is there direct extension of disease into a related structure? Is the disorder vascular? Is the airway compromised? There are many possible clinical problems, and it is important that the clinician formulate a clear question to the radiologist. This is the essence of an effective consultative approach to laryngeal radiology.

Formulating a Diagnosis

Diagnosis of laryngeal disease is really no different from diseases elsewhere in the body.[3] Initially, there is often a "provisional" or working diagnosis; that is, we arrive at the diagnosis based on the best possible clinical, radiologic, pathologic, and other information at hand. The provisional or working diagnosis is a rational guess upon which further management decisions can be predicated.

The pathologist usually provides a *qualitative* diagnosis when, for example, he labels a tumor "squamous cell carcinoma." The radiologist, on the other hand, may suggest a *specific* diagnosis, but more often provides a *differential* and *quantitative* diagnosis. The ability to measure density with CT allows the identification of cystic lesions, such as fluid-filled laryngoceles, or fatty lesions, such as lipomas, and this information can be of great value. If "cystic" disease or "infiltrative" disease or "vascular" disease is detected, he gives real direction to further management. Thus, the roles of the radiologist and the pathologist are complementary.

The radiologist may be able to answer each of four questions:

1. *What is the extent of the disease?* With modalities currently available, the three-dimensional extent of many lesions can be defined. The lesion can be quantified, even in millimeters, utilizing cursor distance measurement with CT or ultrasound.
2. *Is there extralaryngeal extension of disease?* Knowledge of invasion of the laryngeal framework by cancer (T4 cancer) is critical to its proper management. Prior to CT, 50 percent of laryngeal T4 cancer with cartilage involvement was understaged as T3. When the thyroid gland is directly invaded by laryngeal cancer, it is a grave prognostic sign. What has tumor extension done to the adjacent aerodigestive tract?
3. *Is this a local laryngeal manifestation of a systemic disorder* (e.g., lymphoma, sarcoidosis, or systemic lupus erythematosus)? Radiologic imaging can allow an improved understanding of dissemination of local disease, such as N staging the laryngeal cancer with CT and M staging with radionuclide bone scans.
4. *Are there specific anatomic or physiologic deficits related to the laryngeal disorder?* Radiologic imaging can define a foreign body or a specific physiologic abnormality, such as the level of airway obstruction.

Formulation of a laryngeal diagnosis in qualitative and quantitative terms by utilizing radiologic imaging to full advantage helps to eliminate faulty diagnostic impressions (usually failure to recognize disease) and avoids mismanagement of the patient and complications.

The Radiologist as Consultant

Clearly, the radiologist must serve a consultant role. If he is simply a technologist who provides imaging, an unmonitored, undirected study will result. Too frequently, the patient leaves the x-ray department without optimal or maximal information having been obtained. Too often we hear the comment, "If I had only known, I would have studied this area or that area, or continued the CT cuts for another level or two." The radiologist *can* know, if he receives adequate pretreatment information and can direct himself to provide a specific answer to the inquiring clinician in his proper function as a supportive colleague.

In the beginning, there was conventional imaging, which was quite simplistic but functional. It really answered only the most basic of questions: Does disease exist? As clinical methodology advanced (such as improved endoscopes, fiberoptics, cameras), clinical awareness expanded. The physician was no longer content with the simple recognition of disease; he began to understand that it must be quantified in order to evaluate patients and treatment results properly; hence, the evolution of such clinical concepts as TNM staging.

High technology made its own imprint on the present, or second, era. Diagnostic imaging can contribute greatly to appropriate pretreatment staging of a variety of laryngeal disorders.

Finally, there is the clinical evolution that covers these two eras, which ultimately leads to improved patient care through combinations of more effective clinical methods and more effective diagnostic imaging. However, cost and risk factors become significant and must be balanced against a real world in which such matters are eventually weighed against basic humanity.

Historical Perspectives

Conventional Radiology

Soon after its discovery by Wilhelm Roentgen in 1895, the roentgen ray was applied to the study of laryngeal anatomy.[4] MacIntyre,[5] in England, wrote in May, 1896: "I have been able to photograph the larynx in the human subject, the picture obtained showing the base of the tongue, hyoid bone, thyroid and cricoid cartilages with epiglottis." He was describing, of course, the roentgen appearance of the laryngeal structures and adjacent tissues on a lateral view. He further stated, "experimenting on a dead subject, I have also been able to obtain excellent photographs of the presence of foreign bodies in and around the region of the larynx, as well as ossification in the cartilages." MacIntyre was of the opinion that cryptoscopy (fluoroscopy) would be of more importance than photography (radiography). He states: "With regard to the cryptoscope, the light easily penetrates the tissues of the neck and chest. I have seen sufficient of the former to enable me to say that many foreign bodies might be detected in the eye without photography at all." In 1896, Scheier[6] also described roentgen examination of the larynx on a cadaver. He noted that the long exposure time required for photography of the larynx made films on the living patient difficult.

Behn[7] in 1901 made an excellent lateral radiograph of the larynx showing a laryngeal tumor. Movements of the larynx, swallowing function, and ossification of laryngeal cartilages were studied flouroscopically and radiologically by Scheier[8–11] from 1901 to 1911, by Moller and Fischer[12–14] in 1903, and by Frankel[15] in 1908. Thost[16] in 1903 published the first systematic roentgen atlas of laryngeal disease.

In the United States, Iglauer[17] in 1914 wrote on the value of lateral radiography of the larynx in the study of laryngeal disease. He described decalcification of ossified cartilage in laryngeal tuberculosis, a process similar to decalcification and bone resorption in osseous tuberculosis. He also noted associated soft tissue swelling and ulceration and deformity of the laryngeal structures, including the epiglottis. Iglauer also described a more distinct picture of laryngeal calcification and ossification associated with syphilis.

He did not claim originality for these observations but credited Thost with priority. Iglauer also described laryngeal stenosis associated with foreign body, tumor, cicatrices, or external compression. Thost,[16] in 1913, described carcinomatous infiltration of the larynx causing a sievelike appearance of the calcified thyroid cartilage due to cartilage destruction. Coutard,[18] in 1922, emphasized the usefulness of lateral radiography of the larynx in the study of neoplasms.

Hickey[19] in 1928 described the roentgen appearance of the normal larynx using a lateral view and low kilovoltage soft tissue technique. He commented that the anteroposterior (AP) view was not of much use because of the interference of the bony background of the cervical spine.

Coutard and Baclesse[20] in 1932 recommended lateral roentgen examination of the larynx before, during, and after roentgen therapy of the larynx and hypopharynx for epitheliomas. They stressed the importance of radiographic examination for pretreatment diagnosis, as an aid to diagnosis in the patient who is difficult to examine, for study of lesions in the ventricles, preepiglottic space, and sinus of Morgagni, and to evaluate edema of the larynx and cartilage destruction.

Young[21,22] in 1940 and 1942 recommended AP radiography of the larynx with a short 10 cm target skin distance, 45 to 50 kv, 300 ma, and 1/20th of a second exposure time. This technique diminishes the obscuring effect of the cervical spine on the laryngeal airway and soft tissues, and permits visualization of soft tissue masses or cord paralysis.

Gay and Wilkins[23] in 1956 and Gay[24] in 1958 commented on the poor visibility of neck structures with conventional fluoroscopy; they recommended image intensification fluoroscopy, which increased the intensity of the image 200 times over conventional fluoroscopy. Image intensification fluoroscopy could now play a more important role in the study of laryngeal function and laryngeal disease. These investigators pointed out that image intensification fluoroscopy complements conventional radiography and tomography and adds to the diagnostic accuracy of the roentgen study of tumors of the larynx, pharynx, and cervical esophagus. In their routine, a barium swallow examination was used to study the laryngopharynx and cervical esophagus.

Leborgne[25] in 1936, published the first study of AP curvilinear *tomography* of the larynx using his own original equipment. He stressed the value of tomography in the study of cancer of the larynx in a series of articles.[26–29] In France in 1937 Canuyt and Gunsett[30,31] wrote on tomography in the normal and in the pathologic larynx. Leborgne[25,28] stressed the convenience of tomography, which required no patient preparation, and the symmetric structure of the two sides of the larynx surrounding an air-containing lumen, which profiled the normal and the abnormal sides. Howes[32] in 1939, Young[21] in 1940, and Caulk[33] in 1941 in the United States published excellent tomographic studies of the larynx, illustrating the normal and the pathologic larynx, including laryngeal carcinoma, vocal cord paralysis, and laryngocele.

Iglauer[34] and 1926 and Jackson[35] in 1936 studied the larynx by conventional and contrast (Lipiodol) radiography. Iglauer outlined a subglottic laryngeal stricture with Lipiodol. However, Lipiodol was not an ideal contrast medium because it coated the laryngeal mucosa rather spottily. Farinas[36] in 1942 achieved excellent laryngograms in the anesthetized larynx using a pump atomizer that sprayed a 40 percent solution of Neoiodipin through a curved cannula extending behind the epiglottis. Contrast laryngography was not really brought to the fore in the United States until the work of Powers and colleagues[37] in 1957, Ogura and co-workers[38] in 1960, and Medina and co-workers[39] in 1961. These researchers achieved excellent contrast laryngograms using oily propyliodone, a very satisfactory coating agent, after topical anesthesia of the larynx. Barium sulfate in carboxymethylcellulose water suspension had also been used successfully for laryngography and pharyngography.

Khoo and co-workers[40] in 1967 described their technique of contrast pharyngography with liquid barium sulfate after topical anesthesia. This was part of a continuing effort to utilize contrast media to outline mucosal alterations. They used 20 ml of 25 percent liquid barium, suspended with 1.5 percent carboxymethylcellulose, instilled by nasal catheter into the nasopharynx. Combining intensification fluoroscopy, cineradiography, and radiography with submental vertex, lateral, and frontal views, they were able to detect a variety of small mucosal lesions not previously discernible by conventional radiography alone.

Following this development, Zamel and co-workers[41] in 1970 produced excellent laryngograms using powdered tantalum insufflation with or without prior mucosal anesthesia. Subsequently, the possible explosive nature of tantalum caused its abandonment.

By the early 1970s, AP tomography of the larynx was considered the major pretreatment staging examination in the evaluation of laryngeal carcinoma and the best means of obtaining a vertical overview of the soft tissues and (in some measure) the framework of the larynx. Zizmor did much to promote the appropriate role for conventional and tomographic studies.[62]

At the close of the conventional era, clinicians felt that tomography had specific application:◁

1. To demonstrate subglottic extension of tumor
2. To demonstrate obliteration of the ventricle by tumor
3. To show evidence of cartilage necrosis due to tumor, infection, or radiotherapy
4. For comparison of the right and left sides of the larynx
5. As a permanent visual record of the location and extent of tumor at the initial examination
6. To demonstrate regression or extension of tumor during radiotherapy
7. As a valuable diagnostic aid in a patient with a short and thick neck and a backward tilt of the epiglottis making clinical evaluation difficult.

At the same time (the 1970s), many clinicians felt that laryngography did everything that tomography of the larynx could do and, in addition, was valuable in demonstrating anterior commissure and postcricoid lesions that could not be demonstrated by tomography. Laryngeal function and elasticity could be studied fluoroscopically and radiographically as well as by cineradiography and television at that time.

McGuire and co-workers[42,43] in 1965 and 1966 described a practical approach to effective AP diagnostic radiography of the larynx by high kilovoltage and selective filtration using a Bucky technique with 140 kv and 1 mm copper filtration. By this method, the density of the bony background of the cervical spine is diminished. The air within the laryngeal lumen remains a good contrast medium for the soft tissue structure of the larynx. The resultant laryngeal image approaches the quality of AP tomograms. The cords, bands, ventricles, aryepiglottic folds, pyriform sinuses, and subglottic larynx are well visualized. This technique compares favorably with the accuracy of tomography in demonstrating laryngeal lesions, with a much lower roentgen exposure for the patient. McGuire was of the

It was only with the advent of CT and a more critical view of coronal tomography that limitations were recognized. First, there is a normal variation in cord morphology; some vocal cords are just naturally bulkier than others, although symmetry always remains. To assess the ventricles properly, reverse phonation is a particularly useful maneuver; however, many patients have neither the physical capability nor the intelligence to handle this maneuver. Finally, the radiologist's natural desire to create the best contrast between air and soft tissue leads him to pick the midcord level, which may not always be best for the survey in question.

High kilovoltage selective filtration radiography provides a "summary" of the larynx in AP overview; tomography gives a much more discrete sectional evaluation.

Many experienced laryngographers agree that the Valsalva maneuver may successfully coat the undersurface of the vocal cords, giving better definition to subglottic lesions than does high kilovoltage techniques.

opinion that high kilovoltage technique can supersede low kilovoltage tomography. ◁

Thornbury and Latourette[44] in 1967 compared the accuracy of high kilovoltage AP radiography of the larynx with contrast laryngography. They felt that positive contrast laryngography was more accurate than 150 kvp radiography in tumor detection and delineation, except for a few transglottic lesions in which good positive contrast was difficult to obtain. The high kilovoltage technique equaled the accuracy of laryngography in detecting subglottic lesions. ◁ These investigators said that positive contrast laryngography was the procedure of choice in general and that high kilovoltage technique was indicated when:

1. Positive contrast coating of the larynx is unsatisfactory;
2. Airway obstruction by tumor is too great for safe contrast laryngography.
3. Atropine premedication is contraindicated.

This was the comparative status of laryngography and high kilovoltage selective filtration radiography at that time. Fabrikant and co-workers[45] in 1962 described the complete roentgenographic study of the larynx at the Johns Hopkins Hospital and reported the following steps in their examination at that time:

1. AP and lateral radiography for soft tissues of the neck and larynx
2. AP tomography of the larynx
3. Barium swallow with image intensification fluoroscopy and radiography for study of the hypopharynx and cervical esophagus
4. Laryngography

Xeroradiography appeared on the scene in 1970. It relied on a conventional x-ray beam but altered the recording process by using a charged photoconductor for image recording. Holinger,[46] and Noyek and co-workers[47] described its potential role.

Other forms of imaging have been abandoned and become anachronisms. Laryngography, for example, which was held in such esteem that it was ultimately compared to CT when it was first applied to the larynx,[48] has disappeared form the scene. There is now virtually no indication for this study, whereas only 15 years ago it was the prime study for detailing of mucosal abnormality through x-ray examination.

High-Technology Imaging

The impact of high-technology imaging on clinical evaluation has been dramatic. This era began in 1971 with Godfrey Hounsfield's remarkable work with CT at EMI in England. The installation of the first clinical CT unit occurred at the Atkinson Morley Hospital in London in 1973. The past decade has seen the comprehensive advent of CT and the dramatic demonstration of its effectiveness in imaging both soft tissue and laryngeal cartilage framework. Not only has detailed morphologic assessment of the larynx been advanced, but an entirely new perspective to imaging interpretation has resulted. Axial CT examinations exactly match our open operative approaches to the larynx—a pivotal concept in effective imaging and interpretation. The work of Mancuso and Hanafee[48–52] has highlighted this development of CT examination of the larynx.

CT has now been augmented by the development of MRI. Although argument continues that MRI may replace CT, this technique provides another, complementary assessment of the larynx. MRI may (with the use of surface coils and thin sections) yet become the most effective means of imaging laryngeal soft tissues; however, it will more likely complement the framework imaging provided by CT. These high-technology studies may eventually become obligatory in the pretreatment staging of cancer, in the management of trauma, and in other indications.[53-56]

Noyek and co-workers[57] have demonstrated the effectiveness of high-resolution diagnostic ultrasound in appreciating cartilage destruction in advanced laryngeal cancer, when CT imaging has been equivocal. Noyek and colleagues[2,58-61] have also advocated a variety of radionuclide scans for better understanding of physiologic alterations within the larynx.

Contemporary Laryngeal Imaging

Understanding of radiologic findings depends on knowledge of normal laryngeal anatomy and physiology, as well as that of the related upper airway, upper digestive tract, and supporting soft tissue structures. The larynx should be viewed as one anatomic structure in the whole patient, who may present with coincident disease of the upper airway or related systemic disease.

Radiographic Signs and Their Clinical Interpretation

The human eye can discern 16 shades of gray, and it is this capability that allows recognition of altered morphologic features on conventional radiographs and on more advanced studies such as CT, which further expands the gray scale.[59,62-64] Initial attention should be to the air-mucosal interface, regardless of the plane of study. Conventional soft tissue lateral radiograph of the larynx presents the laryngeal air shadow in relationship to the laryngeal airspace above and the tracheal airspace below. Mass lesions are well profiled, and differentiation between sessile and pedunculated lesions may be possible; stenoses or strictures can be identified in the sagittal dimension. The overlapping densities of the thyroid alae and the cricoid cartilage interfere with full airway display.

Many radiologists no longer utilize preliminary radiographs, although distances and topography should be clearly noted both in interpretation and clinical review.

Radiographic findings are heightened in axial display by CT, but the level of airway encroachment must be related to known anatomic landmarks or to preliminary digital radiograph.◁ Once the extent of mucosal disease has been suggested, attention should be directed to other areas of possible mucosal abnormality, whether independent or related.

Next, the framework of the larynx should be assessed. On conventional radiography, this may be quite difficult, since recognition of the cartilaginous framework depends on the density of these supporting structures. This density varies directly with the amount of calcification and ossification within specified laryngeal cartilages. In conventional plain lateral films, the difficulty is compounded by the overlapping images of paired symmetrical structures on either side of the airway. However, tracheal definition can be quite precise, as can the outlining of the cricoid cartilage with its high-rising posterior signet. The paired arytenoid cartilages sitting on the cricoid signet may also be seen.◁ Calcification within the arytenoid cartilages is quite variable, although it tends to be more obvious in women than men at any given age. The cricoid cartilage is usually easy to recognize, since it calcifies even by the early teen years. The thyroid cartilage with its paired alae may be difficult to define, even though it is the most obvious of the laryngeal supporting cartilages by virtue of its size. It tends to calcify and ossify, usually beginning within the second or third decade. Ossification begins in the inferior cornua and progresses in an anterosuper-

The arytenoid cartilages are the most consistently calcified of the cartilages and most readily identifiable on CT examination; they are much less precisely defined on conventional lateral radiographs where the ''arytenoid mass'' is, in reality, the summated image of the paired arytenoid cartilages with surrounding musculature and mucosa.

ior direction. Areas of deficient mineralization may be difficult to differentiate from demineralization by a malignant process.

Generally, the framework can be well-identified in axial display by CT. Cartilage destruction, marrow cavity expansion or encroachment, and joint space disruption (particularly of the cricoarytenoid joints) can be imaged. MRI does not demonstrate the cartilage framework because calcium does not lend itself to this technique. However, the marrow content of the individual cartilages can be appreciated, which may provide improved awareness of thyroid cartilage invasion by carcinoma.

Once the mucosa and framework of the larynx have been examined, physiologic changes should be noted. Extent of airway obstruction and vocal cord mobility can be evaluated through static and dynamic studies. High kilovoltage and selective filtration AP radiography of the larynx still serves as screening examination and may well identify vocal cord paralysis in images comparable to AP tomography. Other physiologic changes such as loss of pliability and distensibility beyond the vocal cord level may also be recognized, especially with contrast examinations and fluoroscopic control.

Finally, attention should be paid to the remainder of the soft tissues of the adjacent head and neck structures for radiographic evidence of abnormality affecting the common carotid arteries, the internal jugular veins, nonenhancing lymph nodes on CT examinations, and the thyroid gland.

Selection of Radiographic Modalities

In choosing an imaging study, the clinician must first ask himself what diagnostic information he would like to obtain. Each study should attempt to answer one or more specific questions, while considering patient risk, cost-effectiveness, and logistic issues. A patient with acute epiglottitis should not have even a simple lateral conventional radiography of the larynx carried out if loss of control of the airway might ensue. On the other hand, no patient with major laryngeal disease such as laryngeal carcinoma or fracture should be managed without documentation and understanding through the best-quality studies available.

Conventional Plain Films

So-called conventional radiography is designed to demonstrate the soft tissues and underlying supporting cartilage, when possible.[62] The major baseline examination is the lateral soft tissue radiograph (Fig. 4–1). This provides an overview of the entire airway, in sagittal display, from the level of the trachea entering the thoracic inlet below to the vault of the nasopharynx above. The radiologist may modify the technique, varying the penetration of the x-ray beam, especially in the search for radiopaque foreign bodies and retropharyngeal or intralaryngeal abscess.◁

In conventional plain film examination, the search for mucosal surface abnormalities is best conducted with low kilovoltage radiographs (even to the point of not visualizing the vertebral column); on the other hand, the search for foreign body and submucosal abnormalities (such as retropharyngeal abscess) is helped by higher kilovoltage studies.

Information may be obtained concerning mucous membrane swelling or distortion. The arytenoids are usually well-profiled, particularly when they are edematous. The cervical spine is routinely evaluated; the soft tissue distance between the anterior aspect of any individual cervical vertebra and the posterior wall of the trachea (as is evident from the air-tracheal interface) should not exceed in distance the height of the body of the cervical vertebra at the same level. Any increase beyond this represents pathologic change and may reflect a variety of soft tissue disorders (retropharyngeal abscess, thyroid mass).

The conventional chest radiograph (both PA and lateral) complements the laryngeal study. Aside from the usual information about the parenchyma and thoracic cage, the tracheobronchial tree is seen in overview and

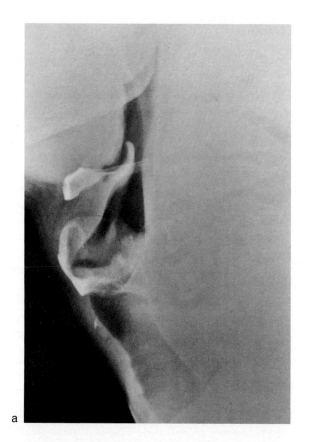

a

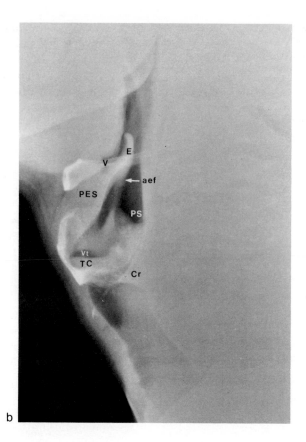

b

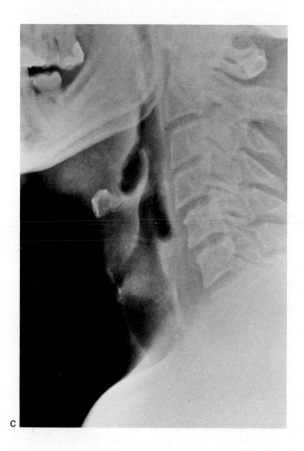

c

Chest radiographs may have intimate relationships to the laryngeal study in certain instances. The cause of recurrent laryngeal nerve palsy, for example, may be demonstrated on chest x-ray, such as hilar metastases or aortic arch aneurysm.

the superior mediastinum can be assessed.◁ Free air may also be noted on conventional radiographs. Interstitial or subcutaneous free air may be seen as a single loculation, as multiple loculated areas, or diffusely, in laryngeal fracture or cricotracheal separation, for example. A multiloculated collection of air is often seen in retropharyngeal abscess. Diffuse air collections may also be seen after tracheostomy.

Xeroradiography

Xeroradiography (Fig. 4–2) relies on the conventional x-ray beam, as does plain film examination.[46,47,65–67] The phenomenon of edge enhancement[68] relates to the developmental processing of the xeroradiogram, rather than attenuation or absorption of the x-ray beam as it passes through the anatomic part under study. An electric charge has been applied

Figure 4–1. Normal soft tissue lateral radiograph of the larynx. **a,** A properly taken soft tissue lateral radiograph shows fine mucosal and framework detail. Air profiles the base of tongue and valleculae. The tip of the epiglottis is clearly detailed. One can follow the laryngeal surface of the epiglottis anteroinferiorly to its petiolus attachment, just below the midlevel of the thyroid cartilage. In the supraglottis, the aryepiglottic folds are profiled (again as overlapping structures) along their posterior borders. The aryepiglottic folds are directed posteroinferiorly toward the arytenoid eminences, which are not seen well. This region approximates the air shadow of the posterior pharyngeal wall, which contacts the posterior surface of the larynx at rest. At the glottic level, the paired, overlapped images of the superior surface of each vocal cord is outlined, as are the air shadows of the air-containing ventricles immediately above. The attachment of the tendinous portion of each vocal cord is profiled anteriorly, right up to the petiolus, at the inner surface of the anterior limit of the paired thyroid alae. The subglottic airspace is not well profiled, although its anterior limit is clearly seen just below the inferior level of the thyroid cartilage, in the region of the cricothyroid membrane. The anterior tracheal wall is profiled down to the level of the thoracic inlet; the posterior tracheal wall is equally well defined, although it is lost superiorly behind the high-rising signet of the cricoid cartilage. The framework of the hyoid bone is detailed above. The thyroid cartilage with its paired alae is defined from superiorly to inferiorly; the inner and outer cortical surfaces of the thyroid cartilage are clear anteriorly. The calcific/ossific nature of the thyroid cartilage is noted. The thyroid cartilage narrows in the region between the lower third and the midpoint as the vocal cords attach to the inner perichondrium. The arytenoid cartilages present overlapping densities that are difficult to define; they sit on the posterior cricoid lamina, which is not fully defined either. However, the downward and forward slope of the cricoid cartilage from its posterior signet toward its anterior ring is evident. The lower surface of the cricoid cartilage is not well defined. The thyroid cartilage begins to calcify and ossify posteroinferiorly; here that relative increase in thyroid cartilage density is observed, although neither the inferior nor superior thyroid cornu are defined. The densities of the individual tracheal rings are noted. With this technique, the cervical vertebrae are not well imaged. However, they are sufficiently well defined, as are the prevertebral soft tissues, to allow normal anatomic definition. The soft tissue distance between the anterior surface of each cervical vertebra and the posterior air profile of the trachea should not exceed the height of that vertebra. Any increase in AP dimension of this soft tissue shadow is pathologic, and usually reflects swelling in relation to the hypopharynx above or the cervical esophagus below (or swelling deep to the prevertebral fascia itself). **b,**The anatomic key to a. E: epiglottis; V: valleculae; PES: preepiglottis space; aef: aryepiglottic fold; PS: pyriform sinus; Vt: ventricle; TC: true vocal cord; Cr: lamina, cricoid cartilage. **c,** Another normal soft tissue lateral radiograph, this time with the technique modified to show more bone detail.

Figure 4–2. Normal lateral xeroradiograph. Note the sharp definition of all structures, from the skin surface to the vertebrae. The air-soft tissue interface and the laryngeal cartilages are all well visualized because of the edge enhancement phenomenon.

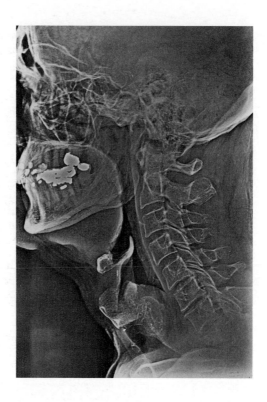

to the photoconductor plate used in place of a standard x-ray cassette so that the beam that reaches it variably discharges the surface in accordance with the tissue densities through which it has passed. Utilizing a toner powder, a blue-white image is created with marked visual differential between tissues.

The xeroradiograph can provide particularly helpful information in foreign body identification and localization and in the assessment of subglottic and intratracheal masses. It is also a good means to follow congenital laryngotracheomalacia, subglottic hemangioma, and strictures, in which lateral xeroradiography may obviate the need for endoscopic follow-up.[69]

On the other hand, the xeroradiograph has high radiation exposure on the order of four times that of conventional plain films, which must be weighed against the value of the information it may provide, particularly in the region of the thyroid gland and in the infant and child. For this reason, the xerotomogram has now been totally replaced by CT in superior mediastinal evaluation.

Coronal (AP) Tomography

In the past, coronal tomography was the pretreatment study of choice for evaluation of the patient with suspected or proved laryngeal carcinoma.[60,70–74] In reality, it provided only limited information, especially when compared with current high-technology imaging (CT, MRI), which has largely replaced it in most centers (Fig. 4–3).

High Kilovoltage Selective Filtration Radiography

This is a focal AP radiograph with definition comparable to but not quite as dramatic as conventional AP tomography. However, it can give excellent morphologic and functional definition of both ventricular bands, both ventricles, and both vocal cords, as well as the subglottic angles. The

Figure 4–3. Normal lateral tomogram of the larynx and trachea. The epiglottis is profiled, as is one-half of the entire larynx. The arytenoid eminence is visualized, as is the air shadow of the ventricle and vocal cord on the imaged side. The anterior and posterior walls of the cervical trachea are displayed from the subglottis above into the superior mediastinum below, behind the manubrium sterni.

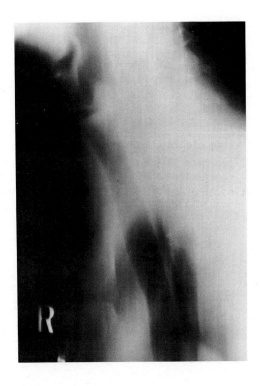

normal subglottic angle lies at approximately 110° it is altered in the presence of tumor infiltration or other mass abnormality. It is an excellent, simple screening examination and may be used in place of more extensive studies.

Contrast Laryngography

Contrast laryngography[37–39,44] is carried out in a variety of views (AP, lateral, oblique) under fluoroscopic control.[75,76] Its main value is for mucosal assessment.◁ Because of CT, laryngography has lost almost all of its usefulness; we have not used it for the past 5 years. However, a contrast laryngogram *might* be of value (Fig. 4–4), when other studies are inadequate in demonstrating the length of long strictures, presuming that the integrity and safety of the airway below the level of the lesion is under control.

Laryngography is to AP tomography what xeroradiography is to the plain lateral film; that is, it provides increased contrast between the air and soft tissues. Although it is of lesser value in assessing deep structures, it allows the radiologist to assess motion during the examination and to record this on cine film or videotape.

The Barium Swallow

The barium swallow examination is designed to study the hypopharynx and upper esophagus. It can, of course, be combined with an upper gastrointestinal examination. Fluroscopy and video control allows detailed review of such studies, and the identification of mass lesions and displacements. The major indication for the examination is in the assessment of patients who have dysphagia accompanying laryngeal symptoms.

In suspected penetrating foreign bodies, the barium examination is best avoided to prevent introduction of contrast material into exposed submucosal soft tissues. Water-soluble contrast agents (such as Gastrografin) can be utilized instead. When nonopaque foreign bodies are suspect, it is best not to obscure the lumen with barium because of future endoscopy. A small pledget of cotton soaked in barium may identify the level of obstruction and assist in treatment planning. The barium swallow examination also plays a role in assessing postsurgical strictures of the hypopharynx and cervical esophagus, particularly after total laryngectomy.

Figure 4–4. Normal
tracheogram. The patient is in
an oblique position "to bring
the trachea off the spine."
Some contrast is seen in the
esophagus immediately
posterior to the trachea. PS:
pyriform sinus.

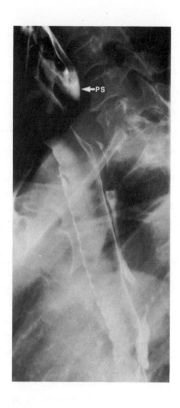

Contrast swallow studies may also permit evaluation of laryngeal aspiration in a variety of postsurgical and neurogenic disorders. It is also the
only realistic way to assess Zenker's diverticulum. Although this is not primarily a laryngeal disorder, it is impossible to consider the larynx without
considering its immediate upper aerodigestive relationships as well. Pharyngeal diverticulae (pharyngeal ears) can be identified on both plain film
or contrast study examination.

Computed Tomography

CT has become the major imaging study for laryngeal evaluation only
within the past 6 years or so.[52,64,77–85] It requires active monitoring by the
radiologist for maximal return. Its value lies in its axial display of all intrinsic and extrinsic laryngeal structures, both soft tissue and framework.
Window manipulations, with high-resolution and extended bone numbers,
allow even more precise definition of laryngeal abnormalities.

A variety of routine studies have been suggested,[59,63,79,85] recognizing
that minimal thickness studies (1.5 mm) give the most precise anatomic
display. However, useful information may be recorded (even allowing for
volume averaging losses) through 5.0 mm or 4.0 mm contiguous or overlapping studies. Further diagnostic information may be obtained both pro-
spectively and retrospectively. In the retrospective "review" situation, soft
tissue and cartilage imaging can be obtained in differing modes. This is of
particular importance in the detection of cartilage destruction by cancer invasion. On critical examinations, it is important that the data recorded on
tape be saved for later manipulation.

The CT examination is currently the most sophisticated anatomic laryngeal study available.[52] The morphologic-pathologic correlates are remarkable.[81–88] It is indicated, in our opinion, in every case of advanced
laryngeal cancer for appropriate pretreatment radiation and surgical planning. Any laryngeal malignancy that cannot be totally defined clinically or

Dr. Harry Shulman debates the concept of enhanced visualization by the mucosal stain about the tumor. He recognizes tumor identification in two ways, by its bulk and by its almost universal increase in density, for reasons ill-understood. However, subtle differences in tissue density can be definably enhanced by contrast medium and this is becoming a rather significant reproducible experience.—AMN

Most lymph nodes do not enhance with contrast. They are usually recognized by the contrast enhancement of the major arteries and veins adjacent, as well as the surrounding fat (within such areas as the parapharyngeal space, for example). However, lymph nodes often stain about their periphery, although the center area of the node is invariably less dense, presumably due to necrosis. This type of lymph node finding is not specific for malignancy, although there is no other inference when a known primary cancer exists. An active inflammatory process can produce a similar structural finding.

This type of study assumes that there is absolutely no change in patient position during the course of the examination. The transition zone is perhaps more accurately determined by the anatomic configuration of the airway at any given level and by an evaluation of the images immediately above and below.

Dr. Hanafee, as of March 1985, indicates that to that point, his experience was based on 27 imaging-clinically correlated cases. He feels that surface coils are essential to provide detail sufficient to match or exceed the information obtainable by CT. He further feels that T1 mucosal lesions do not require any form of radiologic imaging T_1-weighted imaging techniques are best for the larynx, but he notes that T_2-weighted images are exceedingly helpful in studying the related tongue. Finally, he feels strongly that thin sections in the coronal and axial plane make MRI superior to CT in the evaluation of the extent of the disease.

endoscopically should be assessed by CT in order to define its dimensions and deeper extensions.

Intravenous contrast enhancement may permit improved mucosal definition. The relatively hypodense less vascular tumor may be imaged against the normal vascularity of adjacent soft tissues.◁ Contrast enhancement also allows the identification of enlarged, nonenhancing deep cervical lymph nodes and the measurement of their size.◁ Any lymph node greater than 2.0 cm should be presumed malignant. A lymph node between 1.5 cm and 2.0 cm is suspicious.[80,89]

Vascular laryngeal lesions (hemangiomas, arteriovenous malformations) may be identified by dynamic CT study. The most accurate assessment, however, results from angiography (intravenous digital subtraction angiography for screening; arterial studies, with or without digitalization and with or without supraselective catheterization, for exact quantification and election of treatment modalities). Intra-arterial embolization may, of course, be added to the treatment armamentarium.

In any CT examination preliminary digital radiography should be carried out. Prospective slice selections can then be elected both for level and for slice thickness. These can be reviewed against the vertical overview image of the larynx and its regional subdivisions (supraglottis, glottis, subglottis, beyond). We favor scout or preview digitalized radiographs in both AP and lateral dimensions to assure two features: first, on AP examination that the transition from the ventricular band above, to ventricle, to vocal cord is precisely appreciated, millimeter by millimeter, and, second, on lateral preview film that the x-ray beam is directed exactly parallel to the superior surface of the image of the overlapped paired vocal cords. These two maneuvers assure the most valid structural and functional information.◁

Although most studies utilize intravenous iodine-containing contrast materials, other maneuvers may enhance the study as well.[90] The modified Valsalva maneuver allows better definition of both the ventricles and the pyriform sinuses; this can be done quite simply during CT examination by having the patient blow gently against a crimped straw. This increases air pressure between the lips and the closed glottis and may allow display of structures that would otherwise be collapsed and apposing (Fig. 4–5).

Magnetic Resonance Imaging

MRI has come dramatically to the fore in recent years.[53-56,91,92] Only within the past several months, however, have image capabilities come to match those of CT, but without its universal availability.◁

Magnetic resonance (previously called nuclear magnetic resonance) does not depend on x-radiation for its imaging capability. Rather, it depends on the detection of radiofrequency signals by electronic devices, as the random movement of hydrogen atoms (the atomic nucleus has physical properties of charge and spin) is realigned within tissues placed within strong magnetic fields. A magnetic field of 3000 gauss transmits electromagnetic forces in the magnitude of 6000 times that of the earth's natural magnetic field (½ gauss). This results in the polarization of approximately nine per million hydrogen atoms. With relaxation (T_1 and T_2 relaxation times), various levels of radiofrequency signals allow detection by imaging devices because the hydrogen atoms are no longer magnetically aligned. The strength of these imaging signals can be heightened by the use of surface coils, applied specifically to the laryngeal and thyroid regions. All body tissues containing hydrogen atoms give typical signal information that may have both anatomic and biologic significance. Bone is not imaged because of its

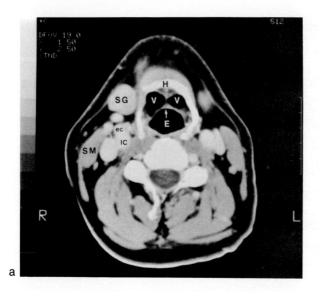

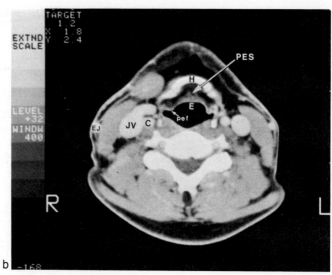

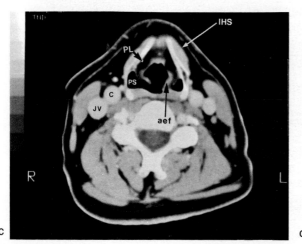

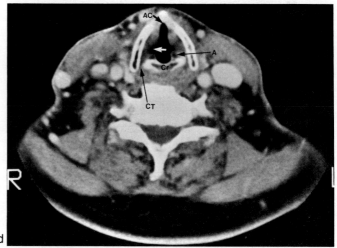

Figure 4–5. Normal CT of the larynx. All images are obtained following intravenous contrast enhancement (infusion plus bolus); all images are 5.0 mm thick. **a,** Section taken just below the upper margin of the epiglottis. E: epiglottis; ec: right external carotid artery; IC: right internal carotid artery; YH: hyoid bone; SG: right submandibular gland; SM: right sternomastoid muscle. V: each vallecula. **b,** A slice just below A. The mainly fatty preepiglottic space (PES) seen between the epiglottis (E) and the anteriorly placed hyoid bone (H). The tripartite nature of the hyoid bone is well seen in this cut. JV: right internal jugular vein, which is usually the larger of the two great veins; EJ: right external jugular vein; pef: pharyngoepiglottic fold. **c,** At the level of the thyroid notch, the infrahyoid strap muscles are well seen. The preepiglottic space extends laterally into the parapharyngeal (PL) space on each side. The fatty nature of this compartment is well seen. PS: right pyriform sinus, (the two pyriform sinuses are more distended than usual); C: right common carotid artery; JV: right internal jugular vein; aef: left aryepiglottic fold. **d,** At the transition from the supraglottis to the glottis, the airway becomes more oval shaped; in the supraglottis the airway has a more pear-shaped appearance. The true cord level is also recognized by the appearance of both the arytenoid cartilages (A: left arytenoid cartilage) and the cricoid (Cr) lamina. There should be no soft tissue in the midline at the region of the anterior commissure (AC). Note the small and symmetrical nature of the space between the posterior portion of the thyroid ala and the cricoid cartilage (CT); this is still above the level of the cricothyroid joint.

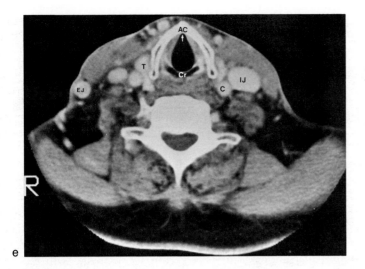

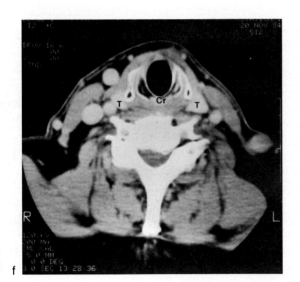

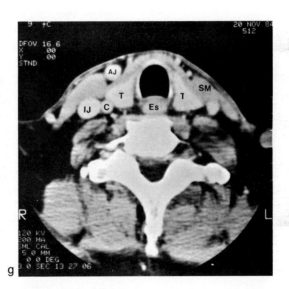

Figure 4–5. (Continued) **e,** This cut is just below the under surface of the true vocal cords (same patient as D). The thyroid cartilage is becoming more U-shaped, and the arytenoids are no longer seen. The signet shape of the cricoid cartilage (Cr) is becoming apparent, as it slopes downward and anteriorly. The anterior commissure (AC) is well visualized (small arrow). C: left common carotid artery; EJ: right external jugular vein; IJ left internal jugular vein. **f,** In the subglottis, the cricoid cartilage is almost completely encompassing the airway and no soft tissue should be evident along any of its internal margins. Cr: posterior cricoid lamina; T: right and left thyroid lobes. **g,** In the upper trachea, just below the cricoid cartilage, the shape of the airway is visualized. There is a natural absence of tracheal ring cartilage posteriorly; this allows the party wall of the esophagus (Es) to bulge forward. T: right and left thyroid lobes; SM: left sternomastoid muscle; AJ: right anterior jugular vein; C: right common carotid artery; IJ: right internal jugular vein.

Dr. Mancuso's belief (October 1985) is that MRI can be equivalent to or even replace CT in the evaluation of primary tumors of the larynx and pharynx. He believes that CT quality images are producible by MRI at all field strengths most of the time. He believes that MRI and CT may be equivalent for evaluating primary site of tumor in the larynx and pharynx. However, he points out that MRI has the potential to be better than CT when multiplanar displays are important, as in assessing laryngeal ventricle involvement or questioning subtle margins at the anterior commissure (where the sagittal view might be helpful). He also points out the potential for MRI to be more accurate in studying cartilage invasion, but he also reflects that there is no clear evidence on this issue at the present time.

calcium content, but nonossified and noncalcified cartilage is seen. However, the marrow content within the bony and cartilage medullary space can be nicely recorded.

Utilizing technologic advances derived from CT imaging, current MRI allows certain particularly favorable imaging opportunities (Fig. 4–6). Images can be derived in all three planes with MRI; the recording of sagittal and parasagittal imaging has particularly useful application to the larynx. Currently, CT allows only axial images; coronal images cannot be recorded directly, but only through the reformation of computer information gathered from axial studies. In thin section examinations, mucosal MRI imaging would seem comparable to CT; however, the soft tissue imaging of the medullary space of the cricoid and thyroid cartilages is very advantageous by MRI.

Guidelines for MRI imaging of the larynx are not well established. In fact, a reasonable approach to CT imaging of the larynx is only just starting to make inroads among clinicians caring for patients with laryngeal disorders. There is little doubt that MRI will have an impact on laryngeal cancer imaging, especially in advanced tumors, where it offers early detection of cartilage destruction due to malignant invasion.◁ Certain tissues about the larynx like the thyroid gland may well be better studied. Currently, extralaryngeal extension of squamous cell carcinoma into the thyroid gland is not readily detected by CT; MRI may improve diagnostic yield in this area.

Angiography

Angiography has made astounding developmental inroads within the past decade.[93–95] Direct arterial puncture techniques have long been supplanted by superselective catheterizations to define specific vascular distribution and compartmentalization. There are now angiographers whose expertise is virtually restricted to the study of vascular anatomy and pathology and to intra-arterial embolization (both as a diagnostic modality and as a "surgical assist").

Digital subtraction angiography by the intravenous route has allowed screening of a host of vascular lesions with a resolution above 1.0 cm. This technology can be applied to laryngeal evaluation, as well as to the assessment of perilaryngeal disorders. Digitalized arterial studies permit the use of lower doses of contrast materials and avoidance of pain from external carotid arterial evaluations, particularly through superior laryngeal artery catheterizations. There are very few lesions that warrant this type of angiographic intervention, but the technology is available to the laryngologist for evaluation of appropriate patients. The major laryngeal vascular disorders that are seen from time to time include arteriovenous malformations (primarily involving the supraglottis and the pyriform sinuses in the adult), subglottic hemangioma in the newborn and infants, and cavernous hemangiomas involving part or all of the larynx, often in young adults.

Diagnostic Ultrasound

Diagnostic ultrasound has had little application to laryngeal evaluation, although we have been primarily interested in it for the past 10 years.[96] Initially, we felt that it might enable us to understand cartilage disorders, before critical CT examinations became available. Now with high-resolution, real-time ultrasound examinations (with small parts 7.5 MHz transducers), it is possible to provide detail of the thyroid alae, uncluttered by unwanted morphologic information.[57]

Diagnostic ultrasound has helped us to recognize thyroid cartilage involvement by malignant extension. Before the CT era, 50 percent of T4 laryngeal cancer with thyroid cartilage involvement was understaged as T3 cancer. Even now, with the sophistication of CT, inadequately monitored studies still yield 30 percent underdiagnosis of T4 laryngeal cancer.[97] Utilizing diagnostic ultrasound to direct CT studies, we are nearly always able to identify those cases in which squamous cell carcinoma of the larynx has extended into the thyroid cartilage.

See Chapter 13.

If we have succeeded in this area, it is because we understand the biologic behavior of glottic and transglottic carcinoma of the larynx.[73,74,98-103] Squamous cell carcinoma tends to extend anteriorly along the involved vocal cord to the anterior commissure region, where it either crosses to the opposite side or buries itself deep to the perichondrium along the lines of insertion of the tendinous vocal cords.◁ The internal perichondrium is deficient at this level, and tumor gains easy access to the thyroid cartilage at this site. Another small group of cancers extend into the cartilage laterally at the junction of the anterior one-quarter and posterior three-quarters of the thyroid ala, at vocal cord level. Finally, some cancers involve the thyroid cartilage at the posterior margin of each thyroid ala by insinuating themselves between the arytenoid cartilage and the thyroid ala.[57] An unexpected use for high-resolution ultrasound is the assessment of vocal cord mobility, since the vocal cords lie within the focal range of the ultrasound transducer held against the larynx.

The ultrasound examination can be carried out in a matter of minutes. The patient requires no preparation, and it is entirely noninvasive. Ultrasound occasionally has other applications, such as in screening of thyroid ala fractures and determination of the need for more extensive investigations with CT. Diagnostic ultrasound also can be useful in detection of external laryngocele.

Radionuclide Scanning

A variety of radionuclide scans are available to the laryngologist for study of laryngeal disorders.[58,60] Details of scan techniques are inappropriate here, but the various radiopharmaceuticals available may provide specific information pertaining to laryngeal disorders.

The radionuclide bone scan[59] with technetium (99mTc) methylene diphosphonate may detect arthropathies, particularly in relation to the cricoarytenoid and, occasionally, the cricothyroid joints. Systemic imaging studies may determine those cases of arthropathy with a systemic basis (such as rheumatoid arthritis). The pertechnetate thyroid scan and the more specific radioiodine (123 I) scan may have roles in evaluating laryngeal disease. Noyek and colleagues[104] described thyroid tumor imaging and the limitations and potentials of radionuclide bone scan.[58]

The gallium (67Ga) citrate scan may have some value in preliminary staging for melanoma and lymphoma. Most of these studies are obtained postbiopsy, since the disease is rarely suspected before endoscopy. Gallium citrate is taken up readily by rapidly dividing cells (both tumor cells and white cells). It is useful in the identification of certain tumors, such as lymphoma, but its uptake by squamous cell carcinoma (and its metastases) is inconsistent. It is effective in assessing the biologic activity of perichondritis, particularly when underlying tumor has been ruled out, and can be important in determining whether infective perichondritis has been eradicated by treatment.

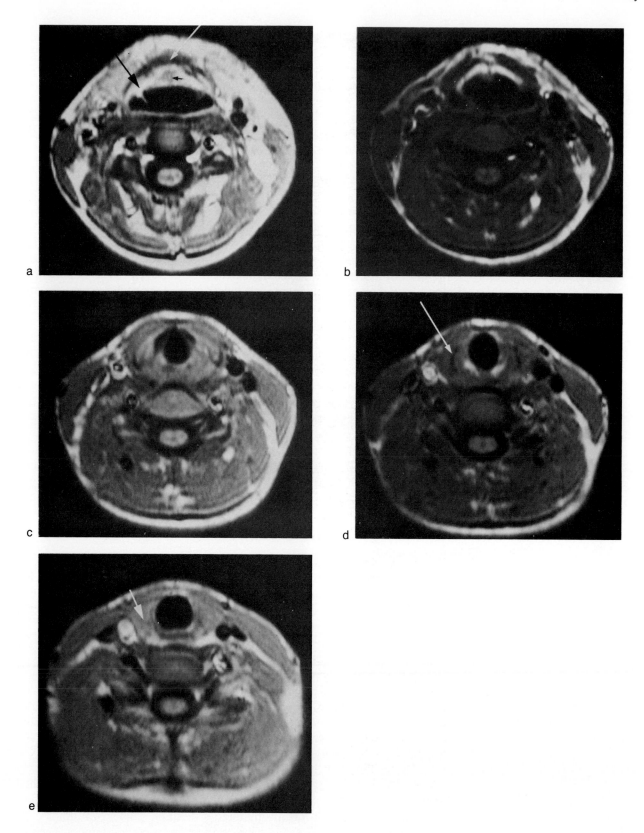

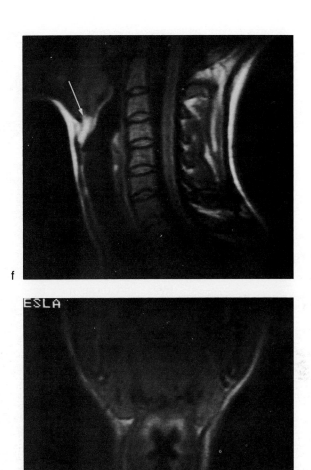

Figure 4–6. Normal magnetic resonance imaging of the larynx. **a,** A series of axial magnetic resonance images are demonstrated utilizing a 0.3 Tesla magnet and a slice thickness of between 4.0 and 7.0 mm. These are T_1 weighted images. A high supraglottic cut demonstrates an absence of signal from the calcified and ossified density of the hyoid bone (upper white arrow). There is some signal from this region due to the presence of marrow or fat. There is a bright signal from the parapharyngeal fat plane (large black arrow). The somewhat reduced signal from the preepiglottic space fat (tiny black arrow) is due to the admixture of cartilage-ligament-seromucous glands in this region. **b,** A somewhat lower MR section in the supraglottis. **c,** An MR cut at the glottic or immediate undersurface vocal cord level. **d,** An MR cut demonstrates the subglottis at the level of the cricoid arch. The cricoid cartilage fat content in its marrow is demonstrated by the presence of a bright signal circumferentially. The posterior portions of the inferior aspect of each thyroid ala are demonstrated by an absence of signal (arrow); no fat content within the thyroid cartilage is apparent on these images. **e,** The lowermost MR cut at the level of the thyroid lobes (arrow indicates right thyroid lobe). The great vessels usually have an absence of signal due to the presence of moving blood. **f,** A midline sagittal image. The epiglottis gives a bright signal, but it is less bright than the fat of the preepiglottic space (arrow). **g,** A coronal MR image. Ventricular band, ventricular and cordal anatomy is well recognized. (Courtesy of Dr. William N. Hanafee, UCLA, Los Angeles, CA).

Radiographic Signs in Laryngeal Disease

Specific radiographic findings can be identified in a variety of laryngeal disorders, ten of which will be discussed.

Congenital Laryngeal Disorders

See Chapter 7.

Congenital disorders of the larynx ◁ and the tracheobronchial tree are relatively common, especially in infants with other major congenital abnormalities. Laryngeal and laryngotracheobronchial hypoplasias and dysplasias may be limited to luminal development or affect the supporting framework structure as well. Some disorders are associated with major agenesis and dysgenesis of the lower respiratory tract and are incompatible with long-term survival.

Laryngeal clefts, however, are occasionally noted as isolated birth defects, and these may be amenable to repair. The major physiologic deficiency appears to be aspiration into the airway rather than primary airway compromise. The actual morphologic deficit should be defined before surgical intervention, utilizing whatever radiologic modalities seem appropriate. Gastrografin and barium swallow studies may demonstrate the size of a cleft, and the exact deficiencies in cartilage development may be assessed through CT. These usually require that the infant be sedated.

Subglottic stenosis may or may not be apparent at birth. *Subglottic hemangioma* and subglottic stenosis may imitate each other and should be differentiated both clinically and radiologically. Congenital laryngeal stenosis and congenital tracheobronchial stenosis[69] may occur over small isolated segments or diffusely (Figs. 4–7 and 4–8). *Tracheoesophageal fistula* is a common neonatal disorder, presenting dramatically; it is beyond the scope of our discussion, but it may be indistinguishable from primary laryngeal dysgenesis initially.

Cysts

Laryngeal cysts are uncommon. The major "cystic" laryngeal disorder is *laryngocele,* and this is discussed in its own section. The most common laryngeal cyst is the *vallecular retention cyst.* Other cystic lesions can

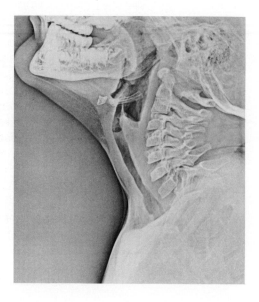

Figure 4–7. Congenital tracheal stenosis; lateral xeroradiograph. A lateral xeroradiograph demonstrates a long congenital tracheal stenosis. (Reprinted with permission from Noyek et al.[69])

Figure 4–8. Tracheal web; soft tissue lateral radiograph. A tracheal web (arrowhead) is clearly demonstrated in a 2-year-old male. (Reprinted with permission from Maguire et al.[42])

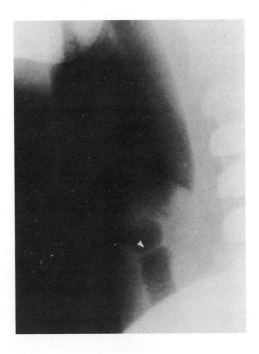

occur from time to time within the larynx. Occasional huge retention cysts arise from the laryngeal surface of the epiglottis (Fig 4–9) or from one of the ventricular bands. These present as large, smooth masses occupying the airway and are often indistinguishable from internal laryngocele or solid soft tissue submucosal masses. CT can clarify the issue and may permit endoscopic treatment rather than an external procedure.

Giant laryngeal cyst of the newborn is an important lesion because it can seriously interfere with the airway. They require immediate attention and usually cannot wait for CT scanning. These youngsters are restless, and CT images are often degraded by motion artifacts; however, once the nature of the lesion is apparent radiographically, treatment can proceed with confidence.

Laryngocele

Laryngocele is a fairly common lesion. It is air-containing and results from expansion of the appendix of the laryngeal ventricle. There are three forms: internal laryngocele (confined solely to the supraglottis of the larynx); external laryngocele (Figs. 4–10 and 4–11), in which the laryngocele herniates through the thyrohyoid membrane to present as a soft tissue compressible mass in the neck, which may or may not be autoinflatable; and mixed internal-external laryngocele.

The classic radiographic appearance of a laryngocele is an air-containing saccular lesion in the supraglottis. Conventional plain films are often inadequate unless the laryngocele is of significant size and contains both an internal and external component, in which case a ''double-bubble'' sign is seen. The internal or external component of the laryngocele was far better visualized on conventional AP tomography. Now, the best definition of laryngocele is obtained with CT scanning. The CT scan easily identifies this air-containing lesion, especially on preliminary digital scout film. The neck of the laryngocele and its point of entry into the ventricle may also be noted.

Another reason for diagnostic imaging in laryngocele is to ascertain if a soft tissue mass lesion has produced the laryngocele by ball-valve effect.

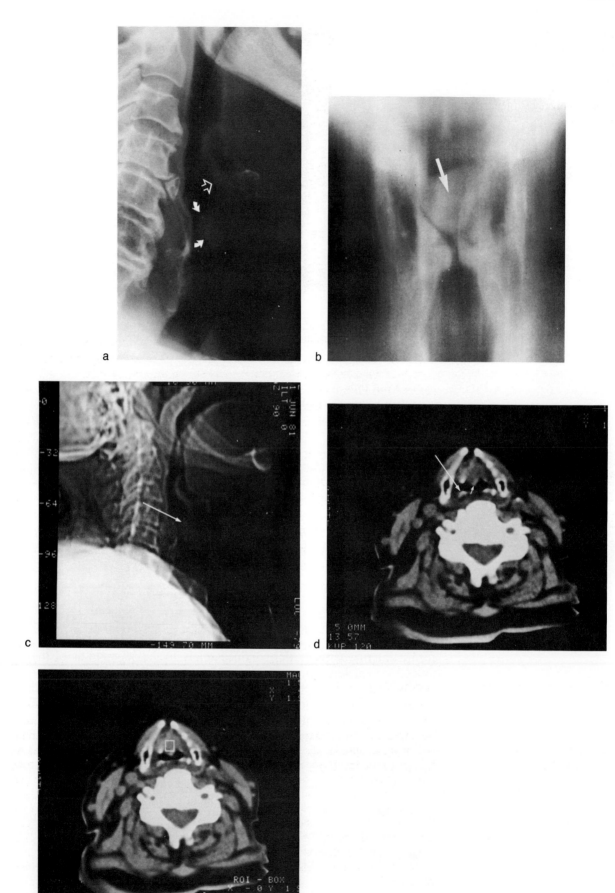

Figure 4–10. Bilateral external laryngoceles. An AP radiograph (postlaryngogram) demonstrates a minimal amount of residual contrast. A modified Valsalva maneuver demonstrates bilateral external laryngoceles (arrows), larger on the right side, in this 18-year-old youth who plays the trumpet. The arrows define the bilateral air sacs.

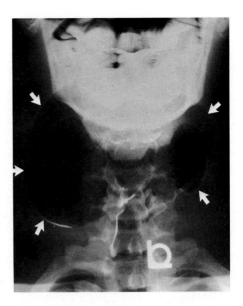

Hounsfield numbers around 0 might indicate clear fluid. Numbers between 0 and 20 suggest that the fluid may be somewhat viscid or contain inspissated matter. Above 20, a complex fluid is present, such as pus.

Squamous cell carcinoma has been identified in conjunction with laryngocele often enough to occasion this concern. External laryngocele may be identified when it is autoinflatable; however, many times it is not. The selective high kilovoltage selective filtration AP radiograph is a good screening examination for laryngocele.

Diagnostic CT imaging can be particularly helpful in fluid-filled laryngocele or pyocele. Fluid-filled laryngocele occurs infrequently, but when it does, this lesion imitates a submucosal soft tissue tumor. It may occur in the absence of previous manipulation, aspiration, or surgery, whereas laryngopyocele almost invariably follows such manipulations and may present in much more dramatic fashion as a large, tender, external neck mass (Fig. 4–12) with or without an inflammatory component within the larynx. CT scanning, especially with contrast enhancement, will demonstrate the fluid-filled nature of the lesion.◁ If there is an inflammatory component, an enhancing "rim-sign" about the infection may validate the diagnosis.

Foreign Bodies

A foreign body in the larynx usually does not require laryngeal imaging. A foreign body may obstruct the larynx in whole or in part or may pass beyond the larynx, impacting within the tracheobronchial tree, or it

◄────────────────────────

Figure 4–9. Large supraglottic cyst. **a,** A soft tissue lateral radiograph, overexposed, demonstrates a normal epiglottis with normal laryngeal surface in its upper portion (hollow arrow). A large rounded mass (curved arrows) projects posteriorly from the base of the epiglottis into the airway. The airway is severely compromised. **b,** An AP tomogram demonstrates the relationship of this large soft tissue density (arrow) to the ventricular bands, ventricles, and vocal cords. The inferior limit of this cyst descends almost to the superior surface of the vocal cords. **c,** A digital preview radiograph, before the selection of axial CT cuts, demonstrates the mass (arrow). **d,** An axial CT cut at the level of the upper portion of the arytenoid cartilages demonstrates the posterior projection of the lesion (tiny arrow) into the airway. The right arytenoid cartilage is indicated by the long arrow. **e,** A cursor measurement of the cyst demonstrates a mean density (arrow) of 45 Hounsfield units. This is compatible with thick fluid within a cyst; it is not, however, diagnostic. (Reprinted with permission from Greyson and Noyek.[60])

Figure 4–11. External laryngocele. An AP xeroradiograph of the larynx demonstrates the wide recording latitude and the phenomenon of edge enhancement on radiologic examination (in a 66-year-old male) of a right external laryngocele. The short arrow demonstrates the external laryngocele, which is herniated through the right thyrohyoid membrane; the neck of the laryngocele at its exit from the larynx is indicated by the long black arrow. h₁: hyoid bone; t: thyroid ala. (Reprinted with permission from Noyek et al.[1])

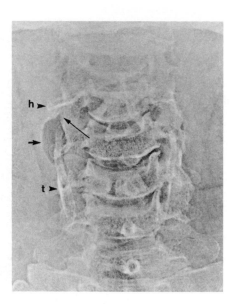

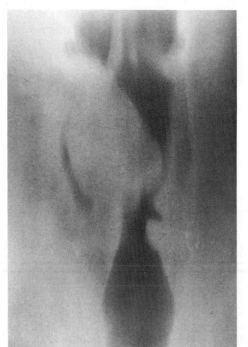

a

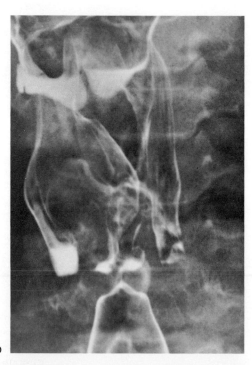

b

Figure 4–12. Laryngopyocele, aryepiglottic fold. **a,** a coronal tomographic cut (in inspiration) demonstrates a large soft tissue density completely occupying the right aryepiglottic fold. It is a laryngocele; an internal laryngocele has become obstructed and infected. The right pyriform sinus is impressed by the laryngopyocele medially; the usual inferior limit of the pyriform sinus extends to the same level as the vocal cords, as normally anticipated. The imaging study does not differentiate the soft tissue density as tumor or a fluid or purulent-filled internal laryngocele. **b,** An AP view of a laryngogram demonstrates the surface contour of the laryngopyocele occupying the right aryepiglottic fold. It otherwise confirms the same morphologic findings as depicted in A. Both these studies quantify the lesion, but do not qualify its nature.

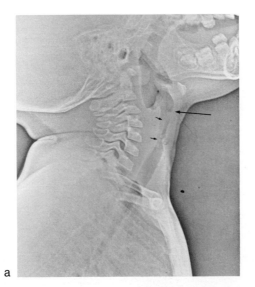
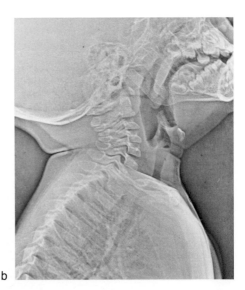

a   b

Figure 4–13. Subglottic plastic foreign body. **a,** A preendoscopy lateral xeroradiograph (in an infant) demonstrates a long, thin, plastic foreign body, longitudinally oriented in the same plane as the subglottis and trachea. The upper tiny black arrow demonstrates the upper limit of the foreign body, lying in the subglottis. Its lower level is indicated by the inferior tiny black arrow; there is tracheal edema and soft tissue inflammatory reaction at this level. The long thin black arrow indicates the level of the glottis. The overlapping ventricular air shadows can be seen. **b,** A lateral xeroradiograph following endoscopic removal of the foreign body. The subglottis and trachea have returned to normal. (Reprinted with permission for Noyek et al[63] and of the late Dr. Paul Holinger, Chicago, IL).

may remain mobile, shifting with respiration or coughing. Thin, somewhat linear, foreign bodies tend to orientate themselves in the sagittal plane within the larynx. This contrasts with similar foreign bodies, such as coins, which lie in the coronal plan when in the hypopharynx or cervical esophagus. Foreign bodies may be multiple (Figs. 4–13 and 4–15).

Opaque objects (such as coins, safety pins) are readily identified and localized by plain film examination. A chest x-ray should always be included as part of the radiographic examination and fluoroscopy might be chosen at times. Foreign bodies of long duration may create false pockets, or become surrounded by granulations. Small sharp foreign bodies can become "buried" and may be impossible to detect on films; very carefully monitored CT examinations can uncover the real abnormality.

Calcified foreign bodies create difficulties on diagnostic imaging when their shadows blend with those of the partially calcified or ossified laryngeal framework. When vertically oriented, a suspected calcified foreign body at laryngeal level may require fluoroscopy to clarify its location, perhaps in conjunction with a minimal barium examination using a barium-impregnated cotton ball. Penetrating foreign bodies produce complications, as do endoscopic manipulations themselves. Conventional plain films and advanced studies, such as CT, may be important in the evaluation of these patients.

Inflammatory Diseases

See Chapter 10.

A commonly encountered inflammatory disease ◁ involving the larynx is *acute epiglottitis* (Fig. 4–16). In children, it produces a classic clinical and radiologic picture; plain lateral x-rays show blunting and edema

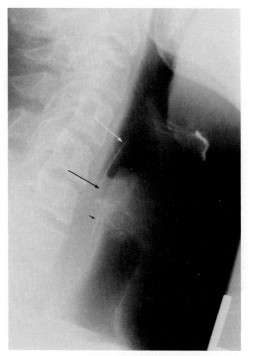 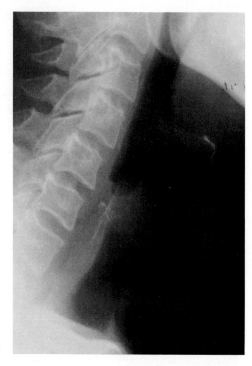

a

b

Figure 4–14. Foreign body (bayleaf) behind larynx. **a,** A conventional soft tissue lateral radiograph demonstrates a foreign body (here a bayleaf) imaged edge-on lying in retrolaryngeal position. The upper limit of the foreign body projects (white arrow) above the arytenoids into the laryngeal introitus. The lower limit of the foreign body is depicted by the long, thin, black arrow, as it lies behind the larynx. The linear density of the foreign body should be differentiated from the calcification of the posterior margin of the nearby thyroid ala. The densities lie in the same direction. **b,** Following endoscopic removal of the bayleaf in this 56-year-old male, the thyroid cartilage image is better appreciated.

Figure 4–15. Metallic foreign body, pyriform sinus. A soft tissue lateral radiograph demonstrates the relationship of a transversely lying foreign body (arrow) to the calcification in the posterior inferior portions of the overlapping thyroid alae in this 37-year-old female who has ingested a small piece of metal in a salad. The foreign body lies in the pyriform sinus; its lateralization is not apparent from a single lateral x-ray.

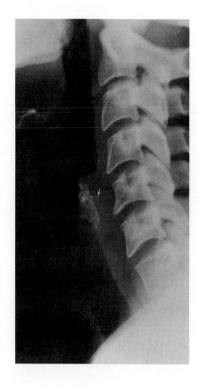

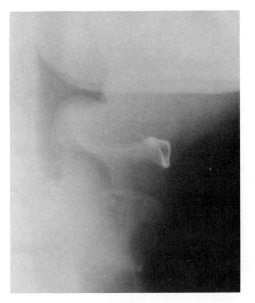
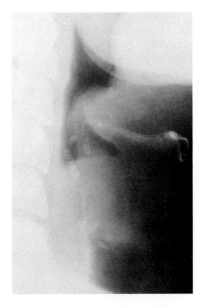

a   b

Figure 4–16. Acute epiglottitis, adult; lateral soft tissue radiograph. **a,** There is edema with blunting of the normal mucosal features. The aryepiglottic folds are swollen as well. the patient is a 72-year-old male. **b,** A less exposed lateral radiograph enhances the appearance of mucosal edema about the epiglottis.

of the epiglottis, primarily of its free margins and laryngeal surface. The valleculae may be elevated at their mucosal surfaces, creating a gentle curve with the outline of the base of tongue rather than the usual sharp angulation. The soft tissue lateral radiograph is not of great importance in the diagnosis of acute epiglottitis; it may be useful, however, in following the resolution of such swelling. Endoscopic and telescopic examinations usually suffice, particularly when the child has been intubated.

Acute epiglottitis is also seen from time to time in the adult, in whom it can be a treacherous disease. The indications for imaging are similar— for pretreatment airway assessment and post-treatment soft tissue response. Allergic *supraglottic edema (angioedema)* (Fig. 4–17) produces epiglottic

Figure 4–17. Acute laryngotracheitis, with laryngeal edema. A soft tissue lateral radiograph demonstrates marked laryngeal edema, involving mainly the posterior wall (black arrows) with severe airway narrowing. The anterior limit of the airway is indicated by the white arrows.

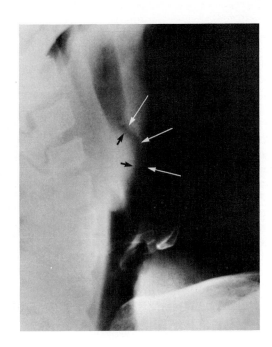

Figure 4–18. Hematoma of
false cord with displacement of
arytenoid cartilage. The left
false cord is widened due to
hematoma (curved arrow) in a
patient who received blunt
trauma to the larynx. The left
arytenoid cartilage has been
displaced medially (small
arrow). (Reprinted with
permission from Shulman et
al.[79])

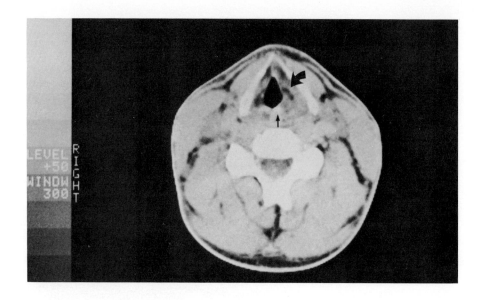

edema as well as swelling of both aryepiglottic folds and arytenoids. No-
dularity and ulceration may be recognized in the supraglottis on radiographic examination. Chronic *fungal infections,* such as blastomycosis,
imitate laryngeal malignancy with gross distortion and infiltration of the
intralaryngeal structures. Diagnostic imaging allows assessment of mucosal involvement and airway compromise. It also permits evaluation of
treatment effectiveness. *Leprosy* produces midline ulceration of the epiglottis, which may be visible on radiographs.

Trauma

The larynx can be the target of a variety of soft tissue (Fig. 4–18) and
framework injuries (Fig. 4–19) through several mechanisms operating acutely
in the short-term and progressively in the long-term. A range of such traumatic lesions is listed in Table 4–1.◁

See Chapter 8.

The larynx is a superficially placed, relatively unprotected organ. It
is, therefore, subject to a variety of injuries from without. It also may be
injured from within. Knowledge of the mechanism of injury permits critical anticipation of possible structural and functional deficits, which in turn
can direct assessment and treatment.

Figure 4–19. Fracture, thyroid
ala. A supraglottic CT cut
demonstrates a fracture (curved
arrow) at the junction of the
anterior three-fourths and
posterior one-fourth of the left
thyroid ala. There is air in soft
tissues of the neck, and an
intralaryngeal supraglottic soft
tissue density (straight arrow),
undoubtedly representing
hemorrhage. (Reprinted with
permission from Shulman et
al.[79]

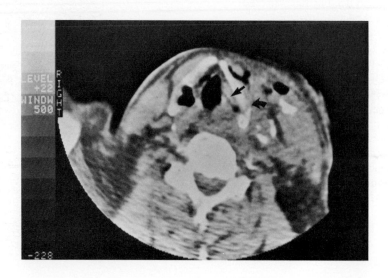

Table 4–1   Trauma to the Larynx

 1. Blunt and penetrating trauma
 2. Prolonged intubation with contact granulomas (see chapter on benign tumors)
 3. Mucosal contusion and hematoma
 4. Cartilage displacements (arytenoid)
 5. Thyroid cartilage fracture (longitudinal)
 6. Cricoid signet disruption (posteriorly with anterior striking injury against cervical spine)
 7. Posterior commissure stenosis and web
 8. Ankylosis of the cricoarytenoid joints
 9. Nonfixation of the cricoarytenoid joints with stenosis of the posterior commissure
10. Thermal burns and chemical inhalations
11. Long-term complications of stricture and stenosis

Regardless of the mechanism, all injured larynges and their immediate anatomic relationships should be examined carefully from the clinical, endoscopic, and radiologic perspective before treatment is begun (presuming no immediate airway compromise or risk to a possibly unstable cervical spine). Conventional plain films provide only limited information; the presence of free air in the soft tissues suggests a fracture (Fig. 4–20), but these films have little localizing value except in discrete penetrating or slash injuries (Fig. 4–21). All laryngeal trauma with an immediate risk to the airway or long-term risk to the airway-voice-swallowing mechanism should be evaluated carefully by CT examination in both soft tissue and cartilaginous modes.[51,52,105] Laryngeal injuries may result in soft tissue involvement and tearing of the mucous membrane and submucosal hematoma.[106] These usually have no long-term significance. However, major soft tissue avulsions may require careful surgical repair after radiologic analysis (Fig. 4–22). This diagnostic imaging may be the only effective means of judging such disruptions in the severely traumatized larynx.

There may be cartilage fractures, avulsions, dislocations, and membranous separations. All of these may be analyzed effectively by CT.[52]

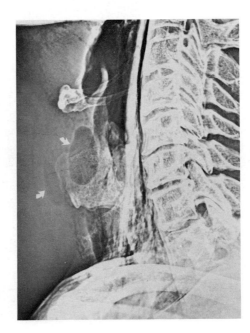

Figure 4–20. Laryngeal fracture with cervical emphysema; lateral xeroradiograph. There is extensive streaking due to cervical emphysema and air in the peritracheal space. Two loculi of pocketed air (arrows) are seen external to the laryngeal skeleton, overlying the thyroid cartilage; the laryngeal fracture that produced these findings is is not visualized by this technique. CT is mandatory for appropriate pretreatment evaluation. (Reprinted with permission from Mancuso and Hanafee.[48])

Figure 4–21. Transection base of epiglottis; soft tissue lateral radiograph. A gaping wound is seen in lateral profile in a 62-year-old male who has attempted suicide with an electric kitchen knife; the knife has entered the larynx through the thyrohyoid membrane just above the superior border of the thyroid cartilage, transecting the epiglottis (arrow). All other vital structures were spared. The patient survived this suicide attempt with surgery and psychiatric treatment.

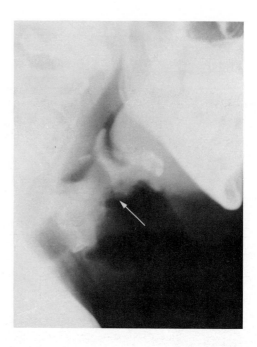

Thyroid cartilage fractures usually involve the thinnest portion of one or both alae, in a longitudinal direction. The fracture usually involves the junction of the anterior one-quarter with the posterior three-quarters of the ala; fracture lines may also run obliquely, isolating either superior or inferior thyroid cornua. The cricoid cartilage is particularly prone to posterior vertical fracture through the signet in compressive or crush injuries. Here, the only complete laryngeal cartilage is splayed and fractured posteriorly by compression against the cervical spine. The arytenoid cartilages are particularly subject to dislocation and may be displaced laterally or medially. The epiglottis, with its elastic consistency, is often transected or avulsed; the axial CT examination allows ready assessment of this type of injury. The larynx can be imaged effectively even when an endotracheal tube has been positioned for airway control or when a tracheostomy has been carried out using nonmetallic tubes. Metal tubes create streaking artifacts.

Direct *recurrent laryngeal nerve damage* may be inferred from radio-

Figure 4–22. Avulsion of epiglottis. A CT scan demonstrates the findings in blunt trauma to the larynx, in which there is massive subcutaneous emphysema and extensive supraglottic hematoma that has severely compromised the airway and necessitated the placement of an endotracheal tube (T). In this section, just above glottic level, the density (arrow) anterior to the endotracheal tube represents inferior displacement of the avulsed epiglottis. There is also a fracture of the thyroid ala anteriorly, just to the left of the midline. (Reprinted with permission from Shulman et al.[79])

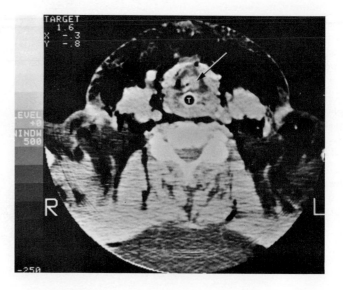

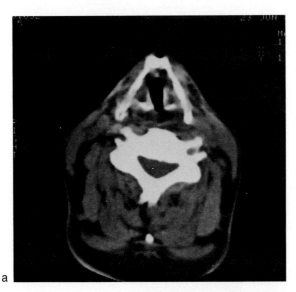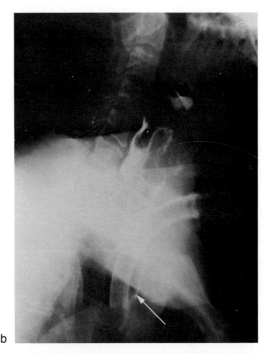

a   b

Figure 4–23. Postradiation laryngeal fibrosis, with glottis fixed in abduction. **a,** A CT scan demonstrates the keyhole shape of the glottis as both arytenoids are fixed in a laterally rotated position. The airway is widely patent. The laryngeal framework is densely ossified or calcified, due to heavy irradiation to the larynx for squamous cell carcinoma some 20 years previously. This 61-year-old male now has recurrent aspiration. **b,** A tracheostomy tube is in position in this oblique contrast study. Contrast has spilled into the larynx and profiles the anterior wall of the trachea (arrow). (Reprinted with permission from Noyek et al.[112]

See Chapter 11.

logic studies, but vocal cord paralysis is best diagnosed by direct observation.◁ CT may have greater value, however, in assessment of delayed neurogenic deficits. Detection of late ankylosis and fixation is a more difficult problem (Fig. 4–23). High-resolution, real-time ultrasound may demonstrate subtle vocal cord movement and allow differentiation from fixation.

The long-term complications of a variety of laryngeal injuries are often segmental or diffuse strictures and stenoses (Fig. 4–24). These are best identified by overview AP tomographic, xeroradiographic, or high-kilovoltage selective filtration studies. Occasionally, laryngography is useful here, if the airway is secure and there is no danger of obstruction (Fig. 4–25).

Benign Tumors

See Chapter 12.

Most of the common benign mass lesions of the vocal cord◁ do not require diagnostic imaging.[59,62,63,79,107–110] However, *contact granulomas* and other large lesions may occasionally warrant such evaluation (Fig. 4–26), if the undersurface of the lesion cannot be visualized and there is fear of airway encroachment during endoscopic manipulations. A good soft tissue lateral radiograph of the larynx can serve to outline the extent and dimensions of these masses.

Viral *papillomas* (Fig. 4–27) in childhood, adolescence, or the adult may require diagnostic imaging to understand their full superior and inferior extent, particularly if they occupy the anterior commissure region. Such imaging might be useful for planning endoscopy. Since these lesions can

Figure 4–24. Total laryngeal
stenosis. A lateral
xeroradiograph demonstrates
total laryngeal stenosis, the
result of infection after a
tracheostomy that involved the
cricoid cartilage. The patient is
a 6-year-old female and a
tracheostomy tube is in situ.
The two arrowheads indicate the
mucosal termination of the
airway through the larynx; the
intervening area is completely
stenotic. (Reprinted with
permission from Zizmor and
Noyek.[119])

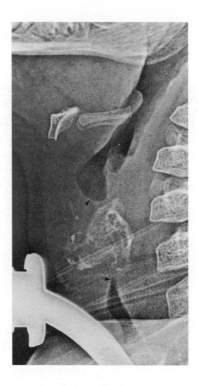

extend into the tracheobronchial tree, the clinician may utilize radiographic
methods to determine these abnormalities, although the flexible telescope
is usually superior to x-ray in this situation.

Larger or submucosal laryngeal tumors should be evaluated by pretreatment CT scan. A thin section axial examination allows full understanding of the configuration of the lesion. The combination of histologic
examination and radiographic quantification may permit realistic approaches either by endoscopy or laryngofissure. It is not the role of radio-

Figure 4–25. Tracheal stenosis.
An oblique view of a
laryngotracheogram
demonstrates a discrete area of
stricture formation at the level
of the thoracic inlet. This has
resulted from the prolonged
contact trauma of the distal end
of a tracheostomy tube against a
denuded surface.

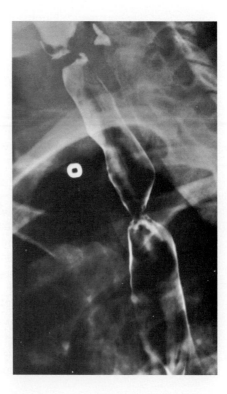

Figure 4–26. Postintubation arytenoid granuloma. Lateral xeroradiograph demonstrates a small pedunculated soft tissue mass whose lower limit is indicated by the tip of the arrow. It actually rises from the vocal process of the arytenoid cartilage, and prolapses for a small distance into the subglottis. Mucosal definition is excellent. Note the outline of the air-filled ventricle and its relationship to the typically posteriorly placed postintubation granuloma. This is a 62-year-old male who has been intubated on three occasions over a period of 2 weeks after a cardiac arrest. (Reprinted with permission from Noyek et al.[47])

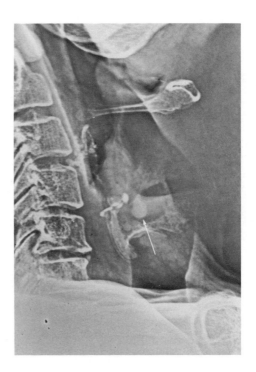

logic imaging to anticipate the pathologist's diagnosis; rather, it is to augment the total clinical picture and help direct appropriate patient management.

Among benign tumors arising from the laryngeal framework, *chondroma* (Fig. 4–28) or *osteochondroma* is the most common. This benign cartilaginous tumor has the biologic capability of ossifying and calcifying.[111] This results in frequent coarse calcifications, readily identifiable on conventional and CT radiographs. The tumor often preserves intact the overlying mucous membrane as it arises. Its most common origin is the inner cortex of the posterior plate of the cricoid signet. As it expands, it encroaches on the subglottic and glottic airway, often producing airway obstruction. It also expands posteriorly or posterolaterally, interfering with the passage of food via the hypopharynx into the esophagus. Axial radiographic studies are important in understanding the extent of the airway compromise and suggesting a preoperative diagnosis. However, chondroma and osteochondroma may coexist with or develop into osteochondrosarcoma. Although the incidence of malignancy in this type of lesion is

Figure 4–27. Multiple papillomatosis. A lateral xeroradiograph profiles multiple collections of viral papillomas at the supraglottic and glottic levels.

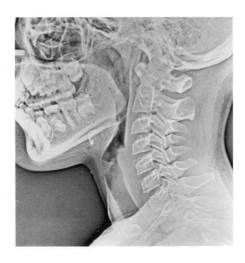

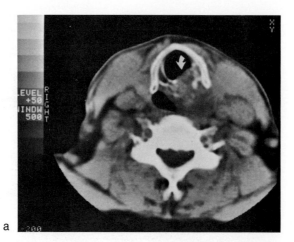 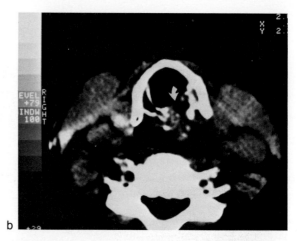

Figure 4–28. Chondroma, cricoid cartilage. **a,** CT scan demonstrates a soft tissue mass arising from the cricoid cartilage, just to the left of the midline. It has a typical origin within the lamina itself. It extends posteriorly and laterally compressing the hypopharynx. There is a minimal anterior encroachment on the airway (curved arrow). **b,** At a lower window setting, extensive calcification can be seen within the mass, indicative of its cartilaginous nature. The curved arrow indicates the same location as in A. (Reprinted with permission from Shulman et al.[79])

We have been impressed that schwannomas have an imaged density less than normal soft tissues, presumably due to the fatty content of such tumors.

fairly high, the biologic behavior of both the benign and malignant tumor is quite similar; only the pathologist can differentiate the two under the microscope, and even then often only with difficulty. Because these tumors can involve the larynx extensively, critical radiographs are important, especially when surgery is being considered.

Neurogenic tumors may also affect the larynx. Schwannoma, for example, may be suspected by its neurogenic density on CT reading.◁ All of these tumors should be quantified as part of the pretreatment investigation utilizing CT or MRI or both. However, the diagnosis is confirmed only by biopsy.

Vascular tumors of the larynx also occur. *Cavernous hemangioma* seems to have a predilection for the aryepiglottic folds and posterior cricoid region; it is a relatively rare lesion (Fig. 4–29). Sometimes these cavernous hemangiomas develop phleboliths with secondary calcification that are visible on x-ray. Laser endoscopy can be quite useful here and should be based on clinical awareness and appropriate diagnostic imaging. Dynamic CT studies may suggest the presence of vascular lesions, which is valuable since they should not be simply biopsied. Digital subtraction angiography may be a useful screening examination to augment CT (and perhaps MRI) studies. We have not utilized supraselective angiography and embolization with these lesions, as it has not proved necessary. *Arteriovenous malformations* may also occur in the larynx with rapid shunting of blood to the venous circulation. Digital subtraction angiography, again by the intravenous route, is a good screening evaluator for these lesions.

Malignant Tumors

See Chapter 13.

Radiologic evaluation of malignant tumors of the larynx◁ is the most important single role for diagnostic imaging.[52,64,112] Among these tumors, squamous cell carcinoma comprises the most common offender (95 percent of cases). Diagnostic imaging provides a baseline examination of any suspected or known malignant tumor of the larynx, in order to allow its more

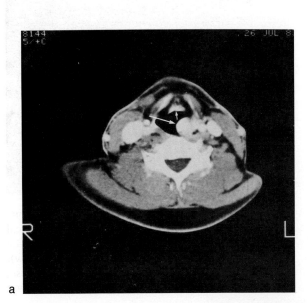

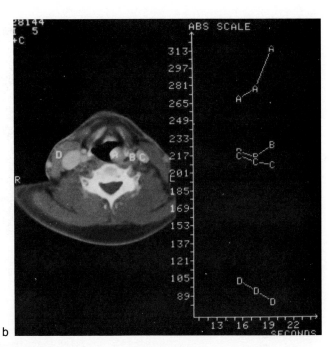

a

b

Figure 4–29. Cavernous hemangioma, aryepiglottic fold. **a,** An axial CT cut demonstrates a contrast-enhancing discrete density, occupying the left aryepiglottic fold and projecting into the airway medially (long arrow). Its relationship to the posterior surface of the epiglottis (small arrow) is well seen. The mass is a cavernous hemangioma and has an apparent vascularity comparable to the great vessels in the neck. The patient is a 53-year-old male. **b,** A dynamic CT scan demonstrates the vascular enhancement in four structures. Note that the sternomastoid muscle is relatively avascular, as anticipated from the scan appearance. The common carotid and internal jugular vein have an almost equal vascularity on this absolute scale. The cavernous hemangioma, however, takes up the contrast enhancement and retains it; this is compatible with the pathophysiology of the cavernous hemangioma. A: cavernous hemangioma; B: common carotid artery; C: internal jugular vein; D: right sternomastoid muscle.

accurate quantification and hence T staging.[49] Any tumor that cannot be fully and clearly T staged by evaluation of its mucosal involvement alone, or by clinical and endoscopic methods, merits radiologic examination. This should be a high-technology, critically directed study, such as CT, MRI, or both.

Axial CT utilizing contiguous or overlapping cuts is the procedure of choice for the larynx.[49,59,113] This evaluation can be augmented by thin section examinations and prospective or retrospective assessment of mucosa or framework. Diagnostic imaging also plays a role in improved N staging[89] of nodal disease of the neck, especially in the difficult-to-examine, heavy-set neck, when palpation of minimally enlarged cervical lymph nodes is difficult. M staging of laryngeal cancers, particularly when systemic metastases are suspect, depends on standard chest radiographs and selective use of other modalities (total body bone scan, liver or spleen scan). Radiographic studies also can play a role in the assessment of coexistent upper aerodigestive malignancies. Finally, diagnostic imagery is important in the follow-up of patients with laryngeal malignancy, particularly for those patients who have been treated primarily with radiation therapy with surgery held in reserve.

Squamous cell carcinoma is the major laryngeal cancer. It comprises the great bulk of our diagnostic concern. All cases of squamous cell car-

Figure 4–30. Supraglottic
carcinoma, involving laryngeal
surface of epiglottis; soft tissue
lateral radiograph. A rather
discrete, somewhat lobulated
mass deforms the laryngeal
surface of the upper half of the
epiglottis. The undersurface of
the mass is indicated by the two
arrows. The radiographic study
gives no indication as to
possible preepiglottic space
involvement, or extension
beyond.

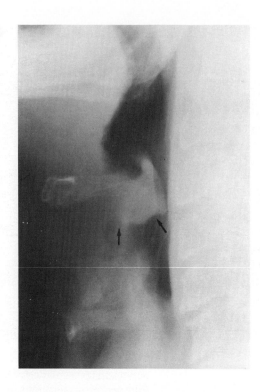

cinoma in which the full extent of the lesion cannot be visualized endoscopically should undergo radiographic quantification. This includes all advanced cancers (T3 and T4), as well as those T2 tumors that do not lend
themselves to clinical, endoscopic and photographic methods alone; in this
instance our major concern lies with soft tissue infiltration. Modern-day
imaging techniques allow superb correlations between pathologic changes
and imaging at both the soft tissue and framework levels. In our experiences, the diagnostic images are rarely wrong; only the interpretations
sometimes go awry.

The soft tissue lateral radiograph provides a baseline examination that
may or may not be relevant (Figs. 4–30 and 4–31). Certainly, bulky supraglottic lesions are nicely visualized in soft tissue lateral profile by conventional radiography or xeroradiography, which may determine the anatomic level of concern for advanced study by CT. Good technique will give
improved visualization over the routine scout or preview radiographs obtained before the CT examination. These conventional films may answer
basic questions about laryngeal involvement. The epiglottis is most amenable to soft tissue lateral imaging. A bulky or deformed epiglottis indicates tumor infiltration. It is difficult to fully determine base of tongue involvement from this view, since only mucosal alterations are seen.

Invasion into the preepiglottic space and base of tongue can be determined by CT, where tissue planes are clearly defined by normal low-density fat. The preepiglottic space and its continuity to the lateral paralaryngeal spaces, which lie on the inner surface of both thyroid cartilages down
to but not beyond the levels of the vocal cords, are imaged well by CT.
These are the natural conduits by which transglottic carcinomas spread and
eventuate.

Soft tissue exophytic masses are well seen, but it is sometimes difficult to differentiate their infiltrative margins. It may be possible to demonstrate secondary mobility defects, due either to vocal cord fixation or to
general loss of distensibility of underlying tissues. Ulcerative lesions are
much more graphic, but again the deep extent of tumor is often not readily

Figure 4–31. Large glottic carcinoma with subglottic extension and airway obstruction. A soft tissue lateral radiograph defines a large ovoid, somewhat lobulated mass projecting into the subglottis (arrow) from the glottic level. Soft tissue definition at the glottic level is usually not so well defined, because of overlying cartilage images. Here the cartilage has largely been demineralized and destroyed. A tracheostomy tube is in place and there is soft tissue granulation above the tracheostomy tube, encroaching on the airway.

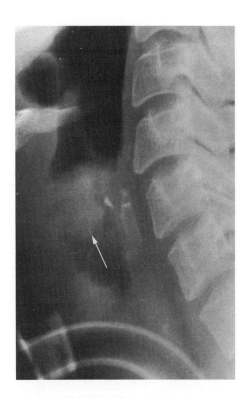

There is a pitfall here: if the images are recorded with the cords in partial or full adduction, an appearance of anterior commissure tumor can be obtained.

recognized unless pathologic-normal tissue density differences are observed. Another key feature is the recognition of those soft tissue tumors that also involve the laryngeal framework. Whereas surgery is often mandatory if cartilage is involved, radiation therapy has the potential of curing even the most extensive soft tissue infiltrations, as long as the underlying cartilage is intact. It is only since entry into the CT era that we can appreciate how often carcinoma of the larynx has been understaged in the past. Conventional AP tomograms give very limited information indeed, except to define the mucosal surfaces of the aryepiglottic folds, ventricular bands, ventricles, vocal cords, and subglottic angles.

In T4 laryngeal cancer, those tumors that extend into and through the thyroid cartilage or that penetrate the cricothyroid membrane also have a predilection to extend directly into the thyroid gland. It is possible to demonstrate such involvement by axial CT examinations, especially utilizing thin section studies, once the site of egress of the squamous cell carcinoma of the larynx has been discovered.

Axial CT can define several major specifics (Figs. 4–32, 4–33, and 4–34). If the fat density of the preepiglottic space is lost and replaced by areas of increased density, it is presumed that tumor has infiltrated the lymph nodes or directly extended into this area. Soft tissue thickening in the region of the anterior commissure on CT is diagnostic of tumor.◁ Detailing of the subglottic region is also possible and the amount of airway compromise can be understood. If the axial sectional examination is matched with an adequate AP or lateral preview study and with clear slice indication, mapping of laryngeal involvement is improved. CT also allows clear definition of the egress of squamous cell carcinoma at the glottic level between the often medially displaced arytenoid cartilage and the thyroid cartilage laterally; here tumor exits the larynx posterolaterally into the pyriform sinus, often amputating a segment of the cricoid cartilage or involving the cricoarytenoid joint as it passes beyond.

An extensive review of the imaging potentials and limitations in de-

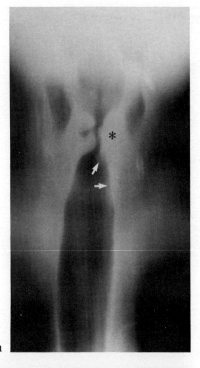

a

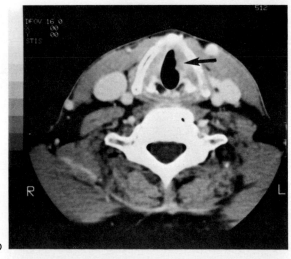

b

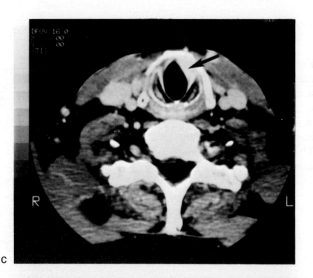

c

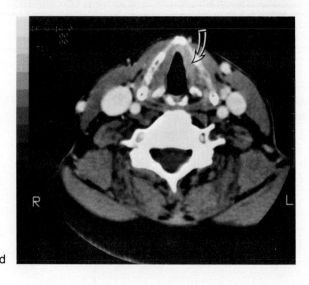

d

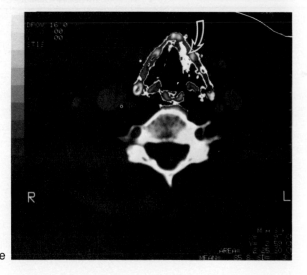

e

Figure 4–33. Transglottic carcinoma. A CT section at true cord level in a patient with a left transglottic carcinoma demonstrates the spread of tumor into the paralaryngeal space (long arrow). The arytenoid is rotated and displaced medially. The tumor also involves the anterior commissure (white arrow) and the inter-arytenoid space posteriorly (arrowhead). Note the deformation and narrowing of the airway in this 59-year-old male. (Reprinted with permission from Shulman et al.[79])

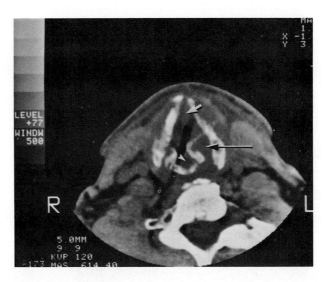

termining cartilage destruction has recently been published by Noyek and co-workers,[57] who found that approximately 50 percent of T4 squamous cell carcinoma with laryngeal framework involvement have been understaged (as T3 carcinoma). Even with "routine" CT examinations, as much as 30 percent of thyroid cartilage invasion remains undetected. These percentages improve as studies are more finely honed.

Figure 4–34. Supraglottic carcinoma, with extension across the midline. A CT slice demonstrates a mass in the supraglottis that exhibits irregular hyperemic streaking. The tumor crosses the midline anteriorly (arrow).

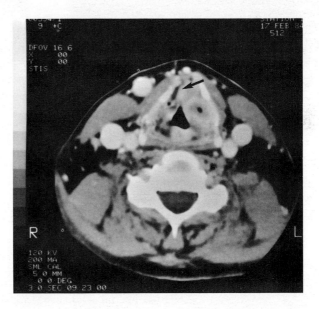

Figure 4–32. Transglottic carcinoma. **a,** A coronal tomogram demonstrates obliteration of the normal glottic contours (asterisk) in the left hemilarynx. There is loss of the subglottic angle (arrow) due to inferior extension of tumor. **b,** A contrast-enhanced CT cut at the level of the vocal cords demonstrates thickening of the left true cord (arrow) with irregularity of its margin. There is soft tissue thickening in the region of the anterior commissure, although no major extension across the midline. **c,** The soft tissue at this level (arrow) is due to subglottic extension. **d,** Cordal level is studied further; the increase in thickening on the left side of the larynx is subtle (open arrow). **e,** Computer enhancement of the difference in density along the anterior half of the left true vocal cord presumably relates to increased vascularity (arrow), a common associated finding in squamous cell carcinoma.

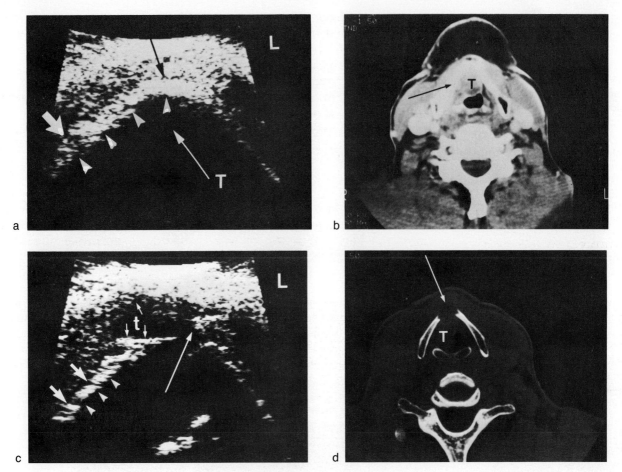

Figure 4–35. T_4 glottic carcinoma with anterior commissure to cartilage extension: the role of high resolution ultrasound in directing the CT examination. **a,** A transverse high resolution 7.5 MHz ultrasound, in supraglottic display, demonstrates intact thyroid cartilage. The right thyroid ala is indicated on its external surface by the heavy white arrow. The three left arrowheads demonstrate the intact internal surface of the right thyroid ala at this level. The anteriorly directed white arrowhead demonstrates the internal surface of the thyroid cartilage just above the intact external surface at the same level. There is not optimal imaging for the left thyroid ala on this photograph; it was well seen on other transducer manipulations. T: the occasional echoes from the tumor mass within the larynx above the vocal cords; L: patient's left. **b,** A routine 5.0 mm CT cut, in axial display, demonstrates the same anatomy as depicted in A from the CT perspective. The intact right thyroid ala is indicated by the black arrow. T: tumor within the larynx. **c,** A 7.5 MHz real-time high-resolution transverse ultrasound image depicts the right thyroid ala and the tumor relationships in the region of the anterior commissure, as tumor extends beyond the larynx into the midline anterior neck soft tissues. The bright ectogonic right thyroid ala is demonstrated on its external surface by the two heavy white arrows, and on its internal surface by the series of three arrowheads. The extension of the laryngeal carcinoma just to the right of the midline is represented by T; its limit of anterior encroachment is shown by the tiny oblique white arrow. The sharp amputation of the right thyroid ala, near the midline, is demonstrated by the paired tiny white arrows. Tumor extends just to the left of the midline, encroaching on the left thyroid ala near its anterior termination (long thin white arrow). **d,** The ultrasound image shown in C generated a retrospective CT examination of the larynx. This resulted in the optimal depiction of cartilage destruction, as shown here. The tumor within the larynx is indicated by T. This CT cut excellently depicts the destruction of both right and left thyroid cartilages anteriorly, at glottic level, matching C. The soft tissue extension is indicated by the long white arrow and the squamous cell carcinoma is shown as a low-density mass exiting the larynx anteriorly. (Reprinted with permission from Rothberg et al.[57])

High resolution *diagnostic ultrasound* (with modern small part 7.5 MHz transducers) can demonstrate fine foci of cartilage involvement. These studies have allowed us to direct CT examinations to suspicious areas (Fig. 4–35). Less costly and minimally time-consuming ultrasound examinations can direct CT studies in patients who might have unsuspected T4 cancer, with virtually 100 percent identification of laryngeal thyroid cartilage involvement. The CT examination (as well as MRI), also allows very clear detection of cricoid cartilage involvement (Fig. 4–36). MRI demonstrates the marrow of these structures as well as other soft tissues to great effect,[114] but it does not show calcified structures themselves. Despite this, the return in definition of cartilage destruction is equal to and may perhaps be even better than that of CT. Knowing the predilection for extension of anterior commissure tumor into and through the thyroid cartilage at the point of insertion of the tendinous vocal cords makes vocal radiographic assessment far more definitive. This area is well-visualized on high-resolution ultrasound◁ and high-resolution CT examinations (Fig. 4–37).

The strength of diagnostic ultrasound lies in its ability to define the integrity or destruction of cartilage independent of its calcium content. However, there is a real limitation; it can define the external cortex when it is invaded by cancer, but cannot clearly define the inner cortex when it alone is involved.

Figure 4–36. Carcinoma of the pyriform sinus with transglottic, cricoid cartilage, and exolaryngeal extension. **a,** A t₁ weighted image at the level of the glottis demonstrates a soft tissue mass (long white arrow) encroaching on the airway (small horizontal arrow). There has been signal alteration from the adjacent right half of the cricoid lamina (small vertical arrow) due to tumor invasion. The tumor also involves the anterior portion of the right thyroid ala (the fat plane is disrupted). **b,** A T₂ weighted image for comparison with A. The images are 6.0 mm thick. Arrow: residual air space; IJ: right internal jugular vein; C; left common carotid artery; SM: left sternomastoid muscle. **c,** Subglottic extension is demonstrated by the two arrows. Cricoid cartilage (Cr) is destroyed by tumor, which is also extended along the posterior pharyngeal wall (Courtesy of Dr. Anthony A. Mancuso, University of Florida College of Medicine, Gainesville, FL.)

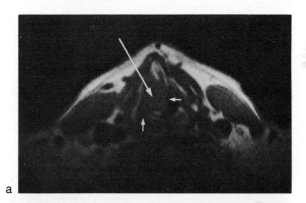

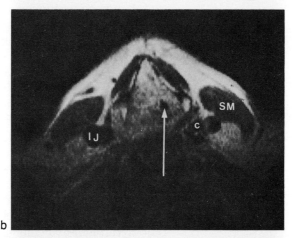

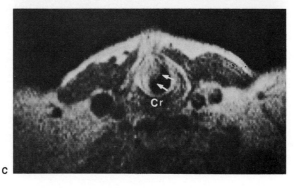

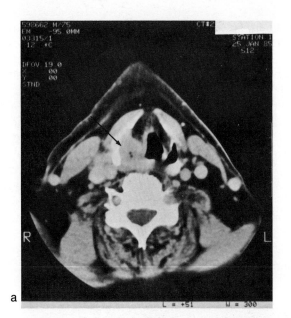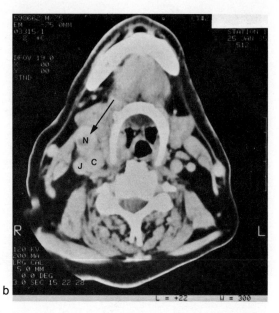

Figure 4–37. Supraglottic carcinoma with lymph node involvement. **a,** On CT, a right-sided mass involves the aryepiglottic fold and obscures the pyriform sinus; it has replaced the paralaryngeal fat (arrow). **b,** At a higher level (2 cm cephalad), there is evidence of metastatic lymph node involvement in the deep cervical chain (arrow). C: common carotid artery; J: internal jugular vein; N: lymph node with central low-density area indicating necrosis.

Diagnostic imaging also can play an important role in N staging and in the follow-up evaluation of patients with treated carcinoma of the larynx, especially when radiation therapy has been used alone.[115] Baseline studies may be performed at the conclusion of radiation therapy treatments (approximately 3 months after initiation of radiation therapy or 6 weeks after its conclusion). This allows an assessment of response, although only histologic examination can confirm the viability or nonviability of tumor. Signs of recurrence of tumor or overt failure of radiation are an increasing soft tissue mass, increasing ulceration, the onset of or increase in laryngeal fixation, or the development of vocal cord paralysis, all of which findings are at the soft tissue level. Recognition of framework involvement not seen previously is virtually diagnostic. The presence of any of these signs of tumor warrant prompt biopsy in order to initiate salvage surgery. Radiologic evaluation may, in fact, be the only way to find early recurrences. Thus directed, deep biopsies may identify persistent malignancy.

Verrucous carcinoma is an uncommon variant form of epithelial cancer, which is relatively insensitive to radiation therapy.[116,117] Only 50 percent of verrucous carcinomas respond primarily to radiation therapy, even when small. These lesions should be quantified by CT examination if any significant infiltration is suspected. Imaging correlations are equally good for these tumors as for squamous cell carcinoma. The follow-up of verrucous carcinoma is particularly deceptive, and critical radiologic imaging should be employed as indicated.

Malignant epithelial tumors of minor salivary gland origin affect the larynx as they do the subglottic region and the trachea. *Adenoid cystic tumor* (formally called cylindroma) is one such lesion with laryngeal predilection. They often present as discrete, dome-shaped soft tissue masses with somewhat sessile base (Fig. 4–38). The subglottis is a favorite site; they tend to involve the party wall common to the trachea and esophagus. Di-

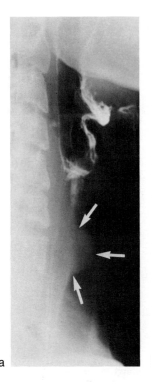
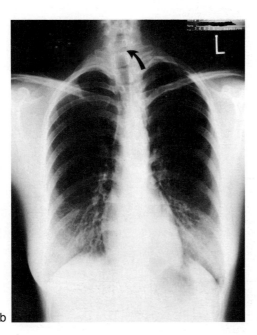
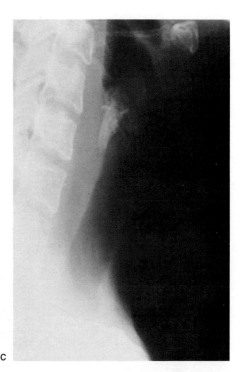

a   b   c

Figure 4–38. Adenoid cystic carcinoma, trachea. **a,** A lateral view of a mini-barium swallow demonstrates the smooth dome-shaped projection of a soft tissue mass, arising from the posterior wall of the trachea and occupying most of the airway (arrows). The party wall seems thickened, and there is suggestion of a somewhat sessile attachment for this adenoid cystic carcinoma in this 22-year-old female. The barium column is unobstructed. **b,** A chest film demonstrates clear lung fields and the soft tissue density projecting into the cervical tracheal airway (arrow). **c,** A soft tissue lateral radiograph 5½ years after surgical debulking and radiation therapy shows normal anatomic relationship of the tracheal airway.

agnostic imaging, both conventional and CT, allows localization and quantification of these tumors. Radiologic imaging is important in follow-up of these difficult patients, in whom long-term survival is not measured in 5-year increments but in terms of 10, 15, or 20 years.

Other malignant tumors can affect the larynx, and diagnostic imaging plays an important role in their management. *Chondrosarcoma* and *osteochondrosarcoma* (Fig. 4–39) has been referred to previously in the discussion on benign lesions. Radiologic imaging allows the quantification but does not define malignancy. Progression of these indolent, slow-growing lesions, however, *does* suggest malignancy. Both benign and malignant cartilaginous tumors can demonstrate varying amounts of fine and coarse calcifications, so that this finding cannot differentiate them.

Other studies can contribute to T staging of laryngeal tumors, whether as pre- or postbiopsy. When *lymphoma* is the diagnosis, radiologic imaging contributes to the appropriate staging process (Fig. 4–40). Often gallium scanning (with gallium-67 citrate) provides an effective overview imaging study before CT of the mediastinum and the abdomen.

Extramedullary plasmacytoma occurs rarely in the upper airway, and especially the larynx. This lesion presents as a soft tissue mass either in the supraglottis, glottis, or subglottis. We have recently encountered a unique case of *multiple myeloma* (Fig. 4–41) with laryngeal involvement in which the cricoid cartilage was expanded by intramedullary tumor; this radio-

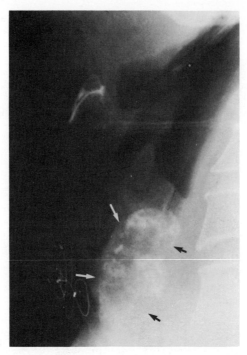
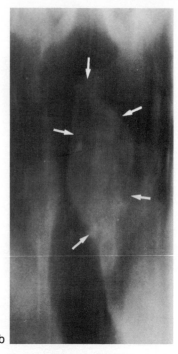

a   b

Figure 4–39. Chondrosarcoma. **a,** Soft tissue lateral radiograph demonstrates a low-grade chondrosarcoma arising from the internal surface of the posterior lamina of the cricoid cartilage (arrows). It extends upward to the level of the arytenoid eminence, encroaching on the laryngeal airway, diminishing it by one-half on its AP dimension. Multiple foci of coarse calcification are present, a diagnostic feature of chondroma and chondrosarcoma. The anteriorly placed wires reflect a previous laryngofissure operation. **b,** A coronal tomogram demonstrates both subglottic and supraglottic extent of the lesions (arrows), as well as several areas of coarse calcification. (Reprinted with permission from Zizmor et al[111] and of Dr. T. D. R. Briant, St. Michael's Hospital, Toronto, Canada.)

Figure 4–40. Lymphoma, epiglottis. A lateral xeroradiograph demonstrates uniform swelling of this structure (arrows) due to the presence of histiocytic lymphoma. The radiographic findings are nonspecific, but inflammatory swelling is not suggested because vallecular definition is preserved. This is a 58-year-old female. (Reprinted with permission from Zizmor and Noyek.[62])

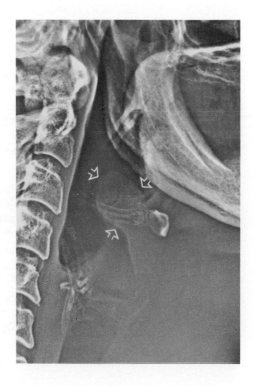

graphic finding led to its recognition as an unusual presentation for multiple myeloma in a patient with past history of skeletal involvement.

Thyroid cancer should be mentioned briefly. Anaplastic carcinoma of the thyroid gland (Fig. 4–42) has a predilection to invade the larynx, often producing cartilage destruction and focal mass deposits within the larynx, usually in the subglottic region. The reader is referred to the work of Noyek and colleagues[104] for details of thyroid tumor imaging.

Arthropathies

See Chapter 9.

The joints of the larynx can be affected by arthropathy; the cricoarytenoid joints are usually involved, often with *rheumatoid arthritis.*◁ Sometimes radionuclide bone scan[58] can be effective in demonstrating an osteoblastic response to the inflammatory joint process, if there is sufficient bone formation in the cricoid lamina and the overlying arytenoid cartilages. Interestingly, the pool phase of the bone scan, which reflects the hyperemia of the inflammatory process, often indicates the primary inflammatory nature of the problem, (e.g., rheumatoid arthritis, as opposed to chronic osteoarthritis or joint ankylosis). The cricothyroid joints may also be involved, but are rarely demonstrated on the bone scan. When the disease is suspected, CT scanning[118] frequently shows the destructive nature of the arthropathy and involvement of the joint space. We have also seen *gout* involving the larynx.[58]

Miscellaneous

The larynx may be involved by a variety of bizarre and unusual diseases.[119] Radiographic information may expand the clinical data base and may even occasionally suggest the diagnosis. A variety of unusual inflammatory diseases have been alluded to previously in the appropriate sections. Some of the autoimmune disorders can affect the larynx, as well, such as systemic *lupus erythematosus.* Subglottic swelling may be seen in this disorder. *Sarcoid* may also affect the larynx, producing unusual morphologic changes, often mimicking other inflammatory or neoplastic processes. When the diagnosis of sarcoid is established, gallium scan may allow determination of biologic activity of disease, as well as demonstrating its response to treatment. It may also show whether other active foci of sarcoidosis exist (such as mediastinum or parotids). *Wegener's granulomatosis* also can affect the larynx, but the radiographic findings are nondescript; however, once the diagnosis has been established, imaging may play a role in following treatment response.

Looking Ahead

If the clinician can envision radiologic imaging as an adjunct to and an important part of his diagnostic armamentarium, he may approach his patients with much more confidence. Radiologic imaging is not everything in diagnosis, nor should it be used in a "shot-gun" approach. Rather, its potentials, limitations, and factors of risk and cost should allow maximal benefit for the patient, the treatment of his disease, and its complications. Much radiologic analysis has been done by rote, in the past, with little regard for how much real information is obtained. Equally at fault were those clinicians who did not think out the best role for diagnostic imaging for each patient.

This situation is changing now. Ground rules are being established for

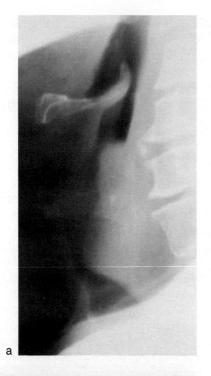

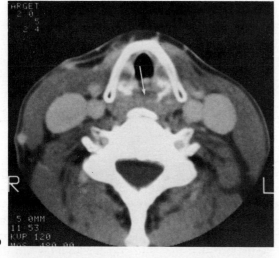

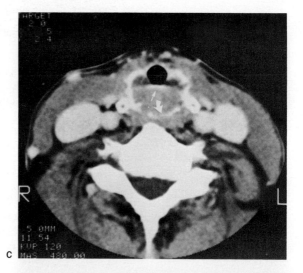

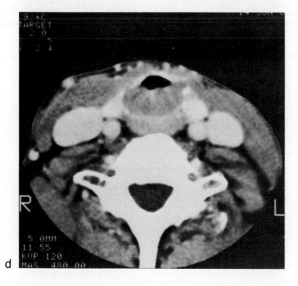

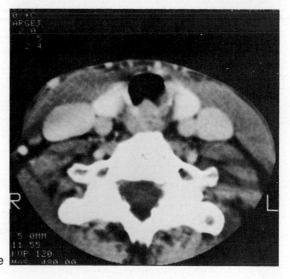

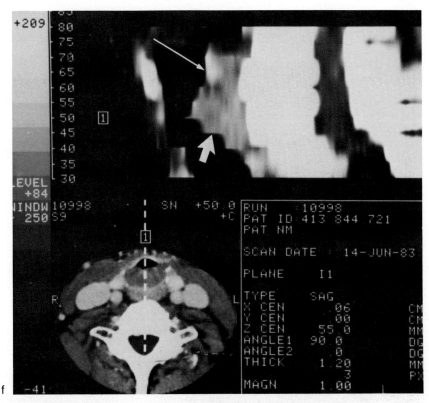

Figure 4–41. Multiple myeloma, cricoid cartilage. **a,** A soft tissue lateral radiograph demonstrates a mass projecting into the subglottic airway in the region of the cricoid signet; there is a small residual anterior subglottic airspace, in this 70-year-old male with previously treated multiple myeloma involving the ribs primarily. **b,** A CT scan demonstrates expansion and bone destruction within the posterior cricoid signet (arrow). The lesion expands posteriorly and laterally on each side, to fill the hypopharynx. **c,** A. CT cut 5.0 mm below B demonstrates intracricoid expansion by a tumor mass. The partially destroyed cortical surfaces are displaced anteriorly (thin white arrow) and posteriorly (thick white arrow). These findings are indicative of an intramedullary mass. **d,** CT cut 5.0 mm below C. The uniform expansion of the cricoid cartilage is well displayed. The smooth encroachment of the hypopharynx posteriorly and on the subglottis and trachea anteriorly are well displayed. **e,** An additional CT cut 5.0 mm below D demonstrates the inferior limit of the tumor, and its relationships. Both thyroid lobes are identified in this intravenous contrast enhanced study. **f,** A sagittal reformation of the axial image data demonstrates the soft tissue tumor mass in midline display (heavy arrow), and its relationship to a portion of the cricoid cartilage above (thin arrow). The plane of the reconstruction is shown in the small axial image below.

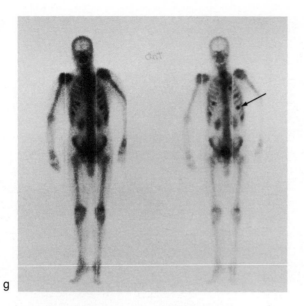

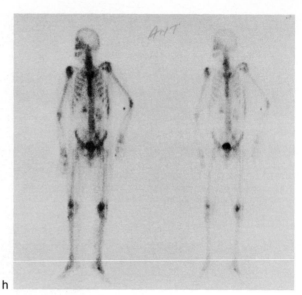

g

h

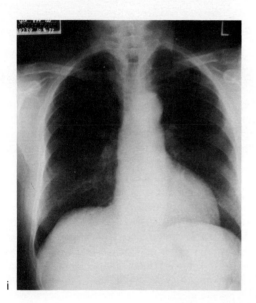

i

Figure 4–41. (Continued) **g,** A whole body MDO bone scan (in delayed phase), demonstrates multiple osteoblastic rib deposits, in anterior display. The patient originally presented with these multiple myelomatous deposits 4 years before his laryngeal involvement. Arrow indicates rib tumor deposit. **h,** A bone scan demonstrates healed rib deposits at the time of presentation with the laryngeal tumor. There is old activity at the distal ends of each clavicle. **i,** A chest radiograph demonstrates clear lung fields at the time of admission with the laryngeal lesion; there is expansion and osteolysis of the distal end of each clavicle; the cortical surfaces are intact in these apparently healed lesions. (Reprinted, in part, with permission from Noyek et al.[112]

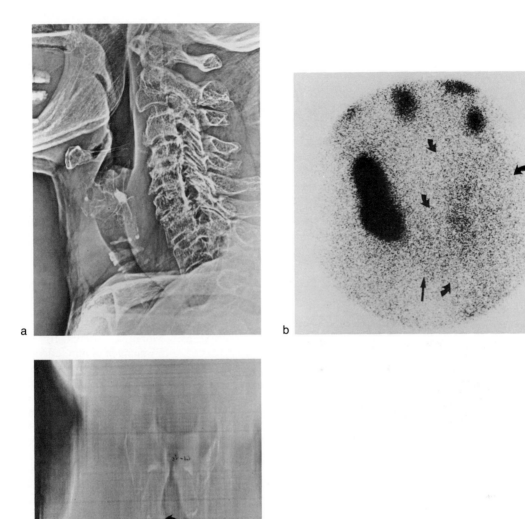

Figure 4–42. Anaplastic carcinoma of the thyroid gland with laryngeal and tracheal invasion. **a,** A lateral xeroradiograph demonstrates annular constriction of the subglottic larynx and trachea by a soft tissue mass, an anaplastic carcinoma of the thyroid gland. Increased soft tissue density is seen both anterior to the trachea and compressing the tracheal air shadow from behind. The patient is an elderly female. **b,** A pertechnetate radionuclide scan demonstrates uptake of the radioactive agent by the right thyroid lobe only. The curved arrows delineate this poorly defined "cold" mass. The straight arrow demonstrates the anterior midline of the neck and the inferior level of midline tumor extension. **c,** An AP xerotomogram (here the patient's left is on the reader's left) demonstrates displacement of the trachea to the right at the level of the thoracic inlet. Note the tracheal relationships relative to the heads of the clavicles; the trachea is displaced by a large soft tissue mass. Two lobulations of tumor are seen within the subglottis (upper curved arrow) and trachea (lower curved arrow). An area of cartilage destruction in the trachea is also defined (straight arrow). (Reprinted in part, with permission from Kirchner et al.[103])

more appropriate radiologic usage. Certainly, the axial display of CT makes laryngeal anatomy and pathology much more understandable to the clinician. It is no longer left to the radiologist alone to interpret overlapping complex shadows, which were easily overread and underread in the absence of experience and clinical correlation.

Certainly, the future should bring us to the understanding that when major disease requires high-technology treatment, that treatment should be supported by high-technology imaging. There should be little place in the future for exploratory operations. Rather, radiologic explorations should replace these surgical ones. Even as CT examinations become more and more reliable, MRI has come upon the scene. Although strong statements have been made to the effect that this might even supplant CT, a more rational look at the future suggests that it will complement CT and augment the rational diagnostic process for all patients. Certainly, this is what should be hoped for.

References

1. Noyek AM, Holgate RC, Wortzman G, et al: Sophisticated radiology in otolaryngology: I. Diagnostic imaging: Roentgenographic (x-ray) modalities. J Otolaryngol, 6 (Suppl 3):73–94, 1977.

2. Noyek AM, Holgate RC, Wortzman G, et al: Sophisticated radiology in otolaryngology: II. Diagnostic imaging: Non-reoentgenographic (non-x-ray) modalities: J Otolaryngol, 6 (Suppl 3):95–117, 1977.

3. Noyek AM: Some comments on the art of diagnosis. Otolaryngol Clin North Am, 2:247–249, 1978.

4. Noyek AM, Zizmor J: The evolution of diagnostic radiology of the larynx. J Otolaryngol, 6(Suppl 3):12–16, 1977.

5. MacIntyre J: Roentgen rays in laryngeal surgery. J Laryngol, 10:231–232, 1896.

6. Scheier M: Ueber die Photographie der Nase und des Kehlkopfes mittels Rontgenstrahlen. Berl Klin Wochenschr, 34:638, 1897. (In Laryngol Gesell 12:1896.)

7. Behn K: Kehlkopf Verknocherung nachgewiesen an lebenden. Fortschr Geb u. Rontgenstr, 43: 1901.

8. Scheier M: Ueber die Ossifikation des Kehlkopfes. Arch Mikroskop Anat, 59, 1901.

9. Scheier M: Zur Verknocherung des menschlichen Kehlkopfs. Schafer-Passow Beitr, 3, 1909.

10. Scheier M: Die Bereutung des Rontgenverfahrens fur die Physiologie der Sprache und Stimme. Arch Laryngol Rhinol, 22:175–208, 1909.

11. Scheier M: Zur Physiologie des Schluckakts. Schafer-Passow Beitr, 4:1911.

12. Moller J, Fischer JF: Ueber die Wirkung der Musculi Cricothyroideus und Thyro-arytenoideus Internus. Arch Laryngol Rhinol, 15:72–76, 1903.

13. Moller J, Fischer JF: Undersogelser over Virkningen of mm. cricothyroideus og thyroarytenoideus internus. Hospitals-Tifends 4R, 11:106–1064, 1903

14. Moller J, Fischer JF: Observations on the action of the cricothyroideus and thyroarytenoideus internus. Ann Otol, 13:42–46, 1904.

15. Frankel E: Uber die Verknocherung des menschlichen Kehlkopfes. Fortschr Geb Rontgenstr, 12:151, 1908.

16. Thost, A: Archiv und Atlas des normalen und kranken Kehlkopfes des lebenden im rontgen Bild. Fortschr Geb Roentgenstr, 31:1–50, 1913.

17. Iglauer, S: Value of roentgenography in the diagnosis of the larynx and the trachea. JAMA 63:1827–1831, 1914.

18. Coutard H: Note preliminaire sur la radiographie du larynx normal et du larynx cancereaux. J Belge Radiol, 13:287, 1922.

19. Hickey PM.: Radiography of normal larynx. Radiology, 11:409–411, 1928.

20. Coutard H, Baclesse F: Roentgen diagnosis during the course of roentgen therapy of epitheliomas of the larynx and hypopharynx. Am J Roentgenol, 28:293–312, 1932.

21. Young BR: Recent advances in roentgen examination of the neck: Body section roentgenography (planigraphy) of the larynx. Am J Roentgenol, 44:519–529, 1940.

22. Young BR: the value of body section roentgenography (planigraphy) for the demonstration of tumors, non-neoplastic disease, and foreign bodies of neck and chest. Am J Roentgenol, 47:83–88, 1942.

23. Gay BB Jr, Wilkins SA Jr: The fluoroscope with image amplifier in the study of the larynx and pharynx. Cancer, 9:1253–1260, 1956.

24. Gay BB Jr: A roentgenologic method for

evaluation of the larynx and pharynx. Am J Roentgenol, 79:301–305, 1958.

25. Leborgne FE: Tomography of the larynx. An Ateneo Clin Quir, June, 1936.
26. Leborgne FE: Tomography, Cancer Laringotomographia. Montevideo, K. Garcia Morales, 1938.
27. Leborgne FE: Laryngeal tomography. An O-R-L Uruguay, 8:169–187, 1938.
28. Leborgne FE: Tomography and cancer of the larynx. Arch Otolaryngol, 31:419–425, 1940.
29. Leborgne FE: Tomographic study of cancer of the larynx. Am J Roentgenol, 43:493–499, 1940.
30. Canuyt G, Gunsett A: La tomographie ou planigraphie du larynx normal: Methode des coupes radiographiques. Soc Laryngol Hop Paris, Proceedings at Brussels, July 19, 1937.
31. Canuyt G, Gunsett A: La tomographie ou planigraphie du larynx pathologique: Methode des coupes ou sections radiographies. Ann Otolaryng, pp 987–994, 1937.
32. Howes WE: Sectional roentgenography of the larynx Radiology, 33:586–597, 1939.
33. Caulk RM: Tomography of the larynx. Am J Roentgenol, 46:1–10, 1941.
34. Iglauer S: Use of injected iodized oil in roentgen ray diagnosis of laryngeal, tracheal, and bronchopulmonary conditions. JAMA, 86:1879–1884, 1926.
35. Jackson C: Value of roentgenography of the neck. Trans Am Laryngol Assoc, 58:112–131, 1936.
36. Farinas PL: Mucosagraphy of respiratory tract. Radiology, 39:84–87, 1942.
37. Powers WE, McGee HH Jr, Seaman WB: Contrast examination of the larynx and pharynx. Radiology, 68:169–177, 1957.
38. Ogura JH, Holtz S, McGavran MH, et al: Laryngograms: Their value in the diagnosis and treatment of laryngeal lesions. Laryngoscope, 70:780–809, 1960.
39. Medina J, Seaman WB, Carbajal P, et al: Value of laryngography in vocal cord tumors. Radiology, 77:531–542, 1961.
40. Khoo FY, Chia KB, Nalpon MSR: A new technique of contrast examination of the nasopharynx with cinefluorography and roentgenography. Am J Roentgenol, 99:238–248, 1967.
41. Zamel N, Austin JHM, Graf FD, et al: Powdered tantalum as a medium for human laryngography. Radiology, 94:547–553, 1970.
42. Maguire GH, Beique RA, Rotenberg AD: Selective filtration: Practical approach to high kilovoltage radiography. Radiology, 85:343–351, 1965.
43. Maguire GH: The larynx: Simplified radiological examination using heavy filtration and high voltage. Radiology, 87:102–110, 1966.
44. Thornbury JR, Latourette HB: A comparison

study of laryngography techniques. Am J Roentgenol, 99:555–561, 1967.
45. Fabrikant JI, Richards GJ Jr, Tucker GF Jr, Dickson RJ: Contrast laryngography in the evaluation of laryngeal neoplasms. Am J Roentgenol, 87:822–835, 1962.
46. Holinger PH, et al: Xeroradiography in otolaryngology. Otolaryngol Clin North Am, 11:445–456, 1978.
47. Noyek AM, et al: Xeroradiography of the Larynx. Otolaryngol Clin North Am, (2):445–456, 1978.
48. Mancuso AA, Hanafee WN: A comparative evaluation of computed tomography and laryngography. Radiology, 133:131–138, 1979.
49. Mancuso AA, et al: The role of computed tomography in the management of cancer of the larynx. Radiology, 124:243–244, 1977.
50. Mancuso AA, et al: Computed tomography of the larynx. Radiol Clin North Am, 16:195–208, 1978.
51. Mancuso AA, Hanafee WN: Computed tomography of the injured larynx. AJR, 133:139–144, 1979.
52. Mancuso AA, Hanafee WN: Computed Tomography of the Head and Neck. Williams & Wilkins, Baltimore, 1982.
53. Hanafee W: Personal communication by letter (AMN), March 15, 1985.
54. Mancuso AA: Personal communication by letter (AMN), Oct. 14, 1985.
55. Stark DD, Moss AA, Gamsu G, Clark OH, Gooding GAW, Webb WR: Magnetic resonance imaging of the neck, Part I: Normal anatomy. Radiology, 150:447–454, 1984.
56. Stark DD, Moss AA, Gamsu G, Clark OH, Gooding GAW, Webb WR: Magnetic resonance imagining of the neck, Part II: Pathologic findings. Radiology, 150:455–461, 1984.
57. Rothberg R, Noyek AM, Freeman JL, et al: Thyroid cartilage imagining with diagnostic ultrasound: Correlative ultrasound/CT/surgical-pathological studies. Arch Otolaryngol, 1986. In press.
58. Noyek AM: Bone scanning in otolaryngology. Laryngoscope, 89 (Suppl 18, No. 9, Part II):1–87, 1979.
59. Noyek AM, Shulman HS, Steinhardt MI, Zizmor J: Radiologic evaluation of the larynx. In Bailey BJ, Biller HF (Eds): Surgery of the Larynx. Philadelphia, WB Saunders, 1985, pp 53–102.
60. Greyson ND, Noyek AM: Nuclear medicine in otolaryngological diagnosis. Otolaryngol Clin North Am, 2:541–560, 1978.
61. Miskin M, et al: Diagnostic ultrasound in otolaryngology. J Otolaryngol, 2:513–530, 1978.
62. Zizmor J, Noyek AMN: An Atlas of Otolar-

yngologic Radiology. Philadelphia, WB Saunders, 1978.

63. Noyek AM, Shulman HS, Steinhardt MI, Zizmor J, Som PM: The larynx. In Bergeron RT, Osborn AG, Som PM (Eds): Head and Neck Imaging, St. Louis, CV Mosby, 1984, pp 402–480.

64. Noyek, AM, Shulman HS, Steinhardt MI: Contemporary laryngeal radiology—clinical perspective. J Otolaryngol, 11:178–185, 1982.

65. Doust DB, Ting YM: Xeroradiography of the larynx. Radiology, 110:727–730, 1974.

66. Hemmingsson A, Lofroth PO: Xeroradiography and conventional radiography in examination of the larynx. Acta Radiol [Diagn] (Stockh), 17:723–732, 1976.

67. Samuel E: Xerography or conventional radiography for laryngeal examination: Can J Otolaryngol, 4:59–63, 1975.

68. Johns HE, et al: Electrostatic methods of imaging in diagnostic radiology. Can J Otolaryngol, 4:102–110, 1975.

69. Noyek AM, et al: Xeroradiography in the assessment of the pediatric larynx and trachea. J Otolaryngol, 5:468–474, 1976.

70. Olofsson J, et al: Radiologic pathologic correlations in laryngeal carcinoma. Can J Otolaryngol, 4:86–96, 1975.

71. Olofsson J, Renouf JHP, van Nostrand AWP: Laryngeal carcinoma correlation of roentgenography and histopathology. A study based on whole organ, serially sectioned laryngeal carcinoma specimens. Am J Roentgenol, 117:526–539, 1973.

72. Bryce DP: Personal communication data from the Conacher Laryngeal Research Laboratory to 1973; quoted in Oloffson J, van Nostrand AWP. Acta Otolaryngol [Suppl] (Stockh), 308, 1973.

73. Olofsson J: Growth and spread of laryngeal carcinoma. Can J Otolaryngol, 3:446–459, 1974.

74. Olofsson J, van Nostrand AWP: Growth and spread of laryngeal and hypopharyngeal carcinoma with reflections on the effect of preoperative irradiation (139 cases studied by whole organ sectioning). Acta Otolaryngol [Suppl] (Stockh), 308, 1–84, 1973.

75. Landman GHM: Laryngography, cinelaryngography, and 70 mm intensifier fluorography in diagnosis of laryngeal cancer. Can J Otolaryngol, 4:74–80, 1975.

76. Landman GHM: Laryngography and Cinelaryngography. Amsterdam, Excerpta Medica Foundation, 1970.

77. Schild JA, Mafee MF: Valvassori, GE, Bardavid W: Laryngeal malignancies and computerized tomography—a correlation of tomographic and histopathologic findings. Ann Otol Rinol Laryngol, 91:571–575, 1982.

78. Hoover LA, Calcaterra TC, Larsson SG, Walter GA: Pre-operative CT scan evaluation for laryngeal carcinoma: Correlation with pathological findings. Laryngoscope, 94:310–315, 1984.

79. Shulman HS, Noyek AM, Steinhardt MI: CT of the larynx. J Otolaryngol, 11:395–406, 1982.

80. Reede DL, Bergeron RT: CT of cervical lymph nodes. J Otolaryngol, 11:411–418, 1982.

81. Mafee MF, Schild JA, Valvassori GE, Capele C: Computed tomography of the larynx: Correlation with anatomic and pathologic studies in cases of laryngeal carcinoma. Radiology, 145:123–128, 1983.

82. Mafee MF, Schild JA, Michael AS, Choi KH, Capek V: Cartilage involvement in laryngeal carcinoma: Correlation of CT and pathologic macrosection studies. J Comput Assist Tomgr, 8:969–973, 1984.

83. Silverman PM, Bossen EH, Fisher SR, Cole TB, Korobkin M. Halvorsen RA: Carcinoma of the larynx and hypopharynx: Computed tomographic histopathologic correlations. Radiology, 151:697–702, 1984.

84. Archer CR, Yeager VL, Herbold DR: Improved diagnostic accuracy in the TNM staging of laryngeal cancer using new definition of regions based on computed tomography. J Comput Assist Tomogr, 7:610–617, 1983.

85. Mafee MF: CT of the normal larynx. Radiol Clin North Am, 22:251–264, 1984.

86. Reid, MH: Laryngeal carcinoma: High-resolution computed tomography and thick anatomic sections. Radiology, 151:689–696, 1984.

87. Archer CR. Yeager VL, Herbold DR: Computed tomography vs histology of laryngeal cancer: Their value in predicting laryngeal cartilage invasion. Laryngoscope, 93:140, 1983.

88. Kavanogh KT, Salazar JE, Babin RW: Bone marrow expansion of the thyroid cartilage: A source of confusion with malignant invasion on CT studies. J Comput Assist Tomogr, 9:177–179, 1985.

89. Mancuso A, et al: CT of cervical lymph node cancer. AJR, 136:381–385, 1981.

90. Gamsu G, et al: CT in carcinoma of the larynx and pyriform sinus: Value of phonation scans. AJR, 136:577–584, 1981.

91. Lufkin RB, Larsson SG, Hanafee WN: Work in progress: NMR anatomy of the larynx and tongue base. Radiology, 148:173–175, 1983.

92. Mancuso, A, Hanafee, WN: Computed Tomography and Magnetic Resonance Imaging of the Head and neck, 2nd ed. Baltimore, Williams & Wilkins, 1985.

93. Freeland AP: Microfil angiography: A demonstration of the microvasculature of the lrynx

with reference to tumor spread. Can J Otolaryngol, 4:111–127, 1975.

94. Holgate RC, et al: Angiography in otolaryngology: Anatomy methodology, complications and contraindications. J Otolaryngol, 2:457–475, 1978.

95. Holgate RC, et al: Angiography in otolaryngology: Indications and applications. J Otolaryngol, 2:477–499, 1978.

96. Kremkau FW: Diagnostic Ultrasound: Physical Principles and Exercises. New York, Grune & Stratton, 1980.

97. Van Nostrand AWP: Personal communication data from the Conacher Laryngeal Research Laboratory to 1985; quoted in Van Nostrand AWP, Lundgren J, Gilbert R: Failure analysis of T3 glottic carcinoma. In press.

98. Kirchner JA: One hundred laryngeal cancers studied by serial section. Ann Otol Rhinol Laryngol, 78:689–709, 1969.

99. Ogura JH: Surgical pathology of cancer of the larynx.

100. Pressman JJ: Submucosal compartmentation of the larynx. Trans Am Laryngol Assoc, 77:165–172, 1956.

101. Pressman JJ, Simon MB, Mondell C: Anatomical studies related to the dissemination of cancer of the larynx. Trans Am Acad Ophthalmol Otolaryngol, 64:628–638, 1960.

102. Yeager VL, Archer CR: Anatomical routes for cancer invasion of the laryngeal cartilages. Laryngoscope, 92:449–452, 1982.

103. Kirchner J, Cornog JL, Holmes RE: Transglottic cancer: its growth and spread within the larynx. Arch Otolaryngol, 99:247–251, 1974.

104. Noyek AM, et al: Thyroid tumor imaging. Arch Otolaryngol, 109:205–224, 1983.

105. Archer CR, Yeager VL: Evaluation of laryngeal cartilages by computed tomography. J Comput Assist Tomogr, 3:604–611, 1979.

106. Greene R, Stark P: Trauma of the larynx and trachea. Radiol Clin North Am, 16:309–320, 1978.

107. Horowitz BL, Woodsen GE, Bryan RN: CT of laryngeal tumors. Radiol Clin North Am, 22:265–279, 1984.

108. Kushner DC, Harris GBC: Obstructing lesions of the larynx and trachea in infants and children. Radiol Clin North Am, 16:181–194, 1978.

109. Momose KJ, MacMillan AS Jr: Roentgenologic investigations of the larynx and trachea. Radiol Clin North Am, 16:321–341, 1978.

110. Bachman AL: Benign non-neoplastic conditions of the larynx and pharynx. Radiol Clin North Am, 16:273–290, 1978.

111. Zizmor J, Noyek AM, Lewis JS: The radiologic diagnosis of chondroma and chondroma and chondrosarcoma of the larynx. Arch Otolaryngol, 101:232–234, 1975.

112. Noyek AM, et al: The radiologic diagnosis of malignant tumors of the larynx. J Otolaryngol, 6:368–373, 1977.

113. Archer CR, et al: Computed tomography of the larynx. J Comput Assist Tomogr, 2:404–441, 1978.

114. Lufkin RL, Hanafee WN: Application of surface coils to MR anatomy of the larynx. AJNR, 6:491–497, 1985.

115. Rideout DF: Appearances of the larynx after radiation therapy. Can J Otolaryngol, 4:98–101, 1975.

116. Abramson AL, Brandsma J, Steinberg B, Winkler B: Verrucous carcinoma of the larynx. Arch Otolaryngol, 111:709–715, 1985.

117. Batsakis JG, Hybels R, Crissman JD, et al: The pathology of head and neck tumors: XV Verrucous carcinoma. Head Neck Surg, 5:29–38, 1982.

118. Charlen B, Brazeau-Lamontagne L, Levesque RY, Lussier A: Cricoarytenoiditis in rheumatoid arthritis: Comparison of fibrolaryngoscopic and high resolution computerized tomographic findings. J Otolaryngol, 14:381–386, 1985.

119. Zizmor J, Noyek AM: Some miscellaneous disorders of the larynx and pharynx. Semin Roentgenol, 9:311–322, 1974.

Chapter 5

Voice Pathology

Melinda Harrison and Harvey M. Tucker

Voice disorders have been considered the stepchild of speech pathology for several reasons: (1) uncertainty as to the speech pathologist's role in treating voice disorders; (2) incomplete understanding of the larynx and voice; (3) limited access for students in training to the full spectrum of voice disorders; (4) rules of treatment differ from those for articulation and language because of the relative involuntary nature of voice production and the lack of fixed standards for normalcy.—After Aronson.[2]

Human phonation can be narrowly defined as that part of the speech act that generates raw sound; yet, *voice* is so much more. Longfellow said, "the human voice is the organ of the soul." It is a window into the individual's personality, intellect, emotional state, and cultural background. As Perkins[1] suggests, voice is an indication of physical health, emotional health, personality, identity, and aesthetic orientation. Voice allows us to communicate deep connotations that go beyond the meaning of the words themselves.

The vocal mechanism is highly complex and must function with exquisitely fine control and coordination. It does not operate in isolation, but functions with the network of physiologic actions responsible for speech production, including those of respiration, resonation, and articulation. Because voice production is primarily controlled reflexively, minor variations in structural, neurologic, or psychologic functions can result in significant alteration.

The diagnosis and treatment of vocal and laryngeal disorders remain something of an enigma,◁ because of relatively limited understanding of the nature of many of the disorders and the complicated interrelationships between structure, physiology, and psychology that impact on voice production. Although firmly rooted in science, the treatment of voice disorders is largely an art, in which individualization of treatment is critical. The therapist must have keen sensitivity, ability to relate well to the patient, facility in making objective judgments, and creativity in developing trial-and-error therapeutic attempts.

A multispecialty clinic is the ideal setting for a comprehensive voice disorders team. In other settings, it is highly recommended that the otolaryngologist identify a nearby speech pathologist with interest or expertise in vocal and laryngeal disorders (or vice versa). Liberal exchange of information is integral to the development of a mutually supportive working relationship.—MH and HMT.

The comprehensive treatment of vocal disorders also requires the close interaction of several disciplines functioning as a team: laryngologist, speech pathologist, neurologist, psychiatrist or psychologist, and internist or family practitioner. The team operates best when referrals are initiated between the members and comprehensive consultation takes place so that full understanding of the problem is facilitated and approaches to treatment are cohesive.◁

General Principles of Phonation

In order to understand disturbances of voice production fully, an overview of basic principles governing normal phonation is necessary. Unfortunately, lack of uniform terminology and definitions preclude easy translation from one text to another (Table 5–1).

Table 5–1   Definition of Terms in Voice Pathology

Aperiodic: vibrations occurring at irregular periods

Diplophonia: phonation at two different pitch levels due to asynchronous vibration of the vocal folds

Elasticity: tendency to return to original shape after deformation under stress

Formant: vocal tract resonance; formants are displayed in a spectrogram as broad bands of energy

Frequency: cycles per second; acoustic correlate of pitch

Fundamental frequency: the lowest frequency component of a complex tone

Glottal attack: a mode of initiation of voicing in which the vocal folds are tightly adducted at onset

Harmonic: an oscillation whose frequency is an integral multiple of the fundamental

Intensity: magnitude of sound expressed in power or pressure; acoustic correlate of volume

Periodic: vibrations recurring at equal intervals of time

Vocal break: abrupt involuntary shift of voice to a higher or lower pitch

Vocal registers: distinctive ranges of phonation, including pulse (lowest down to glottal fry), modal (normally used in speaking and singing), and loft (highest including falsetto)

Voice quality types: breathy (weak, airy voice due to glottal incompetence), harsh (strained voice produced with excessive vocal fold tension), hoarse (rough, raspy voice due to irregular vocal fold vibration)

See also Chapter 2.

For the production of specific types of speech sounds, the air supply must be variable in pressure and quantity. The vocal fold or folds must be able to: (1) limit the flow of air without oscillation of its parts, as for unvoiced sounds; (2) momentarily close the airway without producing sound, as for glottal stops; (3) permit the continuous passage of air while concurrently allowing vibration of the valve elements and the generation of sound, as during aspirate phonation; and (4) interrupt the flow of air intermittently and regularly, as for normal vocal sound.—PG Moore.[4]

Phonation is the physical act of sound production by means of vocal fold interaction with the exhaled airstream. Puffs of air are released within an audible frequency range, including a *fundamental frequency* and its *harmonics*. The harmonics are partial and whole number multiples of the frequency of the fundamental and are resonated primarily in the supraglottic, oral, and nasal cavities. The distribution and relative intensities of the harmonics, therefore, contribute to the individual characteristic quality of the voice.

Normal vocal fold vibration is synchronous and yields a primarily periodic signal. However, some cycle-to-cycle variation or aperiodicity occurs. When *aperiodicity* begins to predominate, a change in vocal quality is observed. Aperiodicity replaces harmonic overtones with noise.

The *myoelastic-aerodynamic theory* of voice production proposed by Vandenberg in 1958 is most widely accepted.[3]◁ It states that the periodic opening and closing of the vocal folds is produced by the mass tension of the folds and the aerodynamic forces exerted on and around them by the exhaled airstream. The vocal folds are approximated by the action of the adductor muscles. As the glottis is narrowed, the airflow moving through it is accelerated. Decreased radial pressure causes the vocal folds to be sucked together, which is called the Bernoulli effect. As a result, subglottic air pressure increases and builds until it overcomes the resistance of the glottis, at which point the vocal folds are blown apart. Tissue turgor and muscular tension help to restore the vocal folds to their adducted position, and the cycle begins again. Phonation, therefore, results from the properties of airflow-air pressure and elasticity of the vocal folds, which is dependent on their length, mass, and tension.◁ Variations in these elements account for intentional and inadvertent alterations in the vocal parameters of *pitch, loudness, quality,* and *flexibility.*

Airflow and *pressure* are influenced primarily by the size of the glottal opening and the tension of the vocal folds. Greater airflow occurs when the vocal folds are incompletely adducted, as in breathy or whispered speech. When the vocal folds are tightly approximated, as in strained voice production, airflow is diminished but air pressure is increased to overcome the tensed folds.

Tension of the vocal folds affects their ability to be displaced. Factors such as shape, density, texture of the mucosa, and tonus of the intracordal structures affect displacement. The greater the tension, the more force necessary to initiate movement.

Mass also influences the force necessary to initiate motion; the greater the mass, the greater the force required. Greater mass results in slower vocal fold vibration or lower pitch. Thus, the longer vocal folds of the male vibrate at a slower frequency, resulting in a lower pitched voice than that of the female. However, as vocal fold length is increased, tension is increased, mass distribution changes, and the result is increased frequency of vibration, resulting in elevation of pitch.

The vocal parameters of *loudness, pitch,* and *quality* are influenced by alteration of these basic principles governing voice. Vocal *loudness* is changed primarily by increase in subglottal air pressure, whereas vocal fold elasticity remains relatively static. *Pitch* is increased by decrease in vocal fold length (except near highest frequency capability) and increase in tension and elevation of subglottal air pressure. Vocal *quality* is determined by the complex interaction of all properties as they affect the vocal fold vibratory pattern.

An understanding of these principles of phonation allows correlation between perceptual and physiologic features of the abnormal voice. When the vocal folds are altered due to a *mass lesion:* (1) pitch is lowered; (2) vocal fold closure is incomplete, allowing abnormal air escape; and (3) tension is increased, requiring greater force to initiate and maintain phonation. When vocal fold motion is altered due to *paresis or paralysis:* (1) closure is incomplete, permitting excessive air escape; (2) turbulence of the airstream results in unwanted noise components (hoarseness); and (3) unequal tension and position of the vocal folds may result in diplophonia. *Increased vocal fold tension,* as seen in *psychogenic voice disorders,* results in decreased compliance necessitating greater force to initiate phonation and hyperadduction of the vocal folds.

Voice Disorders

The comprehensive diagnostic process should include communication between the laryngologist and speech pathologist before informing the patient of the nature of his problem and before treatment is begun. Only in this way can both professionals make maximal contribution to proper patient management.—MH and HMT.

Often valuable treatment time and patient discomfort can be saved by prompt and early referral for voice treatment. The best treatment is preventive, so that additional pathologic changes, effects of learned and habituated miscompensation, and negative emotional reaction can be avoided.—MH.

Voice Evaluation

Patients may be referred for voice evaluation for several reasons: (1) as part of the differential diagnostic process, including recommendations for treatment;◁ (2) for voice therapy as primary treatment; (3) for voice consultation or therapy as part of pre- and postoperative management; (4) to obtain voice recording for medicolegal documentation; and (5) as part of clinical research. Voice evaluation will be particularly important for differential diagnosis when the larynx is apparently normal and the possibility of psychogenic or neurologic origin must be determined. All patients who are undergoing surgical procedures that may alter voice should be seen pre- and postoperatively to assist in adequate return of voice or appropriate adjustment to surgical alterations and to avoid development of poor compensatory behaviors.◁

Typically, laryngologic evaluation is performed before voice evaluation. The condition of the larynx, oral, pharyngeal, nasal cavities, and the head, neck, and chest is of concern to the speech pathologist. Specifically, he or she will need to know the general appearance of the vocal folds, the

I feel strongly that the speech pathologist should visualize the larynx either directly or with the laryngologist. I see no reason why any speech pathologist cannot learn to examine these structures. Use of the fiberoptic scope allows for ease in laryngeal examinations and also allows for videotape recording for review and comparison.—HMT.

presence, size, and location of lesions, and the mobility of the vocal folds.◁ Careful review of the laryngologist's report as well as other medical records should be accomplished before the patient contact.

Comprehensive voice evaluation requires that the speech pathologist identify, analyze, and synthesize the perceptual, acoustic, physiologic, and psychologic factors involved. Without careful consideration of all elements, an incomplete or even inaccurate diagnosis is likely. Such factors as facial and body expression, posture, dress, and grooming can be useful.

Systematic questioning regarding the voice disorder should include:

1. Reason for referral.
2. Onset of the voice disorder: Was the onset gradual or sudden? What were the precipitating or associated factors, such as physical condition, emotional status, environmental influences?
3. Course of the voice disorder: Have there been periods of remission or has the problem been continuous? Does the voice fluctuate in severity and, if so, what are the associated or predisposing factors (i.e., time of day, amount or intensity of use, situational variables)? Has the problem worsened, improved, or stabilized over time?
4. Previous history of voice disorder: Are previous problems similar to the current one? Was the problem previously treated medically, surgically, or through voice therapy and, if so, what was the type and result of treatment? What factors were associated with the onset of previous disorders? Have the vocal problems been episodic?
5. Associated physical symptoms: Are pain, dryness, irritation, muscle tightness or tension present? If so, what is the frequency, intensity, and localization? Are problems noted in breathing, chewing, swallowing, or articulation?
6. Medical history: What are the previous and current medical or surgical problems for which the patient is treated? What medications (dosage and frequency) are used? Has there been previous psychotherapy or pharmacologic treatment of psychologic or emotional problems?◁
7. Exposure to irritants: On what frequency does the patient use alcohol or nonmedicinal drugs or smoke (cigarettes, cigars, pipes, marijuana)? Is the living or working environment dry, dusty, or contaminated with chemicals?
8. Inventory of voice use: What is the typical amount of daily use; purpose of voice use (professional, social); intensity of use (need to project over distance or background noise); need to use voice in an authoritative or influential manner; voice use in stressful situations; amount, manner, and style of singing?

A sign of possible psychogenic component is the patient who provides a copious list of medical conditions and pharmacologic treatments. Often, the conditions are associated with stress, such as ulcers, spastic colon, tension headache. At the initial suggestion that emotional stresses or conflicts may be playing a role in the dysphonia, many patients will vigorously deny or seem very skeptical of the suggestion. Gentle, but persistent questioning will need to continue throughout the interview. Sometimes "planting the seed" about the possible relationship of emotional issues to the voice disorder will stimulate patient reflection and allow for open discussion on a second visit. Some patients react to the initial question by a catharsis of emotion, which may lead to significant improvement of voice.—MH.

During the interview, observations are made about the quality, pitch, loudness, and flexibility of conversational voice. Conditions under which the voice may improve or worsen are noted. Observations of physical signs, including abnormal movement or musculoskeletal tension, are important. It is often helpful if the patient is seen both individually and with a spouse or family member to observe the dynamics of the relationship.

In order to define voice disorders, a description of *normal voice* is necessary first. There is considerable variability and subjectivity within the broad range of "normal." Age, sex, personality, intellect, and cultural biases are all important factors. The characteristics of normal voice include: *quality* pleasant; *pitch level* appropriate to the age and sex of the speaker; *loudness* appropriate, neither too soft nor too loud for the situation; *flexibility* adequate so that pitch, volume, and quality can be altered to allow for intonation and individual expression. Normal voice does not interfere with intelligibility of speech, does not call undesired attention to itself, and does not interfere with occupational or social function.

With these thoughts in mind, a *disordered voice* is defined as one that deviates from the expected in terms of quality, pitch, loudness, and/or flexibility. It may call negative attention to itself and may alter occupational and social performance. The greater the variation from normal, the greater the impact on the individual, although for the professional speaker or individuals whose self-image is highly integrated into vocal function, even minor changes in voice may have disastrous effects. Moreover, voice abnormality must be investigated as a possible indicator of more widespread dysfunction. Often, neurologic or systemic disease, emotional distress, or psychiatric illness may initially be manifested by alteration of voice.

There is no uniform classification of voice disorders in the literature. Previous investigators have classified them in terms of etiology, perceptual features, or kinesiology, such as hyperfunctional or hypofunctional. We will classify voice disorders essentially according to Aronson's[2] system, which is based on etiologic factors. *Organic voice disorders* are those caused by anatomic or physiologic disease of the larynx itself, or by systemic illness indirectly influencing the larynx. *Psychogenic voice disorders* include those that result from psychoneuroses, personality disorders, or faulty habits of voice usage, in which laryngeal anatomy and physiology are essentially normal. The *spasmodic dysphonias, care* of the *professional voice,* and *alaryngeal communication* ◁ are considered separately.

See also Chapter 13.

Voice Examination

Clinical voice examination consists of specific activities, the performance of which allow for judgments to be made about vocal parameters. Audio and videotape recordings are important means of documenting baseline measures for future comparison, allow additional opportunity for evaluation and feedback to the patient, and can provide data for educational and research programs.

Specific examination tasks include the following:

1. Vowel prolongation: Sustained production of "ah" and "ee" is a sensitive means of determining glottal competency. (Breathiness indicates glottal incompetence; harshness indicates overadduction of the vocal folds; hoarseness or noise suggests the presence of a mass lesion or unequal vocal fold tension, respiratory efficiency, vocal pitch and loudness, and rhythmic or arrhythmic fluctuations.)
2. Pitch range. Limitation suggests vocal fold palsy.
3. Loudness range.
4. Glottic coup: Used to judge strength of vocal fold adduction, it consists of sharply produced speech ("uh-oh") and nonspeech activities (sharp cough and throat clearing).
5. Endurance: Having the patient count from 1 to 100 will allow observation of fatigue.
6. Oral reading: Used to judge overall vocal parameters and severity of aberrations.
7. Motor speech examination: Used to determine appearance and strength, range and rate of lingual, labial, palatal, and jaw movements, particularly helpful in revealing neurologic abnormalities. Oral reflexes (gag, palatal, and swallow) are also observed. Evaluation of respiration, resonation, articulation, and prosodic features is completed.

8. Musculoskeletal tension testing (Aronson[2]): Used to reveal areas of pain as an index of abnormal tension and abnormal position of the larynx. Manipulation of the laryngeal area may result in vocal improvement, thus confirming the presence of musculoskeletal tension.
9. Optimum pitch: The ''um-hum'' test, which provides normalization of pitch and can aid in determination of optimal pitch.
10. Stimulability testing: A method to improve performance should be demonstrated by the clinician for each of the voice tasks just listed. The patient should perform several trials in an effort to alter the voice favorably. This provides critical information about presence of behavioral factors and helps determine the direction and prognosis of voice therapy.

Objective Studies

Objective measures should: provide precise measurement, involve minimal or no encumbrance to natural speech, involve minimal hazard to the patient, and provide real-time data. Two additional prerequisites are that they require limited data storage and be cost-effective.—MH

Objective measures of vocal function are usually made for scientific purposes in the laboratory, although some of these measures are relevant to and can be performed within the clinical setting.◁ They can provide baseline data for a variety of specific aspects of vocal function. This can allow reliable and valid measurements and comparisons with postoperative or post-treatment conditions. In addition, they may also help in comparing groups of patients. However, objective vocal measures are not definitively diagnostic of any vocal disorder nor of the nature of the laryngeal abnormality and must be used in conjunction with traditional measures.

Objective techniques may include spectrography, measures of pitch perturbation, and noise-to-harmonic ratio. Aerodynamic studies may include measures of mean airflow rate, maximum phonation time, and subglottal air pressure. Additional methods to observe laryngeal function include high-speed motion pictures, stroboscopy, videofluoroscopy, glottography, electromyography, and flexible fiberoptics[5] with videorecording.

Interpretation

The interpretation of the findings is much like fitting together the pieces of a puzzle. Each piece is examined for its correct place within the whole. Any bit of information that is incongruous or inconsistent must be reexamined. This requires objectivity to avoid under- or overemphasis of any observation, or bias from the interpretations of previous evaluations. It is also important to consider how the patient's vocal behavior during the examination compares with the typical condition, since the patient's level of severity can often be altered within the testing situation compared with normal conversational use.

Analysis and synthesis of all data can lead to such conclusions as type and severity of voice disorder, ability of the patient to alter habitual voice quality despite its anatomic and physiologic condition, consistency of the vocal examination with the laryngeal findings, candidacy of the patient for voice therapy, the patient's incentive or desire for treatment, the need to refer the patient back to the laryngologist for consideration of medical or surgical intervention, and the need for further evaluation, such as trial diagnostic therapy, medical evaluation, or psychologic or psychiatric intervention. It is important that the patient be given a clear understanding of the nature of the vocal and laryngeal disorder, the recommended treatment, an approximation of the time involved in treatment, and the prognosis.

Treatment

I have observed that some patients who have had voice therapy previously are unable to explain the goals and objectives of treatment and at best recall an isolated "exercise." They often feel that voice "exercises" are similar to gymnastics in that frequency equals mastery without conscious alteration of behavior. It seems highly unlikely that therapy will be effective unless the patient has full understanding of the desired changes and his responsibility in developing behavioral control.—MH.

The goals of therapy may include one or more of the following:

1. To obtain additional information through a period of trial diagnostic therapy.
2. To reacquire normal vocal function.
3. To develop maximal compensation for permanent loss of vocal function.
4. To augment for functional losses.
5. To assist in accommodation to or control over environmental factors that precipitate or worsen voice disorders.

Successful voice therapy requires the patient's awareness and desire to accomplish a change in vocal quality.◁ The patient may not fully appreciate the various steps involved in voice therapy, but a commitment to working openly and actively in trying to accomplish the recommended changes must be made. If it is determined that the patient is not actually interested in changing vocal behavior and is only following the advice of the referring physician, spouse, family, or friends, the therapy is not likely to be successful.

The immediate goal of voice therapy is to produce a voice in the most efficient manner possible regardless of what acoustic inadequacies impinge on the auditory system. By-products of effortless phonation include: reduction in compensatory strain, gradual remission of the pathologic features and gradual habituation of improved voice.—Eugene Batza, Ph.D.

The aim of therapy for voice disorders is to evoke a conscious behavioral change over an activity that is normally highly involuntary and nearly reflexive.◁ To this end, the patient must be motivated and open to altering a very individual and personal aspect of himself. Often, he is rightfully concerned about voice therapy necessitating a change in personality, against which there may be considerable resistance. The doubtful eye cast on voice therapy may be justifiable when intertwined in a network of psychologic factors, including secondary gain.

A logical, stepwise program, based on physiologic and acoustic principle can avoid some of the mystique of voice therapy. Aronson[2] has stated that the trial-and-error system and continued need for intensive counseling makes voice therapy seem to be an "art." However, Moore[4] indicates that voice therapy begins at the level of speech in which the patient *can* achieve the desired change. This behavior is then stabilized and serves as a framework on which more difficult skills can later be added.

In addition to necessary technical expertise, the speech pathologist must often be able to serve the role of counselor. Because so many primary or secondary psychologic factors are involved, the clinician must become an active and nonjudgmental listener. This will allow the patient the freedom to discuss anxieties, stresses, angers, and fears openly.

Specific Treatment Techniques

Voice Rest

Historically, voice rest has been recommended in the treatment of organic and psychogenic voice disorders, often for protracted periods. Contemporary thinking has shifted from the use of vocal rest so that now it is most often recommended only for brief periods postoperatively or after severe vocal trauma. *Lengthy voice rest is inadvisable* because of the potential loss of muscle tonus and subsequent vocal weakening, which can add yet another physiologic abnormality. Moreover, the psychologic impact of voice rest can worsen or initiate psychogenic disturbances.

Modified Voice Use (Vocal Hygiene)

As a substitute for voice rest, modifications of the amount, intensity, and stress of voice can be recommended in the early postoperative course or as one of the steps in treating disorders resulting from vocal abuse. In addition, patients who are chronic vocal abusers need to acquire lifelong modifications in voice use. Typically, improved voice use is present at first, but as the patient reacquires more normal vocal function, less dramatic strategies can be permitted.

Relaxation Techniques

When tension is severe enough to alter voice measurably the advice to "just relax" is not sufficient. Specific techniques to modify tension include: (1) progressive relaxation, in which individual muscles are alternately voluntarily contracted then relaxed; (2) chewing method (Froeschels[6]) in which a chewinglike motion with wide-open, slow, and relaxed oral excursion attempts to release tension; (3) digital manipulation (Aronson[2]) in which the extrinsic laryngeal muscles and laryngeal cartilage are progressively kneaded or rubbed and the larynx is progressively lowered to a more normal position in the neck; (4) electromyographic feedback (Prasek et al[7]) that heightens awareness and perception of laryngeal muscle tension.

Establishing Easy Initiation of Phonation

Boone[8] described the "yawn-sign" and "aspirate 'h' " techniques as a means of eliminating hard glottal attack. Both are directed toward maximizing airflow during voice initiation to control vocal fold hyperadduction. Directing the patient's attention to more efficient respiratory control over voice production, particularly speaking at the top of the exhalatory cycle and monitoring continued, smooth flow of air during voice production is also an effective strategy.

Respiratory Control

There is lack of agreement about the role of respiratory control in normal voice production. Most often, faulty breathing techniques during phonation are secondary to tense glottal constriction, improper phrasing, and inefficient control of subglottal air pressure to vary pitch and volume. Respiratory efficiency is also altered in cases of abnormal vocal cord movement. Therapy is directed toward controlled, steady inhalation and exhalation. Abdominal breathing is particularly important for the professional singer or speaker, or the individual with frequent need to speak loudly, but may not be critical to the individual with less demanding vocal needs.

Optimum Pitch

Aronson[2] suggests that optimum pitch usually appears when the vocal mechanism becomes physiologically normalized. It may occasionally be necessary to modify pitch individually, for which he recommends the "um-hum" method.

Effort Closure Techniques

Most frequently applied to unilateral vocal cord paralysis, Froeschels and co-workers[9] advocate strong glottal closure by pushing or lifting while phonating "ee." Effort closure can also be accomplished by coughing, throat-clearing, or grunting. Change of head position or digital pressure to the affected side can also be useful.

Organic Voice Disorders

Congenital Disorders of the Larynx

As discussed in Chapter 7, congenital laryngeal disorders may result in weak, hoarse, muffled, stridorous, or absent cry. Depending on the pathologic condition, the vocal and laryngeal abnormality may persist beyond infancy into childhood. If the vocal abnormality is severe, and especially if tracheotomy is required, significant impact on development of communication can result. The effects of severe restriction or total lack of phonation have been observed in a small group of children by Tucker and colleagues.[10] Receptive language development in a group of nonvocal children was generally adequate, but there was severe restriction in expressive language. Compensatory, essentially self-generated pharyngeal and buccal speech and gestural communication was observed, but allowed only a limited growth of expressive skills.◁ Early, systematic intervention for teaching techniques, such as sign language, use of artificial laryngeal devices, communication boards, and esophageal-pharyngeal or buccal speech has been advocated by Kaslon and associates.[11] Voice therapy to develop normal or best phonation and speech therapy to develop articulation and language skills are usually necessary after decannulation. More extensive clinical experience with this population is needed to determine the most effective methods of augmenting communication function, while stimulating oral-motor and expressive language development.

In several cases of severe congenital papillomas, we have observed compensatory phonation on inhalation, ventricular phonation, and/or forceful whispered speech.—MH and HMT.

Acquired Voice Disorders

Mass Lesions

The vocal deviations associated with mass lesions are not usually distinguishable from one another on the basis of perceptual or acoustic variables. In general, examination of the voice reveals the following aberrations: vocal pitch is depressed (due to the additional bulk of the vocal folds), vocal quality is breathy and hoarse (due to the alteration in shape and incomplete glottic closure), and often harsh (due to the increased tension and excessive approximation of the vocal folds). Pitch and phonation breaks may occur, especially at the upper end of the pitch range and flexibility in pitch and volume change may be noted.

Trauma

Diffuse trauma to the larynx due to crushing or penetrating wounds may result in edema, hematoma, fractures, dislocations, lacerations, and paralysis. Focal trauma resulting from laryngeal intubation may cause paralysis or arytenoid granuloma. The characteristics and severity of the dysphonia depend on the nature and extent of vocal fold disruption.

Endocrine Disorders

The characteristically low-pitched, coarse voice of *hypothyroidism* results from the effects of myxedema of the vocal folds. It may lead to breathy vocal quality and insufficient loudness. *Virilization* due to androgenic hormones in females may result in low-pitched voice and hoarseness.

Chronic Irritation

Chronic irritation occurs from environmental factors, such as excessive smoking and alcohol use. Constant vocal abuse and coughing are additional predisposing factors. Benign laryngeal changes may include chronic *laryngitis, hypertrophy, leukoplakia,* or *polypoid degeneration.* The formation of a discrete lesion may occur in the form of a vocal fold *nodule* or *polyp,* typically at the junction of the anterior and middle one-third of the vocal folds or a *contact ulcer* at the tip of the vocal process of the arytenoid. Malignant changes, most often *squamous cell carcinoma,* may arise on the vocal folds or in surrounding laryngeal structures.

The treatments available for carcinoma of the larynx frequently result in alteration of vocal function, ranging from mild to severe. Even "conservative" management with *radiation therapy* can alter vocal fold mass and elasticity, which may have an effect on voice quality.◁ *Surgery* frequently has a much more significant impact on communication. Partial laryngectomy always affects vocal function, the degree depending on the extent and location of resection. After standard hemilaryngectomy or subtotal laryngectomy with epiglottic reconstruction, the voice ranges from moderately to severely breathy secondary to glottic incompetence. Standard supraglottic laryngectomy usually has little lasting impact on voice except for harshness and low and restricted pitch. With an extended supraglottic resection involving one or both arytenoids and part of a vocal fold, the impact on voice quality is greater. Moderate to severe breathy, hoarse dysphonia may result.

Voice therapy for partial laryngectomized patients involves strategies to improve glottic competence, including vocal adductory exercise and maximizing respiratory efficiency. Use of a voice amplifier for voice projection may be advisable in some cases.

In a study of voice following radiation therapy, quality was observed to be rough and hoarse, due to increased vocal fold stiffness and decreased compliance as well as reduced glottic closure. Often after termination of radiation treatment, voice improvement was noted (Stoicheff and colleagues[12]). Voice therapy facilitated improvement in some cases.

Neurologic Diseases

Fine, highly organized neurologic control is essential for all laryngeal functions. Phonation, range, and strength of vocal fold adduction and abduction, adjustments of vocal cord tension and length, maintenance and controlled adjustment of subglottic air pressure, and all other contributory factors must be coordinated, timed, and precisely executed. When disruption in the central or peripheral nervous system occurs, this fine control is often altered. There may be a change in vocal function and other aspects of speech, including respiration, resonation, and articulation. Such dyscoordination in speech is called *dysarthria.*

Darley and associates[13,14] identified acoustically different dysarthrias and their associated dysphonias caused by damage to specific regions of the nervous system. Flaccid, spastic, ataxic, hypokinetic, and hyperkinetic dysarthria results in a distinctive alteration of speech because of the separate and unique physiologic responsibilities and neurologic function of their associated sites of lesion. The dysarthrias that most frequently result in vocal or laryngeal aberrations are discussed:◁

1. Flaccid dysarthria or dysphonia. Flaccid dysphonia results from damage to the tenth cranial nerve, producing paralysis or paresis on a temporary or permanent basis. Damage can be unilateral or bilateral and may result in a variety of findings. When damage occurs in the brainstem, at a level above the separation of the pharyngeal, superior laryngeal, and recurrent laryngeal branches, the vocal fold will assume an abducted position and palatal weakness will also be present. When damage is unilateral, voice is weak and breathy and volume is limited. Hypernasality and nasal emis-

Aronson[2] classifies the dysarthrias/dysphonias in terms of constancy of symptoms: (1) Relatively constant neurologic voice disorders—flaccid, spastic, mixed flaccid-spastic, and hypokinetic; (2) arrhythmically fluctuating neurologic voice disorders—ataxic, choreic, and dystonic; (3) rhythmically fluctuating neurologic voice disorders—palatopharyngeal myoclonus and essential (voice) tremor; (4) paroxysmal neurologic voice disorders—Gilles de la Tourette; and (5) neurologic voice disorder associated with loss of volitional phonation—akinetic mutism, apraxia of speech, and dysprosody of pseudoforeign dialect.

sions are also present. Bilateral damage at this level will result in essentially whispered speech, with greater degrees of hypernasality and nasal emission.

Unilateral lesions of the recurrent laryngeal nerve result in immobility in a paramedian position, because the intact cricothyroid muscles act as adductors and pull the vocal folds closer to midline. There is moderate breathiness and hoarseness with limited vocal volume. Diplophonia and pitch breaks may occur because of unequal tension on the vocal folds. Involvement of the superior laryngeal nerve alters pitch range due to inability to adjust vocal fold length. Bilateral peripheral damage results in paramedian paralysis, which allows for near normal voice production but with compromise of airway and inspiratory stridor.

Voice therapy for flaccid dysphonia due to unilateral vocal fold paralysis strives for development of compensatory overadduction of the intact vocal fold. In addition, modification of respiratory control, particularly increased subglottic air pressure, is helpful. A voice amplifier may be necessary in cases in which vocal projection is important, particularly at the beginning of treatment. Teflon® injection or vocal fold medialization may be recommended, particularly if results of voice therapy are suboptimal.◁ Additional voice therapy may be beneficial after these procedures to ensure maximal vocal adjustment and function.

See Chapter 11.

Flaccid dysphonia also occurs in myasthenia gravis, a neuromuscular disease that results from reduction of available acetylcholine receptors at the neuromuscular junction, perhaps on an autoimmune basis. Clinical features include weakness and easy fatigability. Often the earliest sign of myasthenia gravis is vocal weakness. Laryngeal examination is frequently negative, but critical observation after extended phonation may reveal mild bilateral weakness or vocal fold bowing. In most cases, as the disease progresses, changes in resonation and articulation also become apparent, resulting from observable palatal, lingual, and labial weakness.◁

Myasthenia gravis focal to the larynx producing breathiness and weakness without resonatory and articulatory changes is seen on rare occasions.—Nieman and colleagues.[15]

Medical treatment of myasthenia gravis with anticholinesterase drugs or thymectomy is often quite effective in eliminating vocal and speech symptoms. Although not substantiated in the literature, voice consultation may be helpful to ensure maximum vocal efficiency and to encourage voice conservation measures, such as limited use of loud volume, reduction of ambient background noise, and intermittent, brief periods of voice rest.

2. Spastic dysarthria or dysphonia. Spastic dysarthria or dysphonia results from a lesion in the pyramidal system. In cases of unilateral dysfunction the resultant dysarthria or dysphonia is mild. However, bilateral corticobulbar tract damage causes abnormally tense muscle tone that results in harsh, strained-strangled vocal quality, low pitch, monopitch, reduced loudness, and monoloudness. In its most severe form, initiation of voice may be delayed and accompanied by considerable effort due to hyperadduction of the true and false vocal folds. Associated abnormal speech characteristics include hypernasal resonance, distorted articulation, and overall slow rate of speech production. Pseudobulbar signs, such as inappropriate crying and laughing, may be present. Motor examination will typically show fairly normal movement or perhaps hyperadduction of the true and false vocal folds. Palatal elevation will be limited. Lingual and labial movements will be slowly produced with restricted range. However, the motor examination may seem disproportionately mild to the severity of the voice and speech impairment.

Voice therapy for spastic dysarthria or dysphonia typically focuses on all aspects of speech production. Goals include improving the initiation and maintenance of continuous voicing and reducing the excessive muscular effort associated with speech.

Despite the deteriorating nature of motor neuron disease, we have found early use of a palatal lift (to elevate the soft palate) and hard palatal reshaping (to lower the hard palatal vault) prosthesis to aid overall speech production. The maxillofacial prosthodontist and speech pathologist must work closely together to custom-contour the prosthesis. In amyotrophic lateral sclerosis severe physical limitations may necessitate the use of adapted nonvocal communication.—MH and HMT.

Early signs of hypokinetic dysarthria usually consist of breathy voice quality and reduced loudness. In the absence of other clinical signs, such patients are frequently misdiagnosed as "functional."—AE Aronson.[2]

3. Mixed flaccid-spastic dysarthria or dysphonia. Mixed flaccid-spastic dysarthria or dysphonia is most commonly seen in motor neuron disease or amyotrophic lateral sclerosis, which is a degenerative disease of bilateral corticobulbar tracts and lower motor neuron nuclei. Either spastic or flaccid components may predominate. Thus, the laryngeal examination may show normal movement, hyperadduction, or hypoadduction of the vocal folds. Complete vocal fold paralysis, however, is uncommon. Pooling of saliva in the pyriform sinuses and velopharyngeal incompetence resulting from weakness or limited range of motion are frequently noted. Lingual and labial movement is weak and restricted in range. Tongue fasciculations and atrophy are common, particularly as the disease progresses. Associated vocal alterations include excessively strained harsh quality, breathiness, restricted pitch, volume variability, and audible inhalation. A characteristic "wet hoarseness" results from pooled pharyngeal secretions. Additional dysarthric features include hypernasal resonance, nasal emission, distorted articulation, slow rate of speech production, and monotonicity.

Because the disease is progressive, normalization or even significant improvement of vocal production are not realistic goals of therapy. However, prompt initiation of treatment directed toward maximizing vocal and speech efficiency as progressive alterations in speech occur is desirable. The use of a palatal lift, a palatal reshaping prosthesis, or both, may improve resonatory and articulatory deviations.◁ When intelligibility of speech becomes restricted, primary or augmentative use of nonvocal communication systems should be provided.

4. Hypokinetic dysarthria. Hypokinetic dysarthria, most commonly seen in Parkinson's disease, results from involvement of the basal ganglia. Vocal deviations include breathiness, restricted loudness, monopitch and tremor, which are the result of rigidity and slowness of movements.◁ Additional variations of speech production include imprecise articulation, rapid rate, especially in short rushes, and palilalia, which is stuttering-like repetition of syllables, words, or whole phrases. Laryngologic findings may include mild glottic incompetence or bowing of the vocal folds, according to Hanson and colleagues.[16] Restricted range and rate of lingual, labial, and jaw movements result in masked facies. Treatment for Parkinson's disease most often consists of drug therapy with L-dopa. Voice and speech therapy is directed toward maximizing vocal fold adduction, increasing vocal volume by increasing respiratory drive, and controlling palilalia by use of pacing techniques. Patients are often able to alter speech in structured context, but may lack carryover into spontaneous speech.

Hypokinetic dysarthria may also be present in Shy Drager syndrome, which is a rare disorder that is characterized by progressive autonomic system failure. Because the lesions extend beyond the extrapyramidal system, subsequent development of bulbar and cerebellar signs become apparent. Ward and co-workers[5] observed progressive abductor paresis of the larynx and respiratory failure in patients with Shy Drager. The severity may eventually necessitate tracheotomy.

5. Hyperkinetic dysarthria. Two general forms of hyperkinetic dysarthria or dysphonia have been identified, emanating from lesions in the basal ganglia. Chorea, characterized by quick, jerky, and irregular movements, results in the following vocal deviations: sudden forced inspiration or expiration, harsh vocal quality, excess loudness variations, strained phonation, monopitch and monoloudness, reduced stress, transient breathiness, and voice arrest.[16,17] The slower form, dyskinesia or dystonia, is evident from repetitive, slow, writhing movements. Orofacial dyskinesia or vocal dystonia are terms that indicate involvement of the speech mecha-

The adductor laryngeal spasms that occur in dystonia may sound similar to those of spasmodic dysphonia. The presence of involuntary lip, tongue, and facial movements may clinically distinguish dystonia.—MH and HMT.

nism only. Vocal characteristics include harsh and breathy vocal quality, in addition to adductor and abductor laryngeal spasms.◁ Treatment of hyperkinetic dysarthria is minimally effective. A major goal in treatment is to minimize the amplitude of involuntary movements by enhancing respiratory, phonatory, and articulatory efficiency.

6.   Essential voice tremor. Essential voice tremor can appear as an isolated finding or in conjunction with tremor in the upper limbs, head, face, neck, chest, or diaphragm. If autosomal dominant inheritance can be proved, it is called heredofamilial tremor. The disorder does not have a uniform site of lesion in the central nervous system. Characteristically, this intention-type tremor is an arrhythmic quaver occurring at a frequency of 4 to 8 Hz. The tremor is most noticeable on sustained phonation of ''ah.'' Aronson and Hartman[17] indicated that essential (voice) tremor can mimic spasmodic dysphonia because the adductor phase of the vocal fold tremor oscillation can occur with such great amplitude that the folds hyperadduct against each other, momentarily arresting the exhaled airstream. The entire larynx may oscillate superiorly and inferiorly if the extrinsic laryngeal muscles are involved.

Diagnostic differentiation between spasmodic dysphonia with or without secondary essential (voice) tremor, and primary essential (voice) tremor is critical to treatment planning, since recurrent laryngeal nerve lysis will not help in essential tremor. Tremor on sustained ''ah'' and signs of tremor in other body parts suggests a diagnosis of essential tremor. Treatment for essential tremor consists primarily of drug therapy. According to Hartman and associates[18] propranolol hydrochloride therapy has produced only equivocal results in reducing voice tremor. Sorenson and colleagues[19] reported success in one patient treated with metoprolol tartrate therapy. Alcohol (ethanol) has been reported to lessen the amplitude of tremor.

7.   Palatopharyngolaryngeal myoclonus. Palatopharyngolaryngeal myoclonus, a slow form of vocal tremor, consists of rhythmic or semirhythmic involuntary movements of the soft palate, pharyngeal walls, laryngeal musculature, eyeballs, diaphragm, and tongue. Rhythmic movements of the vocal folds can cause phonatory interruptions that are often not apparent in conversational speech but are noticed only on vowel prolongation.

Voice therapy for neurogenic dysphonias resulting from involuntary vocal fold movements (i.e., chorea, dystonia, tremor, and myoclonus) is often either ineffective or untested,[2] especially if the problems are severe. However, consultation regarding the nature of the disorder and utilization of the best possible vocal control to prevent inadequate or overcompensation may be helpful. The possibility that patients will exacerbate the amplitude of involuntary movement by reactive hyperadduction can therefore be minimized.

8.   Afferent sensory dysphonia. Ward and co-workers[5] described a disorder in which dysphonia was felt to be secondary to afferent sensory dysfunction. They felt that the aberrations arose from failure to override primitive reflexes due to faulty integration of sensory and proprioceptive control of the larynx. In these cases, the presence of a primitive, hyperresponsive gag reflex inhibited initiation of laryngeal closure for phonation.

Psychogenic Voice Disorders

Psychogenic voice disorders are that group of vocal aberrations in which the laryngeal function is normal, or the severity of the dysphonia is disproportionate to the laryngeal findings. The etiologic bases of these disorders

We support Aronson's[2] belief that the term "psychogenic" means that the voice disorder is due to one or more types of psychologic disequilibrium that interfere with normal volitional control over phonation.—MH and HMT.

The patient with psychogenic voice disorder is most often unaware of the emotional aspects of his dysphonia. The approach we find most successful is for the laryngologist to lay the framework of laryngeal normalcy upon which the speech pathologist can discuss behavioral and emotional issues.—HMT and MH.

Vocal fold bowing may be seen in psychogenic dysphonias. Hyperkinetism may eventually lead to hypokinetism.—Luchsinger and Arnold.[21]

Improvement in physical function by rehabilitation training is indirect psychotherapy. When the vocal mechanism is used in a more normal and effortless manner, patients are able to deal with emotional problems with greater confidence and security.—After Brodnitz.[22]

See also Chapter 9.

include stress, emotional conflict, personality disorder, or psychiatric illness.◁ The tremendous sensitivity of the vocal mechanism to even minor variations in physical and emotional health explains the large population of patients with psychogenic voice disorders seen in an active voice clinic. Vocal deviations may range from mild dysphonia to complete aphonia. Greene[20] reports that psychogenic dysphonia is seven times more common in women than men.

Identification and treatment of psychogenic voice disorders remain an enigma to many laryngologists and speech pathologists. All too frequently, patients present to the clinic after treatment for such entities as laryngitis, allergic conditions, and other upper respiratory conditions, which have often included medication, such as antibiotics or antihistamines, or protracted voice rest. Another frequent diagnosis is one related to "nervous condition" for which tranquilizers or advice for the patient to "learn to relax" are recommended.◁ These approaches are often ineffective and promote the "doctor shopping" practice that is pervasive in this population.

The effective treatment of suspected psychogenic voice disorders begins with a thorough laryngeal examination. Findings may include a benign vocal lesion, such as vocal nodules, mild inflammation, bowing of the vocal folds, or normal-appearing vocal folds.◁ In the absence of laryngeal disease, the differential diagnosis will include neurogenic versus psychogenic etiology. The voice evaluation, with a careful and sensitive investigation of psychologic or emotional factors, aids in the diagnosis. Treatment involves restoration of normal voice with discussion and resolution of pertinent psychologic factors.◁

Psychogenic Voice Disorders Associated with Benign Laryngeal Disease

Vocal nodules, polyps, and contact ulcers are often the direct or indirect result of psychogenic factors.◁ Each type of lesion will be discussed with reference to individual features, but an underlying theme of excessive or stressful voice use and tense, aggressive compulsive personality characteristics is common.

1. Vocal nodules, children. Vocal nodules are seen in both children and adults and are felt to result from vocal abuse and misuse. It is clear that psychologic factors play an important part in their development.

Vocal nodules in children are fairly common and are seen in males more often than females. Barker and Wilson[23] suggested that children who develop nodules are louder and more talkative and have a greater incidence of emotional reactivity, hyperactivity, and family problems. Aronson[2] details many associated personality traits of children with vocal fold nodules: aggressiveness, hyperactivity, nervousness, tenseness, frustration, or emotional disturbance.

Frequent vocal abuses in children include yelling, using loud conversational voice, making unusual vocal noises, or singing at a loud or high-pitched level. Voice characteristics include breathy and harsh and hoarse quality, pitch breaks, and loud volume. Musculoskeletal tension is often present.

Treatment of vocal nodules in children requires joint efforts by the patient, parents, siblings, friends, and school teacher to aid in altering environmental or situational conditions that precipitate vocal abuse, including advantageous seating in the classroom and reduction of noise at home. Behavior management approaches toward modifying vocal abuses, especially use of positive reinforcement, may be helpful. Individual patient counseling and sometimes also family counseling are needed to resolve the potential emotional stress issues. Therapy for alteration of vocal misuse often emphasizes the elimination of hard glottal attack, reduction of habitual vocal volume, and modification of musculoskeletal tension.

Conservative, nonsurgical treatment for vocal nodules in children is advocated. Because of the behavioral and motivational factors that are frequently involved, therapy may be long-term in this population. Surgical removal is justified *only* when the severity of the vocal nodules interferes with communication or when successful alteration of behavior has not resulted in their resolution.

2.   Vocal nodules, adults. Adults with vocal nodules display many of the same features as do children. Characteristics of vocal quality, including breathiness, hoarseness, harshness, pitch breaks, and loud volume, are essentially the same. Etiologic factors of emotional stress are similarly observed. Occupational factors are also noted in many individuals who, for example, speak in environments with loud ambient noise levels, who speak to groups without the aid of amplification, who teach or sell a product, who raise young children at home, or who sing. Smoking and use of alcohol can be predisposing factors.

Just as for children, therapy involves reduction of vocal abuses, development of appropriate methods of voice production, and resolution of emotional stresses. Although complete voice rest is not advocated in the treatment of vocal nodules, significant modification of amount and intensity of talking is warranted, at least initially. Elimination of singing is advised even for the professional singer. Often this initial period of modified voice use will allow for a reduction or perhaps even elimination of the nodules within several weeks. As the nodules resolve, the patient is taught appropriate methods of voice production, with emphasis on easy initiation of phonation, adequate breathing control for speech, and normalization of laryngeal tension. Occasional alteration of habitual speaking pitch is necessary, although this is somewhat controversial.[9,24,25]

In our experience, voice therapy for vocal nodules in adults is typically short term. Given adequate patient insight and motivation, at least partial resolution occurs within 6 to 8 weeks. If not, surgical removal is seriously considered, followed by additional postoperative therapy.— MH and HMT.

Surgical removal of vocal nodules may be necessary if behavioral methods are not completely successful.◁ This can occur despite the patient's best effort to control abuse and misuse, especially if the nodules are fibrotic. Adequate preoperative and postoperative voice therapy should allow the best opportunity for the patient to reacquire normal voice after surgery, most often within a 6- to 8-week period. The ultimate goal for such patients is acquisition of normal quality and function of voice, without the need to become a lifelong "vocal cripple."

3.   Vocal polyps. Development of vocal polyps can result from inflammatory, allergic, immunologic, and traumatic causes. Kleinsasser[26] estimated an 80 to 90 percent incidence of vocal polyps in smoking individuals. The traumatic causes primarily involve vocal abuse. Essentially, vocal characteristics are similar to those associated with vocal nodules. One exception is the excessively low-pitched characteristic of massive polyps. Another is the intermittent vocal disturbance characteristic of the pedunculated polyp. When such a polyp moves onto the free edge of the vocal fold, phonation may be momentarily halted, following which normal or near normal voice reappears.

Intractible postoperative dysphonia or delayed recovery of normal voice does occur sometimes and may be the result of a disturbance of the mechanoreceptor reflex system (Greene[20]) or failure of the reflexogenic phonatory control systems to adapt to alterations of vocal fold mass (Wolfe and Ratusnik[27]).

Vocal polyps are typically treated with surgical removal. Vocal consultation and recording is important both preoperatively and postoperatively, both to confirm vocal status before surgical intervention and to ensure elimination of vocal abuses and reacquisition of normal phonation.◁

4.   Contact ulcers. The most frequent presentation of contact ulcers occurs in a male, between 40 and 50 years of age, working in a high-pres-

sure job that requires considerable use of voice, particularly in an authoritative or influential manner. Smoking, use of alcohol, air pollution, and extremes in temperature and humidity are contributory. Gastric reflux may be an important etiologic factor also.[28]

The patient may complain of musculoskeletal pain and dryness and often experiences pain on swallowing. He may also be aware of heartburn and gastric reflux. Voice evaluation reveals excessively low vocal pitch with accompanying low laryngeal position in the neck. Glottal fry phonation may intermittently occur, with reduced subglottal air pressure and respiratory drive. Harsh vocal quality and loud volume are the result of musculoskeletal tension and tight approximation of the vocal folds. Very frequent, strenuous throat-clearing is prevalent.

Voice therapy is directed toward eliminating excessive and intense voice use initially, to assist in healing of the ulcerated areas. Concurrently, reduction in musculoskeletal tension and elevation of laryngeal position is advised. Often vocal pitch will elevate spontaneously with this maneuver, but the patient must be counseled to accept the normal, albeit higher vocal pitch. Overall respiratory and glottal efficiency should be established to eliminate harshness and glottal fry. Environmental irritants, such as smoking and use of alcohol, should be at least minimized. Strenuous throat-clearing must be eliminated. Surgery and appropriate medication are necessary if conservative measures fail.

Psychogenic Dysphonia without Laryngeal Disease

1. Musculoskeletal tension dysphonia. Excessive hypercontraction of the extrinsic and intrinsic laryngeal muscles as a reaction to emotional stress underlies virtually all psychogenic voice disorders. However, the specific term ''musculoskeletal tension dysphonia'' is used to describe the vocal abnormality directly attributable to tense, rigid laryngeal musculature in the absence of significant vocal lesions. The disorder may emanate from primary emotional stresses varying from suppressed conflict to cancerophobia. Habitual hoarseness after laryngitis or vocal fold surgery for secondary gain or miscompensation may also be a factor.[29] Musculoskeletal tension dysphonia has also been reported in the presence of hyperventilation syndrome.[20]

Musculoskeletal tension may be observable, especially in the strap and jaw muscles. Aronson[2] suggests physical manipulation of the larynx to evaluate for discomfort or pain that occurs secondary to elevation of the larynx and hyoid bone. Additional sensations may include chest and cervical tightness, pain radiating to the ear, and globus, which is a foreign body sensation in the throat.

Characteristics associated with musculoskeletal tension dysphonia include harsh, rough, and strained vocal quality and restricted pitch and volume range. Breathy vocal quality may also be present, especially when vocal fold bowing occurs after long-term dysfunction. In severe cases, intermittent aphonia may also be observed.

Treatment involves counseling as well as techniques to improve vocal quality. Often, as critical emotional issues are discussed, voice improves dramatically. Patients are sometimes unwilling to discuss emotional issues, especially at the outset. In such cases, direct voice therapy, particularly digital laryngeal manipulation and easy onset of voice production will often result in rapid voice improvement. However, if the underlying emotional factors are never acknowledged, the risk of recurrence is high. Therefore, gentle persistence in probing for emotional conflict and providing counsel-

See also Chapter 9.

Aronson's[2] criteria for conversion reactions are: (1) Specific physical symptoms or syndromes that cannot be traced to anatomic or physiologic disease; (2) unconscious simulations of illness that the patient is convinced is of organic origin; (3) serves the psychologic purpose of enabling the patient to avoid awareness of emotional conflict, stress, or personal failure that would be emotionally intolerable if faced directly; and (4) can occur in any sensory or voluntary motor system. It is important to understand that the problem is not malingering (willful use of an abnormality for personal gain) or a fabricated dysfunction.

We consider treatment of the conversion disordered patient a near-emergency and initiate the voice evaluation immediately after the laryngologic examination whenever possible.—MH and HMT.

ing about the etiologic factors of the dysphonia are important for a lasting resolution.

2.   Dysphonia plicae ventricularis. Voice produced with the false vocal folds results in excessively harsh, low-pitched, strangled, or groaning quality. It is produced with extreme effort and is often a feature of severe musculoskeletal tension dysphonia. It is also observed in adductor spasmodic dysphonia. In addition, it may serve as a compensatory means of vocalization for those individuals with organically (most often neurologically) based limitations of true vocal fold function.

When dysphonia plicae ventricularis is used as a compensatory means of vocalization, treatment may not be appropriate. However, when it occurs as a result of musculoskeletal tension, techniques to encourage laryngeal relaxation are useful. If hypertrophic ventricular folds are persistent, surgical reduction with the laser may be helpful to prevent apposition of the false cords.◁

3.   Conversion voice disorders. Conversion reaction is a loss of voluntary control over normal sensory or motor function as a consequence of environmental stress or interpersonal conflict.[2]◁ Freud first explained the idea of conversion as a mechanism whereby an unbearable idea is rendered innocuous by having its energy transmuted into some bodily form of expression.

Vocal manifestations of conversion reaction can include muteness, aphonia, and dysphonia. These terms depict essentially a range of abnormality, from no speech production to articulation with no sound to whispering to various degrees of dysphonia. In all forms, conversation reaction results from the inability to express emotions, such as anger, fear, or grief, a breakdown in communications, and fear or shame in verbalizing feelings.

The onset of conversion reaction may be very sudden or may follow an upper respiratory infection or a lengthy period of voice rest. The patient may report a previous history of similar episodes with spontaneous recovery. A critical feature is that the patient indicates no insight into the possibility that emotional factors may be responsible for the vocal abnormality. In fact, the patient frequently has many theories regarding the possible organic contributions to the problem.

Treatment involves voice therapy to restore vocal function and counseling regarding the emotional issues involved. The voice therapy must be prompt and is usually quite short-term.◁ Direct voice therapy, especially in the case of aphonia, should aim to establish some form of vocal sound. This may involve involuntary throat-clearing or cough, which demonstrates the ability of the vocal folds to adduct. Gradual modification of this gross sound with encouragement for continued gains in voluntary control of vocalization will often lead to rather rapid normalization of voice production. Improvement in voice production depends on the ability of the patient to accept the change, which can be facilitated by a nonjudgmental and depersonalized approach to therapy. The reacquisition of more normal voice production provides an excellent starting point from which to discuss the underlying emotional issues. Following such a treatment session, a catharsis of the repressed emotion often results. However, there are cases in which, despite improvement in vocal function, the patient may continue to deny the possibility of emotional factors.

Referral for psychologic or psychiatric counseling is often appropriate and should be decided on an individual basis. For some patients, the resolution of the vocal dysfunction and emotional catharsis may be sufficient, but this depends on the depth of the emotional problem involved. Any uncertainty about the patient's psychologic and emotional status should initiate a referral for evaluation.

4. Mutational falsetto. Mutational falsetto is the failure to undergo expected change in voice that accompanies adolescence. The deviation from normal voice is not usually the result of a structural or physiologic abnormality of the larynx. ◁ Although the disorder has not been well identified, the underlying psychologic features seem to related to self-identification and resistance to normal transition into adulthood.

This disorder occurs from midteens up to the 50s or 60s. The voice is characterized as weak, hoarse, thin cracking, and high-pitched and gives an impression of immaturity and femininity. The laryngeal examination is normal.

Voice therapy for mutational falsetto is rapid. A sudden drop in vocal pitch is achieved by sharp glottal attack on high lung volume. Habituation of the lower pitch usually occurs in two to three sessions.

Aronson[2] discusses several factors other than psychologic that may be attributed to mutational falsetto: delayed maturation in endocrine disorders that alters timing of voice change, severe hearing loss, neurologic disease, and general debilitating disease associated with poor respiratory status.

Adductor Spasmodic Dysphonia

Adductor spasmodic dysphonia is a relatively uncommon but often severely disabling voice disorder that has received considerable attention in recent literature. Originally described by Taube in 1871 as a "spastic form of nervous hoarseness," the disorder is a squeezed, strained, choked, staccato, stuttering-like, jerky, grunting, groaning, effortful, pinched, and grating phonation caused by hyperadduction of the true and false vocal folds. Why the abnormality is observed in propositional speech, but often not during singing, laughing, crying, speaking in off-the-cuff utterances, and when speaking in an angry or high-pitched voice, has remained a mystery throughout the years. Despite variable levels of severity, the disorder often creates disastrous occupational, social, and emotional effects.

Previously, the etiology of spasmodic dysphonia was felt to be entirely psychogenic because of the discrepancy between speaking voice and the appearance of the larynx and because of the high incidence of traumatic or emotionally stressful events occurring at or around the time of onset. However, treatment with psychotherapy, hypnotism, biofeedback, and use of tranquilizing drugs has been consistently unsuccessful, thus strongly challenging the psychogenic theory.

Neurologic origin of adductor spasmodic dysphonia has been postulated in more recent years. Rabe and colleagues[30] concluded that spasmodic dysphonia was due to extrapyramidal lesions of possible postencephalitic etiology, after noting such signs as voice tremor, head and hand tremors, facial and tongue twitches, and hyperreflexia. Spasmodic dysphonia has been reported in association with other neurologic disorders and sites of lesion, specifically in the peripheral nervous system and brainstem. In addition to the extrapyramidal system, other neurological lesions have been suggested, specifically in the peripheral nervous system and the brainstem. ◁ In cases in which neither a psychogenic nor neurogenic cause can be reasonably concluded, the disease is labeled idiopathic.

Aronson[2] regards adductor spasmodic dysphonia as a voice sign of any one of several different causes: psychogenic, neurologic, or idiopathic. It is important to bear in mind that differentiation of clinical features and etiologic bases is far more than a semantic debate, since the treatment may widely differ, depending on the cause.

Onset of spasmodic dysphonia is typically in the fourth and fifth decades, although a range from teenage years to the 70s is reported. Male to female rations range from 1:1 to 1:4. The disorder usually is manifested as

Dysfunction of the peripheral nervous system was suggested when histopathologic studies of resected recurrent laryngeal nerves showed evidence of demyelinated nerve fibers in reports by Bocchino and Tucker[31] and Dedo, and Izdebski.[32] However, Ravits and colleagues[33] did not support this finding and further suggested that a peripheral nerve lesion would likely produce flaccidity, not spasticity, and would not allow for periodic normal voice production. Schaeffer[34] found evidence of brainstem dysfunction in visceral afferent-visceral efferent, subcoritcal-visceral efferent, and special somatic afferent pathways, suggestive of both somatic and visceral disease— HMT.

a mild hoarseness that is intermittent and fluctuates in severity. Most often, the severity and consistency increase over a period of a year to two, with gradual development of the characteristic strained, spasmodic quality. Few cases of spontaneous remission have been reported.

Both medical and psychologic factors have been associated with onset of the disease, including upper respiratory infection, cold, sore throat, or "flulike" symptoms. Psychologic factors included death of a relative, divorce or marital conflict, unremitting work stress, and continuous pressure.

Laryngologic examination in patients with adductor spasmodic dysphonia is usually normal, but occasionally hyperadduction of the true and perhaps false vocal folds may be observed. Rhythmic oscillations of the vocal folds are suggestive of associated vocal tremor.

The purpose of voice evaluation for suspected adductor spasmodic dysphonia is to confirm the diagnosis and to determine the type, if possible. To date, there are no clinically conclusive tests for confirmation. Therefore, signs and symptoms are observed but leave room for doubt regarding the cause of the problem.

Vocal characteristics of all types of adductor spasmodic dysphonia include strained, harsh vocal quality, random adductory voice arrest, usually intermittent glottal fry phonation, limited vocal volume in contextual speech (often with preserved ability to yell loudly), and restricted pitch range and variations. Voice arrest is most noticeable on vowel-initiated words, stressed syllables, or speech at loud volume. Typically, falsetto voice and vowel prolongation are produced more normally than other voice tasks. Severity may fluctuate according to the nature of the task. Associated signs of the considerable effort during voice production include facial grimace, eye blinks, and obvious extrinsic laryngeal, cervical, and chest muscle tension.

Neurogenic adductor spasmodic dysphonia is most easily recognized when tremor of the voice, head, lips, mandible, velum, pharynx, thorax or upper extremities is observed. Voice tremor is most noticeable on vowel prolongation and may be unrecognized in contextual speech, particularly when sharp adductory voice arrests are frequent. Lingual tremor may be noticed on prolonged "s." The presence of uncontrolled, involuntary movements of the head and neck or any other body musculature suggests dystonia.

Psychogenic adductor spasmodic dysphonia occurs from conversion reaction or musculoskeletal tension. Although presence of emotional stress or trauma at the onset and throughout the course of the vocal aberration does not definitively conclude a psychogenic cause, these factors must be carefully investigated. Wide variations in severity or lengthy periods of return to normal voice are suggestive of psychogenic origin. Voice improvement as the result of disclosure of emotionally laden information or during trial diagnostic voice therapy also is consistent with a psychogenic cause.

Voice therapy for adductor spasmodic dysphonia historically has been disappointing. Very little is offered in the literature to explain this fact. Therapy is most often recommended in the early stages, regardless of the cause, as a trial diagnostic procedure as well as treatment. Only in the most severe and long-standing cases, or if neurologic origin is firmly established, should voice therapy be dispensed with. Therapy goals include musculoskeletal tension reduction, establishing easy initiation of vocalization with adequate respiratory airflow and pressure, and elevation of vocal pitch, including elimination of glottal fry.

Surgical lysis of one recurrent laryngeal nerve for spasmodic dysphonia was first introduced by Dedo in 1976. The goal of the procedure is to prevent tight apposition of the vocal folds by paralyzing one of them and thus improving transglottic airflow. Results of this surgical procedure have been variable. In all reports, nearly 100 percent of patients experience marked or complete reduction of vocal strain and spasm and the accompanying physical effort immediately after surgery. Initially, voice tends to be breathy, hoarse, sometimes diplophonic, and uncontrolled. Intermittent strain and spasm sometimes persist as a result of habitual overeffort. Rhythmic vocal tremor is not altered by surgery. Voice typically becomes stronger over time, although most often not to complete recovery. Postoperative therapy is recommended to develop maximal control and eliminate patterns of vocal hyperadduction. Persistent restrictions in vocal loudness and control are often observed.

Of 306 surgically treated patients, 10 to 15 percent developed recurrent spasticity, usually 6 to 18 months postoperatively. Recurrence was related to presurgical severity.[35] A 3-year follow-up study of 33 patients showed a 65 percent failure rate to presurgical severity or worse. Vocal tremor was thought to be related to recurrence of spasticity patients.[36] Long-term results of 22 patients showed recurrence of some spasticity in 55 percent, not related to presurgical severity but did seem to be associated with vocal tremor.—MH and HMT.[37]

Recurrence of presurgical voice characteristics has been reported to varying degrees, although most often less severe than presurgically.◁ The pathophysiology of recurrence of spasticity has not been firmly established, but may involve overcompensation of the mobile cord[35] or regeneration of nerve potentials in the sectioned vocal fold.[38,39]

Further surgical procedures to modify voice include laser thinning, in the case of recurrence of spasmodic quality. Teflon injection has been utilized to improve glottic closure in persistent breathiness.

The diagnosis and treatment of adductor spasmodic dysphonia remains an enigma. Patients should receive comprehensive consultation regarding the nature of surgical intervention and its potential results. The profound emotional, social, and occupational implications of this disorder may warrant careful but aggressive treatment in the highly motivated and thoroughly educated patient.

Abductor Spasmodic Dysphonia

"Abductor spasmodic dysphonia" is a term used to identify a distinctive voice in which normal or hoarse voice is suddenly interrupted by brief moments of breathy or whispered segments. Abductor spasms are often triggered by voiceless consonants in initial positions of words.

Onset of the disorder is essentially the same as that of adductor spasmodic dysphonia; nonspecific hoarseness gradually progressing to abductor voice breaks occurs over several months. It may be associated with upper respiratory tract infection, emotional stress factors, or have no identifiable associated factors. Severity fluctuates with stress, fatigue, or vocal demands.

Aronson's[2] early data suggest that abductor spasmodic dysphonia may also be subdivided into psychogenic, neurologic, and idiopathic types. The neurogenic type described by Hartman and Aronson[41] was the abductor dysphonia of essential voice tremor. A psychogenic type associated with conversion reaction has also been described.[2]

The goal of voice evaluation is similar to that of adductor spasmodic dysphonia, in which possible etiologic factors are investigated. Thorough history and trial diagnostic voice therapy are the key ingredients. Voice therapy should aim toward development of better timing of voice initiation after unvoiced consonants. The success of therapy to date has been equivocal at best. On an experimental basis, Teflon injection of one or both vocal folds to narrow the glottis is suggested by Aronson.[2]

Voice Disorders of Professional Users

Although many of the vocal aberrations encountered are similar to those previously described, special consideration is necessary in the management of the professional voice user. This is particularly true for the actor or singer, whose voice is utilized during a performance in a manner that far exceeds the vocal demands and precision of other individuals. Singers are often concerned over very subtle and often nearly imperceptible vocal or laryngeal alterations. Their problems must be approached with great understanding and sensitivity, often on a semiemergency basis. Expedient and skillful treatment of the current complaint as well as investigation of previous problems and "trouble-shooting" to prevent future difficulties are all important components of patient management. A close working relationship among patient, laryngologist, speech pathologist, and voice teacher is critical to successful treatment of the professional. The experienced, well-trained singer usually has considerable insight into the vocal mechanism and often can provide information that points directly to the nature and source of the problem. The novice or amateur singer, on the other hand, may have only a vague awareness of the factors associated with his complaints. A complete history is essential to management. Specifically, it is important to determine if the problem is acute, chronic, or an exacerbation of a recurrent problem. Through careful interview, what may have initially seemed to be a new, acute problem may actually be found to have prior roots, although perhaps in a somewhat different manifestation.

The singer most frequently seeks treatment because of a change in the singing voice. Such alteration may include an actual change in vocal quality or even in an inability to sing, but more frequently involves one of the following: Inability to sing either extreme of the pitch range, discrete vocal or pitch break anywhere within the pitch range, limitation in control of volume, reduced endurance resulting in early fatigue, loss of full timbre or resonance, and inability to develop full singing voice. This latter is most often seen in voice students. Hoarseness may be a symptom, usually after a performance. The patient may sometimes present with a change in singing voice with little or no change in speaking voice or vice versa.

Alterations in vocal function may be accompanied by sensations of pain or discomfort, laryngeal fatigue, throat dryness, or excessive secretions. Otolaryngologic findings most often include vocal fold edema and inflammation or vocal nodules. Vocal fold hemorrhage or mucosal disruption are more serious conditions that are fortunately rare. The cause of the singer's complaints can include those common to any vocal or laryngeal disorder. Medical or physical, environmental, and behavioral factors may be involved singularly or in combination.

Medical factors often include conditions directly related to the head and neck, such as upper respiratory infection, sinusitis, allergies, or postnasal drip. Reflux laryngitis, resulting in chronic arytenoid and vocal fold irritation, may be present. Hormonal causes are most often experienced by females. Effects of menstrual cycle, particularly in the premenstrual period, pregnancy, and birth control pills may result in vocal fold edema. Any other medical illnesses or conditions affecting general health may have a deleterious effect on the finely tuned singing voice. Effects of aging are noticed particularly in the adolescent male, during which time the rapid growth of the larynx affects vocal control, and in the elderly singer, due to changes in muscle mass and condition of vocal fold tissue.

The singing voice is particularly susceptible to environmental conditions. Dust, pollutants, smoke, and extremes of temperature or humidity are examples of mucosal irritants that may have a deleterious effect on vocal function. Dryness is often experienced during travel on airplanes and in hotels. Singers are strongly encouraged to refrain from smoking, but singing in smoky environments cannot always be avoided. Poor room acoustics or excessive background instrumental volume can also contribute to the development of poor vocal technique. ◁

Behavioral factors relate to the manner in which the voice is produced

Rock singers, in particular, are subject to all of these factors, and yet are least likely to have good technical training to fall back on. If these performers are serious about a professional career, they must be willing to obtain professional training and to learn good vocal hygiene to spare their "instrument" for performances.—HMT.

and how it is utilized. Methods associated with dysfunction may include singing without adequate warm-up, singing with faulty or underdeveloped techniques, singing for excessively lengthy time periods, and pushing the voice past its comfortable and natural pitch and volume range. Faulty singing technique, most often noted in the novice or amateur singer, often involves inadequate or inappropriate respiratory support, excessive laryngeal tension, and deficient resonatory focus in the supraglottic, oral, and nasal cavities. Musculoskeletal tension, due to performance anxiety, stress, or other emotional conflicts is a common factor influencing vocal function. Even the most well-trained singer faces the possibility of alteration of the voice due to behavioral factors, because of the need for exquisite conditioning and control to maintain performance level skill, much as is true for the professional athlete. Therefore it is not surprising that singers often develop voice-related problems at peak points of their career, when extensive rehearsal, need for precise control, and stress are often at inflated levels.

Dissociation of singing and speaking voices is probably the most common cause of disorders in the excellent singer. Singers, especially those who are amateur or semiprofessional, tend to have difficulty acknowledging their own limits, and their dissatisfaction may lead to pushing the voice past its comfortable pitch and volume range.—RT Sataloff.[42]

Speaking voice misuse or abuse often occurs in the singer, frequently without recognition. Particularly at risk are singers who also direct choirs or teach vocal music to groups, because of the need to raise speaking volume over distance and background noise.◁

Treatment of disorders in singers requires careful consideration of all factors involved in the nature and cause of the problem. Treatment is often intensive, but it must also be conservative, so that development of further problems can be avoided while function is restored. All treatments must be considered within the context of the singer's performance schedule, so that a balance between resolution of the problem and maintenance of schedule can be accomplished whenever possible.

The importance of the singer's voice in his long-term career plans, the importance of the upcoming performance, and the consequences of canceling the concert must be seriously considered. In the frequent borderline conditions, the condition of the larynx must be weighed against other factors affecting the singer as an artist.—RT Sataloff.[42]

Modification of singing schedule is often necessary or advisable. In the presence of a hemorrhagic polyp or mucosal disruption, absolute voice rest (cancellation of performance) is essential until the condition is resolved. When edema or inflammation, such as an acute laryngitis, severely alters the voice, rest is strongly advised. With less severe or acute vocal conditions, such as mild edema or early vocal nodules, restriction of singing is preferred but is not as critical.◁ Under any of these conditions, speaking voice should be kept to a bare minimum. Following any modification of voice use, gradual resumption of use with careful reconditioning will be necessary.

Use of humidification and large intake of fluids is recommended for any condition causing dryness, irritation, or excessively thick secretions. It may be advisable for singers to limit the intake of milk products that can lead to copious secretions and resultant excessive throat-clearing. Pharmacologic treatment of infections includes the use of antibiotics. Antihistamines for the treatment of allergies should be very sparing to avoid excessive drying. Use of corticosteroids to treat inflammation should be short term and limited to those cases in which performance is mandatory. Mild diuretics may be prescribed for premenstrual fluid retention. Antacids may be helpful in treating reflux esophagitis, in addition to elevating the head of the bed and dietary restrictions.◁

One of the greatest problems faced by the clinician caring for performers is medication abuse. Careful investigation of current medications and education in drug management are essential.—Schechter and Coleman.[43]

Voice therapy for singers involves evaluation of vocal abuses and misuses. Depending on the nature of the vocal deviation, therapeutic techniques are applied in a manner similar to those described previously. In particular, singers are prone to musculoskeletal tension, which is treated through physical manipulation and relaxation. Musculoskeletal muscle condition may be maintained through stretching, strengthening, and conditioning exercise of the entire body.

See Chapter 9.

Surgical intervention for vocal fold lesions such as polyps should be considered *only* when all conservative measures have been exhausted.◁

When function of singing voice is not negatively affected by small residual nodules, surgical intervention should be avoided. Laser removal of the lesion should be performed only when chronic alteration of vocal function cannot be controlled behaviorly, with no guarantee that full vocal quality will be restored. Redevelopment of singing voice after surgery requires careful, systematic conditioning that often takes up to 6 months or more.

Management of Dysphagia

The specialist who works most actively with the dysphagic patient may be a speech pathologist, occupational or physical therapist, dietician, or nurse, depending on the clinical setting. It is our feeling that the speech pathologist is the preferred therapist because of strong background in anatomy and physiology of the upper aerodigestive tract, as well as close working relationships with otolaryngologists.—MH and HMT.

In keeping with the major thrust of this text, only those aspects of swallowing that primarily affect the larynx will be discussed. Other aspects will only be highlighted. Complete discussions of all aspects of swallowing can be found elsewhere.[44] Interest in evaluation and treatment of swallowing disorders has become widespread only in recent years. Best management of these problems must involve specialists from several disciplines, including speech pathologists, laryngologists, neurologists, gastroenterologists, dieticians, nursing staff, occupational therapists, and physical therapists.◁ The goal of any such program is the evaluation and treatment of dysphagia. The two major concerns of patients with dysphagia are aspiration, leading to potential pulmonary complications or airway obstruction, and inadequate nutritional status. These concerns necessitate expeditious but also judicious patient care.

Swallowing disorders are usually the result of neurologic or anatomic dysfunction. They can occur at any age, present acutely or gradually, and range in severity from minor alteration in dietary intake to a life-threatening condition.

Basic physiology of swallowing must be understood before considering its various dysfunctions. Logemann[44] divides the act of deglutition into four phases: (1) the oral preparatory phase that includes bolus placement and mastication; (2) the oral phase, when food is voluntarily propelled posteriorly until the swallowing reflex is triggered; (3) the pharyngeal phase when the reflex swallow carries the bolus through the pharynx; and (4) the esophageal phase, in which esophageal peristalsis carries the bolus through the cervical-thoracic esophagus and into the stomach.

In the oral preparatory phase the bolus is masticated as necessary, then pulled together between the tongue and the hard palate. Although these actions are voluntary, they are most often at a minimally conscious level. Adequate bolus preparation requires adequate saliva. The larynx and pharynx are at rest during this phase. The tongue then begins to move the bolus posteriorly to the oropharynx by pushing against the hard palate. When the bolus reaches the area of the anterior faucial pillars, the swallow reflex is triggered, following which involuntary action takes place without interruption in movement of the bolus until completion of the swallow. These involuntary actions include (1) elevation and retraction of the soft palate, anterior movement of the posterior pharynx, and medial movement of the lateral pharyngeal walls to accomplish *velopharyngeal closure;* (2) initiation of *pharyngeal peristalsis* by the pharyngeal constrictors to move the bolus rapidly through the pharynx; (3) *superior-anterior movement* of the *larynx;* (4) tight *closure* of the larynx at all three levels (epiglottis, false vocal folds, and true vocal folds); (5) *relaxation* of the *cricopharyngus* to allow passage of the bolus into the esophagus. The movement of the bolus into the pharynx is aided by negative pressure that results from laryngeal elevation. Without prompt triggering of the swallow reflex and controlled and coordinated execution of these involuntary activities, normal swallowing cannot take place.◁

Timing is critical in normal swallowing. The oral and pharyngeal phases typically take only 1 second each. When the timing is significantly delayed, laryngeal closure may not be coordinated, which can result in aspiration.—J Logemann.[44]

Neurologic control of swallowing involves both sensory and motor components. The swallow reflex is triggered through receptors in the fauces, tonsils, soft palate, base of tongue and posterior pharyngeal wall, and sensory impulses reach the medullary reticular formation in the brainstem through the seventh, ninth, and tenth cranial nerves. Efferent function is mediated through the ninth, tenth, and twelfth cranial nerves. Cricopharyngeal sphincter relaxation occurs reflexively when the bolus reaches the posterior pharyngeal wall. Cortical input to the control of swallowing is not well understood but is thought to play a role also.

Dysfunction at any level of the alimentary tract can result in dysphagia. At the level of the larynx, causes of dysphagia can be either direct or indirect. A direct effect results from disturbance to the larynx itself, from anatomic or neurologic alterations. An indirect one occurs when abnormality at another level affects laryngeal closure, so that the airway remains unprotected in the presence of a bolus remnant. In either case, aspiration may result.

Aspiration may occur at three separate junctures: before the swallow, during the swallow, and after the swallow. Aspiration may occur before the swallow due to reduced tongue control, which allows the bolus to fall over the base of the tongue and thus into an unprotected airway. This can also follow if sensory impairment results in delayed or absent triggering of the swallow reflex. Aspiration during the swallow results from insufficiently tight closure of the laryngeal sphincters or from reduced laryngeal elevation. Aspiration after the swallow can be caused by inadequate pharyngeal peristalsis or cricopharyngeal hypertonicity. In either case, remnant of the bolus remains in the pharynx after the swallow is completed and can be sucked into the airway as the larynx relaxes.

A variety of neurologic conditions can affect laryngeal control during swallowing. In the case of a cerebral vascular accident, tumor, or trauma in the brainstem, subcortex, or bicortical areas, the major disruptions in swallowing include *delayed triggering* of the swallow reflex and *cricopharyngeal dysfunction.* Isolated *unilateral vocal fold paralysis* may result in incomplete laryngeal elevation and closure, but typically aspiration is minimal in these cases. Degenerative disease such as *myasthenia gravis* may result in disruption of the swallow reflex, reduced pharyngeal peristalsis, dysfunction of the cricopharyngus, and incomplete laryngeal closure, all of which typically become more prominent with fatigue. In *amyotrophic lateral sclerosis,* premature swallow, delayed or absent swallow reflex, reduced pharyngeal peristalsis, cricopharyngeal hypertonicity, and reduced laryngeal closure may be noted. In *Parkinson's disease,* delayed swallowing reflex and reduced pharyngeal peristalsis are seen most often.

Anatomic causes for dysphagia often include surgical excision of structures due to cancer. Standard *hemilaryngectomy*◁ typically involves removal of the true vocal fold, the ventrical and false vocal fold, but excludes the arytenoid cartilage and preserves the hyoid bone and epiglottis. Most investigators have reported rapid reacquisition of swallowing function postoperatively. However, when the resection extends to the arytenoid cartilage, the risk of permanent aspiration is reportedly much higher.◁

Supraglottic laryngectomy includes removal of the epiglottis, aryepiglottic folds, and false vocal cords and may require removal of one or both superior laryngeal nerves. The hyoid bone may or may not be removed. Postoperatively, difficulty in swallowing can persist for several weeks, particularly for liquids. Dysfunction occurs because of lack of bolus control at the base of the tongue, reduced pharyngeal peristalsis, and cricopharyngeal dyssynergia and aspiration primarily due to limitations in lar-

See Chapter 13.

Aspiration to some extent, even when not clinically apparent, has been demonstrated in hemilaryngectomized patients. The issue of how much aspiration is tolerable has not been answered.[45] *Several patients with hemilaryngectomy have been reported who were unable to regain the ability to swallow liquids.—MH and HMT.*

See Chapter 13.

Flores and coworkers[47] found myotomy to be helpful when performed primarily but not as a secondary procedure.

yngeal elevation and closure. Swallowing is facilitated by development of the compensatory "supraglottic swallow."◁

When "standard" supraglottic laryngectomy must be extended superiorly or inferiorly, or includes the pyriform sinus, chances for prolonged dysfunction are increased. When part of the base of the tongue is removed, laryngeal elevation may be further compromised and a precipitous drop from the tongue to the airway can result. Supraglottic laryngectomized patients with base of tongue extension have a greater that 50 percent chance of significant aspiration.[46] When the resection includes part of one vocal fold or arytenoid, laryngeal closure may be compromised and may lead to chronic aspiration because compensatory vocal fold adduction cannot be developed. Patients with extension to all or part of the arytenoid cartilage spend a minimum of 2 months and more frequently 6 to 12 months attempting rehabilitation. Some patients never regain swallowing function. The characteristics that are associated with the best prognosis for rehabilitation after supraglottic resections include mobile tongue base, larynx able to rise far enough to meet the tongue base, resected hyoid bone, and capability for bilateral approximation of the vocal fold. There is controversy about the value of cricopharyngeal myotomy at the time of surgery, but most agree that it is useful when the hyoid or arytenoid cartilage must be sacrificed.◁

Total laryngectomy may result in dysphagia due to reduced pharyngeal peristalsis, anatomic structure of the pharynx, or development of a scarband that provides a pocket for food collection in the upper pharynx. Dysfunction of the cricopharyngus is also a possible cause.

Thorough evaluation is necessary in order to determine the nature and cause of the swallowing disorder, including clinical and radiographic swallowing assessments and laryngeal examination. Esophageal manometry can provide important information in some cases. This clinical swallowing evaluation should involve review of general medical condition, mental status, presence of tracheotomy tube or nasogastric tube. Onset, course, description, and location of dysfunction are important historical concerns. Oral-motor and sensory examinations are necessary to identify anatomic abnormalities, range and strength of motion, and presence or absence of normal and abnormal reflexes. Basic assessment of vocal quality, particularly noting breathiness, wet hoarseness, and glottic insufficiency, is performed. Secretions in the posterior oral cavity and the patient's ability to clear them voluntarily should be noted.

Clinical observations of food intake must be performed with caution, particularly if the degree of dysphagia is severe enough to warrant the use of alternative feeding. Attention is directed to the timing and completeness of oral transmission, time necessary to trigger the swallow reflex, extent of laryngeal movement during swallowing, presence of coughing or throat clearing either during or subsequent to swallowing, and voice quality after completion of a swallow. These observations are made separately for liquid, paste, and solid consistencies.

Tracheotomy tubes often are a disturbance to swallowing and must be considered at the time of the evaluation. The tracheotomy tube may inhibit laryngeal elevation, may impinge on the tracheoesophageal party wall and obstruct bolus passage, especially when an inflated cuffed tube is used, and may allow leakage of air, thus interfering with necessary elevation in subglottic pressure. If the cuff must be inflated to restrict aspiration of saliva and food, swallowing rehabilitation should be deferred. Whenever possible, the tracheotomy tube should be occluded digitally or plugged during swallows, to minimize leakage of subglottic air pressure. If swallowing intervention is initiated after removal of the tracheotomy tube (which is preferable), time for complete closure of the site should be allowed.

Radiographic assessment to compliment clinical evaluation is usually necessary to identify silent aspiration as well as to determine with greater precision the location of abnormality and how varied consistencies and technique affect swallowing function. A modified barium swallow is recommended to minimize aspiration, in both the lateral and anteroposterior planes. Liquid, paste, and solid consistencies in very small amounts are all utilized to judge their potential effects.

Esophageal manometry can identify disruption in peristalsis through the pharynx and esophagus and to diagnose disorders in the upper or lower esophageal sphincters. It is performed with pressure transducers that are passed into the esophagus and record changing pressures at various levels during swallowing. Manometry may substantiate cricopharyngeal dysfunction and is particularly useful in diagnosing achalasia, diffuse spasm of the esophagus, aperistalsis, and other unclassified motor disorders of the esophagus.

Therapy for swallowing disorders follows similar principles to those for voice disorders, aiming for development of conscious voluntary control over a mechanical activity that is normally unconscious and reflexive. The goal is timely and adequate intake of food without aspiration. The patient should be sufficiently alert to be able to cooperate and medical status must not be so tenuous that even mild aspiration cannot be tolerated.

General Therapy Techniques

1. Posture and positioning. When laryngeal closure is a factor, the patient should be positioned upright or with the head slightly forward of midline. With unilateral laryngeal or pharyngeal involvement, tilting the head toward the stronger side or turning the head toward the affected side is suggested.
2. Supraglottic swallow. Whenever laryngeal closure must be maximized, this strategy may be effective. It involves tight breath-holding during the swallow, followed by throat-clearing and second swallow.
3. Multiple swallows. Swallowing several times per bolus can aid pharyngeal transmission and prevent aspiration when bolus retention occurs. Interspersing frequent throat-clearing between active swallows is also recommended to clear the airway.
4. Improved timing. Voluntary holding of the bolus in the oral cavity before activation of a conscious, voluntary swallow may aid in triggering the swallow reflex. This is particularly helpful when lengthy reflex delay is unrecognized by the patient and may thus alleviate premature additional intake of food.
5. Controlled bolus size. Small bolus size may limit aspiration, particularly when pharyngeal peristalsis is reduced and laryngeal closure is incomplete.
6. Variation in texture, taste, and temperature of the bolus. Varying these aspects of substances may provide additional stimulation when the swallow reflex is delayed. Also altering consistency may aid in pharyngeal transmission of bolus remnants.

Techniques to aid preparation for swallowing, even when patients are not yet candidates for oral intake, are also very helpful. They may include the following: (1) Stimulation of swallow reflex: use of a wet, iced cotton swab or small laryngeal mirror to stimulate the area of the anterior faucial pillars is suggested. This may then be followed by introduction of a very small amount of liquid to stimulate a swallow reflex; (2) oral exercises: increasing range and strength of tongue mobility can help in controlling premature bolus transmission; (3) laryngeal adduction exercise.

A swallowing disorder may represent significant nutritional and medical risk to the patient. In addition, it can severely affect the patient emotionally and socially, because eating represents the natural and gratifying fulfillment of a basic need. The challenge of treating the dysphagic patient lies not only in managing the physical factors, but also in providing necessary emotional and psychologic support.

References

1. Perkins WH: Vocal function: A behavioral analysis. In Travis LE (Ed): Handbook of Speech Pathology and Audiology. New York, Appleton-Century-Crofts, 1971.

2. Aronson AE: Clinical Voice Disorders, 2nd ed. New York, Thieme, 1985.

3. Vandenberg J, Moolenaar-Bijl AJ: Cricopharyngeal sphincter, pitch, intensity and fluency in oesophageal speech. Pract Otorhinolaryngol, 21:298–315, 1959.

4. Moore PG: *Organic Voice Disorders*. Englewood Cliffs, NJ, Prentice-Hall, 1971.

5. Ward PH, Hanson DG, Berci G: Observations in central neurologic etiology for laryngeal dysfunction. Ann Otol Rhinol Laryngol, 90:430–441, 1981.

6. Froeschels E: Chewing method as therapy. Arch Otolaryngol, 56:427–434, 1952.

7. Prasek RA, Montgomery AA, Walden BE, Schwartz DM: EMG biofeedback in the treatment of hyperfunctional voice disorder. J Speech Hear Disord, 43:282–294, 1978.

8. Boone DR: The Voice and Voice Therapy. Englewood Cliffs, NJ: Prentice-Hall, 1971.

9. Froeschels E, Kastein S, Weiss DA: A method of therapy for paralytic conditions of the mechanisms of phonation, respiration and glutination. J Speech Hear Discord, 20:365–370, 1955.

10. Tucker HM, Rusnov M, Cohen L: Speech development in aphonic children. Laryngoscope, 92:566, 1982.

11. Kaslon KW, Grabow DE, Ruben KJ: Voice, speech and language habilitation in young children without laryngeal function. Arch Otolaryngol, 104:737–739, 1978.

12. Stoicheff ML, Ciampi A, Passi JE, Frederickson JM: The irradiated larynx and voice: A perceptual study. J Speech Hear Res, 26:482–485, 1983.

13. Darley FL, Aronson AE, Brown JR: Differential diagnostic patterns of dysarthria. J Speech Hear Res, 12:246–269, 1969.

14. Darley FL, Aronson AE, Brown JR: Clusters of deviant speech dimensions in the dysarthrias. J Speech Hear Res, 12:462–496, 1969.

15. Neiman RF, Mountjoy JR, Allen EL: Myasthenia gravis focal to the larynx. Arch Otolaryngol, 101:569–570, 1975.

16. Hanson DG, Gerratt BR, Ward PH: Glottographic measurement of vocal dysfunction, Ann Otol Rhinol Laryngol, 92:413–420, 1983.

17. Aronson AE, Hartman DE: Adductor spastic dysphonia as a sign of essential (voice) tremor. J Speech Hear Disord, 46:52–58, 1981.

18. Hartman DE, Overhold SL, Vishwanat B: A case of vocal nodules masking essential (voice) tremor. Arch Otolaryngol, 108:52–54, 1982.

19. Sorenson P, Paulson D, Steiness E, et al: Essential tremor treated with propranolol: Lack of correlation between clinical effect and plasma propranolol levels. Ann Neurol, 9:53–57, 1981.

20. Greene M: The Voice and Its Disorders. Philadelphia, JB Lippincott, 1972, p. 130.

21. Luchsinger R, Arnold GE: Voice-Speech-Language. Belmont, CA, Wadsworth Publishing, 1965.

22. Brodnitz FS: Psychological considerations in vocal rehabilitation. J Speech Hear Disord, 56:21–26, 1981.

23. Barker KD, Wilson FB: Comparative study of vocal utilization of children with hoarseness and normal voice. Paper presented at the convention of the American-Speech-Hearing Association, Chicago, 1976.

24. Fisher HB, Logemann JA: Objective evaluation of therapy for vocal nodules: A case report. J Speech Hear Disord, 35:277–284, 1970.

25. Reed CG: Voice therapy: A need for research. J Speech Hear Disord, 45:157–169, 1980.

26. Kleinsasser O: Pathogenesis of vocal cord polyps. Ann Otol Rhinol Laryngol, 91:378–381, 1982.

27. Wolfe VI, Rotusnik DL: Vocal symptomatology of postoperative dysphonia. Laryngoscope, 92:635–643, 1981.

28. Kambič V, Radsel Z: Acid posterior laryn-

gitis. J Laryngol Otol, 98:1237–1240, 1984.

29. Kaufman JA, Blalock PD: Classification and approach to patients with functional voice disorders. Ann Otol Rhinol Laryngol, 91:372–377, 1982.

30. Rabe E, Brumlik J, Moore P: A study of spastic dysphonia. Laryngoscope, 70:219–245, 1960.

31. Bocchino JV, Tucker HM: Recurrent laryngeal nerve pathology in spasmodic dysphonia. Laryngoscope, 88:1274–1278, 1978.

32. Dedo HH, Izdebski K: Intermediate results of 306 recurrent laryngeal nerve sections for spastic dysphonia. Laryngoscope, 93:9–16, 1983.

33. Ravits JM, Aronson AE, DeSanto LW, Dyck PJ: No morphometric abnormality of recurrent laryngeal nerve in spastic dysphonia. *Neurology* (New York) 29:1376–1382, 1979.

34. Schaeffer SD: Neuropathology of spasmodic dysphonia. Laryngoscope, 93:1183–1204, 1983.

35. Dedo HH, Izdebski K: Problems with surgical (RLN section) treatment of spastic dysphonia. Laryngoscope, 93: 268–271, 1983.

36. Aronson AE, DeSanto LW: Adductor spastic dysphonia: Three years after recurrent laryngeal nerve resection. Laryngoscope, 93:1–8, 1983.

37. Harrison M, Tucker H: Unpublished data, 1986.

38. Fritzell B, Feuer E, Haglund S, Knutsson E, Schiratzki H: Experiences with recurrent laryngeal nerve section for spastic dysphonia. Folia Phoniatr, 34:160–167, 1982.

39. Wilson FB, Oldring DJ, Mueller K: Recurrent laryngeal nerve section: A case report involving return of spastic dysphonia after initial surgery. J Speech Hear Disord, 45:112–118, 1980.

40. Dedo HH, Izdebski K: Evaluation and treatment of recurrent spasticity after recurrent laryngeal nerve section. Ann Otol Rhinol Laryngol, 93:343–345, 1984.

41. Hartman DE, Aronson AE: Clinical investigations of intermittent breathy dysphonia. J Speech Hear Disord, 46:428–432, 1981. 43:282–294, 1978.

42. Sataloff RT: Professional singers: The science and art of clinical care. Am J Otolaryngol, 2:251–266, 1981.

43. Schechter GL, Coleman RF: Care of the professional voice. *Otolaryngol Clin North Am,* 17:131–137, 1984.

44. Logemann J: Evaluation and Treatment of Swallowing Disorders. San Diego, College-Hill Press, 1983.

45. Schoenrock LD, King AY, Everts EC, Schneider HJ, Shumrich DA: Hemilaryngectomy: Deglutition evaluation and rehabilitation. Trans Am Acad Ophthalmol Otolaryngol, 76:752–757, 1972.

46. Logemann JA, Bytell DE: Swallowing disorders in three types of head and neck surgical patients. Cancer, 44:1095–1105, 1979.

47. Flores TC, Wood BG, Koegel L, Levine HL, Tucker HM: Factors in successful deglutition following supraglottic laryngeal surgery. Ann Otol Rhinol Laryngol, 91:579–583, 1982.

Chapter 6

Laryngoscopy, Endoscopic Surgery, and Special Techniques

The vast majority of so-called primary care physicians do not include visualization of the larynx in their "complete" physical examinations. If one considers the potential for earlier detection of significant disease, it is apparent that mastery of mirror laryngoscopy should be required in all medical curricula.—HMT

The otolaryngologist-head and neck surgeon is able to visualize and, when necessary, manipulate the larynx and adjacent structures. As a result, he can usually ascertain the cause of voice and airway symptoms by indirect mirror laryngoscopy, without the need for radiologic intervention, anesthesia, or direct laryngoscopy.[1] Skill in this necessary technique will, therefore, be essential to all other aspects of diagnosis and management of laryngeal disorders.

Indirect Examination

Mirror Laryngoscopy

The *materials* required for mirror laryngoscopy include head mirror and light source or headlight, laryngeal mirrors (no. 5 or no. 6 in adults), a mirror warmer, gauze pads, and, occasionally, a topical anesthetic. The patient sits in a straight-backed chair raised to place his head at the same level as the examiner's, who may carry out the procedure in either a sitting or standing position. A head mirror (or electric headlight) is positioned firmly, as close to the examiner's nose or eyeglasses as possible, and focused so that the light is directed exactly wherever the examiner looks. If a head mirror and movable lamp are used, the bulb should be positioned at or slightly above the level of the patient's and examiner's heads and as close to the patient as possible (Fig. 6–1). This provides as acute an angle between the light source, the head mirror, and the point of examination as possible and will thus achieve the brightest and most sharply focused illumination.

Best visualization can be had if the patient assumes a *"sniffling" position* (Fig. 6–2), with the head extended on the neck and the neck flexed forward on the torso. This creates the straightest possible line of sight between the uvula and the plane of the glottis. The procedure is briefly explained to the patient, reassuring him that he will be able to breathe without difficulty throughout. The confidence and positive attitudes presented by the examiner are very important in relaxing the patient and permitting a successful examination. The patient is asked to extend his tongue, which is gently wrapped with a gauze pad. Using his left hand, the examiner grasps the tongue between his thumb (above) and second finger, (which protects

Figure 6–1. Proper positioning
of the patient, head mirror, and
the light source provides
optimal illumination.

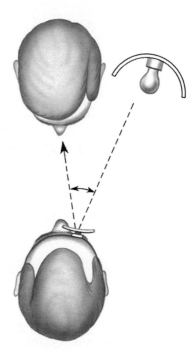

the undersurface of the tongue from the lower teeth) and pulls it out and
down, having placed his index finger against the upper teeth and lip to stabilize them (Figs. 6–3 and 6–4). The patient is asked to inspire, a maneuver that elevates the palate, depresses the tongue, and dilates the faucial
pillars, thus providing the widest possible opening for placement of the
mirror.

An appropriately sized mirror is grasped in the right hand between the

Figure 6–2. The ''sniffing''
position.

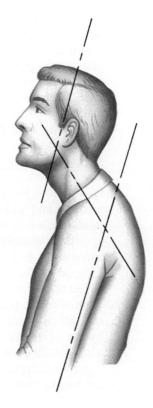

Figure 6–3. Proper position of hand while grasping patient's tongue.

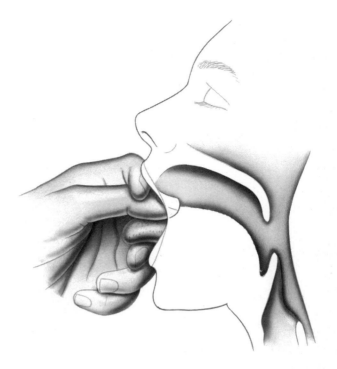

thumb and first two fingers, much as if it were a dart to be thrown. With experience, the examiner will be able to estimate how much of the length of the mirror must be available to reach the posterior palate and still permit proper positioning of the right hand during the examination. The position of the patient is checked and the mirror is warmed using an alcohol flame, by dipping it into hot ceramic beads, hot water, or, if nothing else is available, by holding the glass surface of the mirror to the exposed light bulb, so that it will not be fogged by the patient's breath. Immediately after warming and checking the temperature against the back of the examiner's hand, the mirror is inserted into the patient's mouth and its posterior surface is brought smoothly into contact with the soft palate and uvula. In an essentially continuous motion, the soft palate is displaced posteriorly and superiorly toward, but not touching, the posterior pharyngeal wall

Figure 6–4. Note use of second finger as a roller or fulcrum over which the upper surface of the patient's tongue can be ''rolled'' out to flatten its surface.

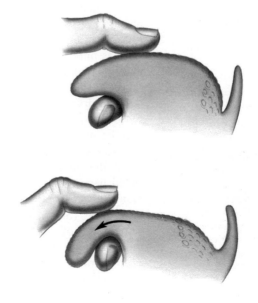

Figure 6–5. Position of laryngeal mirror against soft palate, but not touching the posterior pharyngeal wall.

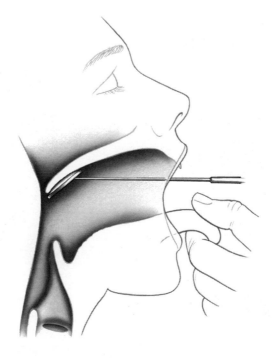

No receptors for the physiologic gag reflex are situated anterior to the tonsillar pillars. Therefore, if care is taken to avoid touching the posterior pharyngeal wall or the posterior tonsillar pillars with the mirror or by displacement of the uvula, any gagging that may occur will be of psychological origin. Such gagging always fatigues if the examiner persists judiciously. Moreover, the first stages of regurgitation, should they occur, can usually be anticipated and aborted by quickly removing the mirror and pushing the chin upward smartly to close the mouth and extend the head. With attention to detail of technique and good rapport, it should be possible to examine at least 80 to 90 percent of all patients without anesthesia, and most of the rest with light topical anesthesia.—HMT

Mirror examination provides only a two-dimensional view of the larynx. As a result, it is easy to be misled regarding the position of structures relative to each other or to the apparent plane of the glottis. With experience, rapid, very slight changes in the position of the mirror can be substituted for depth perception by providing slightly different angles of observation. Slight differences in color can also alert the examiner that the two vocal folds may be at different levels.[2]—HMT

(Fig. 6–5). If properly done, the little finger of the hand holding the mirror can be rested against either the patient's cheek or the fingers of the examiner's other hand holding the tongue, thus creating a single unit of the patient's head, the examiner's hands, and the mirror. Once a good position has been achieved, only the reflecting surface of the mirror should be moved, and that only by minimal rotation to obtain the proper angulation for fine adjustment of the view of the larynx. In this manner, most patients can be successfully examined without recourse to topical anesthesia.◁

In most cases, if the mirror has been properly placed, the epiglottis and vocal folds will be immediately in view (Fig. 6–6a and b). At most, minor adjustments in positioning of the mirror should be required. The base of tongue, supraglottic larynx, pyriform sinuses, and postcricoid areas should be visualized first. Thereafter, the false and true vocal folds can be observed, first in quiet respiration, then during deep inspiration, and finally during phonation.

Orderly examination of the peripheral structures and in the same sequence every time, before observing the vocal folds themselves, may avoid missing minor but important findings in other areas. Obvious mass lesions, such as tumors, polyps, or papillomas, should not distract the observer from gaining maximum information by carrying out a full examination of the other, perhaps less obvious structures. It is also important to record color, unusual dryness, the presence or absence of secretions, and aberrations in normal motion or position, as well as the more obvious mass lesions that may be present.◁

Local anesthesia should rarely be required, but, when it is, it may make the different between a successful examination and a totally frustrated patient and examiner. Personally, I have used Cetacaine[r] spray, but many other preparations are available for this purpose that will serve satisfactorily. (See also Anesthesia for Direct Endoscopy.) In some patients, 5 to 10 mg of diazepam (Valium) given intravenously will ablate the gag reflex enough to permit examination when other techniques have failed.[3] Such intravenous medications should not be given, however, unless the physician is prepared to monitor the patient adequately until they wear off

Figure 6–6. **a,** View of larynx
at rest. **b,** Mirror view of larynx
during vigorous inspiration.

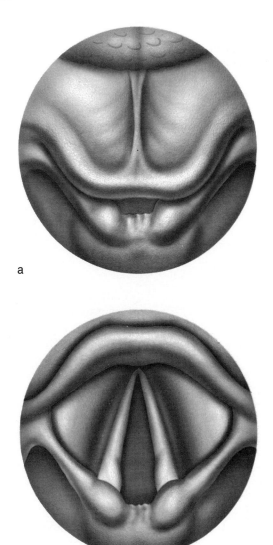

a

b

or to intubate and support circulation intravenously, if necessary. Finally, there are occasional patients who simply cannot or will not cooperate for an indirect examination under any circumstances. In these cases, only flexible, fiberoptic laryngoscopy or direct laryngoscopy under general anesthesia will suffice.

Telescopy and Fiberoptic Laryngoscopy

In recent years, various angulated *telescopes* with integral light sources have been developed to permit visualization of the larynx. They have the distinct advantages that they magnify the larynx, permit photography or videotaping, and can sometimes be coupled to an observer's port for teaching purposes. Their disadvantages include significant expense, more time required for examination, more frequent need for anesthesia than for mirror examination, and interference with development of indirect mirror laryngoscopy skills. However, if properly used as an *adjunct* to mirror laryngoscopy, telescopes can provide additional valuable information and documentation.

The *flexible, fiberoptic laryngoscope* has most of the same advantages and disadvantages as telescopes, but it is clearly superior in allowing visualization under circumstances in which mirrors or telescopes may fail.

Anesthesia and decongestion of the nostril through which the scope will be passed is generally required, and the picture, although quite satisfactory, is usually smaller and less sharp than that which can be provided by telescopy because it is obtained via a fiberoptic bundle. However, with its flexible tip, the fiberoptic laryngoscope can "get past" an overhanging epiglottis or other obstruction to direct visualization and can be used in patients who are unable to sit up, open the mouth, or extend the head. In these latter circumstances, it may be the only way to visualize the larynx. The well-prepared otolaryngologist-head and neck surgeon must master mirror laryngoscopy, but should also have the equipment and capability to perform fiberoptic laryngoscopy and telescopy when those techniques are called for, if only to permit photographic documentation.

Direct Examination

Although indirect manipulation and biopsy of the larynx are possible using appropriately curved instruments and under local anesthesia, with the common use of general anesthesia for operative laryngoscopy this technique has generally fallen from favor. When indirect laryngoscopy is inadequate, if palpation is required to distinguish paralysis from fixation, or when biopsies or removal of lesions are required, *direct laryngoscopy* is usually carried out.

Anesthesia for Direct Endoscopy

If properly applied, excellent *local anesthesia* of the pharynx, larynx, esophagus, and adjacent structures can be obtained that will permit most rigid endoscopic procedures (bronchoscopy, laryngoscopy, esophagoscopy) to be carried out without difficulty or significant discomfort to the patient. Examination, palpation, biopsy, and most endoscopic surgical procedures that require no more than 5 to 10 minutes can be undertaken in this manner. The major *limiting factor* is not the adequacy of the local anesthesia, but the discomfort from pressure of the instruments on the teeth and other oral structures, as well as the difficult position that must be maintained during the examination. Operative procedures, such as laser surgery and endoscopic arytenoidectomy, generally are not attempted under local anesthesia, but most other endoscopic procedures can be. In addition to Teflon[r] injection, which should almost always be carried out with the patient awake,◁ the effort to be more cost effective is providing an impetus to return to local anesthesia for the bulk of adult endoscopic procedures.

See Chapter 11.

Premedication is commonly used, but I have generally found it to be unnecessary. A common regimen consists of: pentobarbital 150–200 mg, orally 1 hour before the procedure; meperidine hydrochloride 50 to 100 mg and hydroxyzine 25 to 50 mg, intramuscularly on call to the operating room; and atropine 0.2 to 0.4 mg, intramuscularly on call to operating room. (The atropine should be deleted if bronchoscopy to obtain secretions for culture or cytology is intended.) The exact dosages are determined by the weight and age of the patient. Such premedication usually results in the patient sleeping quietly on entering the operating room. Usually, he can be aroused to take part in the procedure and then falls back to sleep afterward. There is also usually some degree of amnesia. However, I have found that if good rapport has been established, premedication really adds little to the patient's comfort and may interfere in his ability to cooperate. It also results in an unnecessarily long stay in the recovery room.

The *technique* of *local anesthesia* that I use is modified from that described by Jackson.[4] The *materials* needed include: Cetacaine spray; tetracaine 0.5 percent solution;◁ a control syringe with a malleable cannula; gauze pads; laryngeal mirrors; hot water or other means to warm the mirror; and a headlight.

The patient sits on the operating room table, legs over the side and feet resting on a stool. A nurse stands behind the patient to help stabilize him. The posterior pharynx is sprayed with Cetacaine to obtain initial topical anesthesia. After 1 or 2 minutes, the patient is asked to extend his tongue, it is wrapped with a gauze pad and the patient holds it with his right hand. The malleable cannula is bent at its tip to approximately a 90° angle and the surgeon draws 0.5 to 1.0 ml of tetracaine solution into the control syringe. The patient opens his mouth and pulls his tongue out and down. The examiner uses a warmed laryngeal mirror in his right hand to visualize the larynx and the cannula is inserted using the left hand. The tip of the cannula, which can now be seen in the mirror, is aimed at the glottis and the patient is asked to inspire. At precisely that moment, the contents of the syringe is discharged into the trachea, between the abducted vocal folds. If successful, the patient will immediately cough, thus creating an aerosol and distributing the anesthetic over all the laryngeal and hypopharyngeal surfaces. Frequently, the first application of anesthetic is really all that is required, but, in some cases, two or three further applications are necessary. Successful anesthesia has been achieved if the patient no longer coughs or gags when anesthetic is sprayed on the vocal folds. It is not necessary to place cotton pledgets soaked in anesthetic into the pyriform sinuses, as is suggested by some investigators when using this technique. Precisely the same approach will provide adequate anesthesia for both bronchoscopy and esophagoscopy, since little or no anesthesia is required within the esophagus itself and additional solution can be instilled into the trachea and bronchi through the bronchoscope, if needed. Although no further anesthesia than that provided by this technique is generally necessary, infiltration of the superior laryngeal nerves using lidocaine injection has also been recommended.[7]

General anesthesia for endoscopy requires confidence and close cooperation between the endoscopist and the anesthesiologist, since they will be in competition for control of the airway. It is essential for the anesthesiologist to know that the surgeon is able to restore airway control at any time during the procedure. If any mechanical problem exists that may interfere with intubation, the otolaryngologist must discuss it with the anesthesiologist, so that he is forewarned of the problem or plans can be made for other means of obtaining an airway.◁

For most endoscopic procedures under general anesthesia, a small bore endotracheal tube with a large, soft cuff is satisfactory. In general, the smallest tube possible to permit adequate oxygenation and removal of carbon dioxide should be used. Such an approach, using a tube as small as 5.5 to 6.5 mm outer diameter in adults can provide safe ventilation for at least 1 hour.[8] Alternative techniques include Venturi jet insufflation,[9] placement of a small bore catheter for mass transfer ventilation, and the use of the Carden tube.[10] If laser surgery is contemplated, the endotracheal tube should be wrapped with metallic tape over its entire length from the balloon to the point at which the filler channel leaves the body of the main tube (see later).

The usual conduct of anesthesia for endoscopy includes intravenous

"Pontocaine (tetracaine) . . . is at the same time the most effective and most toxic of the 'caine' drugs after cocaine itself. It is effective, however, in dilute solutions and therefore can be used safely, provided it is applied accurately and the total dose used at any one time does not exceed the maximal recommended dose of 80 mg."[5] I do not exceed 8 ml of 0.5 percent solution so that not more than half the recommended dose is used in any individual case. Experience with more than 1000 cases using this technique has failed to reveal a single true toxic reaction.[6]—HMT

It is often possible to intubate with a bronchoscope when an endotracheal tube will not suffice. If need be, tracheotomy can then be carried out as a semielective procedure. The decision to gain control of the airway by any means other than normal intubation should be made in consultation with the anesthesiologist, but remains the ultimate responsibility of the otolaryngologist.—HMT

induction with thiopental sodium, use of a paralytic agent, placement of topical anesthesia before intubation to minimize cardiac arrhythmia in response to laryngotracheal stimulation, and maintenance of anesthesia with halothane, nitrous oxide, and oxygen.

Selection of Laryngoscopes

There are several types of laryngoscopes available (Fig. 6–7), which suggests that each of them has certain advantages over the others. However, there are only three basic types in common usage. These include the slide laryngoscope, the anterior commissure type, and the suspension type.

The *slide laryngoscope* is designed to visualize the vocal folds by placing its fluted tip into the valleculae, pressing forward against the base of the tongue, and lifting the epiglottis to permit passage of a bronchoscope under direct vision (Fig. 6–8) I have found it equally useful for wide-field, overall examination of the hypopharynx, base of tongue, and epiglottis, before resorting to the narrower view provided by the anterior commissure laryngoscope.

The *anterior commissure laryngoscope* is designed to visualize the glottis and other endolaryngeal structures by lifting the epiglottis with its

Figure 6–7. Various laryngoscopes. Each type has its special advantages and must be available in order to obtain adequate exposure, depending on the needs of the particular case.

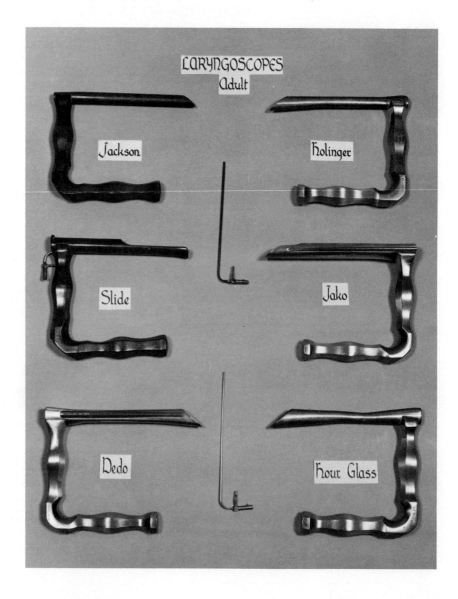

Figure 6–8. **a,** Slide laryngoscope in position in vallecula. Only the epiglottis is seen clearly. **b,** Advancement of the laryngoscope into vallecula flips epiglottis upward to expose the vocal folds.

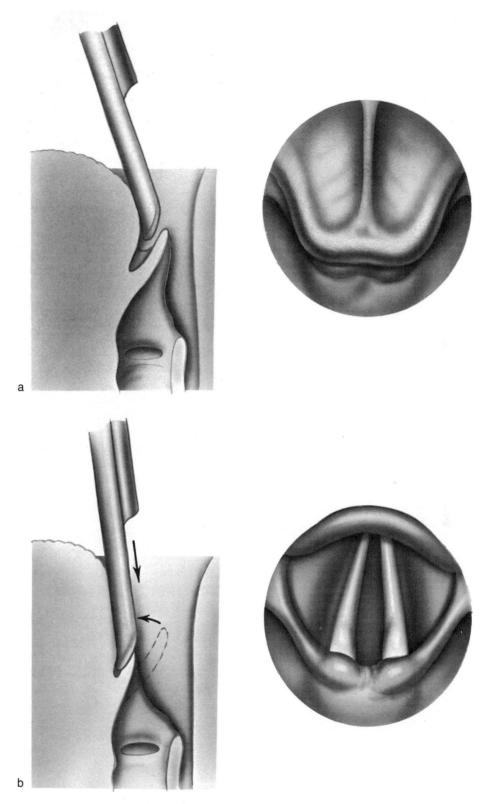

tip. It is also useful for examination of the pyriform sinuses, postcricoid area, cricopharyngeus, valleculae, and base of tongue. The original straight design of Chevalier Jackson was improved in the modification of Paul Holinger by raising the tip and enlarging the proximal end. In this manner, two routes of straight-line access are provided, thus permitting simultaneous, unobstructed visualization while suctioning or other instrumentation is carried out. The Holinger anterior commissure laryngoscope is the "work-horse" instrument in my hands.

The *suspension type* permits mechanical positioning of the laryngoscope, so that the operator can use both hands for instrumentation. It is also commonly used with the microscope for microlaryngoscopic or laser procedures. Since such procedures are usually carried out under general anesthesia, larger lumen scopes can be tolerated than would be possible with the patient awake, thus affording a better view and more working space. The two types of suspension laryngoscope that I have used are the Dedo and Jako. Either of these can be suspended using the Lewy arm, which I prefer, or any of the other apparatuses available. The suspension arm can be rested on a pad placed on the patient's chest or on a padded Mayo stand. Generally speaking, if the larger Jako laryngoscope can be inserted safely, it should be used. However, in children, females, and some males with narrower larynges, its tip is too broad and the narrower Dedo laryngoscope is preferrable.

Patient Positioning

The patient is placed close to the head of the table in the "sniffing" position. This can best be achieved by placing a roll under the shoulders and a "doughnut" under the head. When suspension laryngoscopy is not anticipated, a good alternative is for the surgeon to sit sideways on the head of the table with his right leg resting on the floor. The patient's head can then be placed on the operator's left iliac crest, so that by leaning forward the patient's head can be forced into the "sniffing" position. If general anesthesia is being employed, the endotracheal tube is positioned on the left side and taped so that it does not interfere with opening of the patient's mouth.

Insertion of the Laryngoscope

The laryngoscope is grasped in the surgeon's right hand, the mouth is opened with the left hand, and the tip of the instrument is placed well behind the tongue under direct vision. The entire laryngoscope is displaced toward the patient's feet, thus using the muscular base of the tongue as a pad while opening the mouth widely (Fig. 6–9). If properly done, this maneuver will expose the tip of the epiglottis resting against the posterior pharyngeal wall (Fig. 6–10). The laryngoscope is transferred to the examiner's left hand and the right index finger is placed between the upper teeth and the undersurface of the laryngoscope.◁ The peculiar, bulbous design of the handle of most Jackson-type laryngoscopes has been developed to favor correct positioning of the left hand while holding the instrument during examination (Fig. 6–9). The bulge in the middle of each of the two right-angle limbs of the handle should rest, respectively, against the head of the second metacarpal and the muscular pad overlying the fifth metacarpal. This seemingly awkward hand position prevents the application of excessive pressure on the laryngoscope and favors proper displacement of the oral and laryngeal structures by the instrument without "levering" against the teeth. The right thumb is placed against the lower lip of the proximal opening of the laryngoscope and is used to guide it. The instrument is brought as far to the right of the patient's oral commissure as possible and is placed lateral to the upper teeth. By avoiding insertion of the laryngoscope in the midline over the upper incisors or alvolar ridge, the line of vision between the oral commissure and the plane of the glottis is made as straight as possible.

Many surgeons recommend the use of a rubber mouth guard to protect the upper teeth. In my opinion, such an implement not only may fail to protect the teeth, but may even lend itself to causing damage. Although it may be true that a rubber guard can prevent minor chipping of the upper incisors, it will also transmit any force applied to it to the teeth, almost without attenuation. With the teeth covered, the examiner may be lulled into a false sense of security, whereas, if the teeth are left exposed and are protected during insertion by the examiner's finger, it is much less likely that excessive force will be applied.—HMT

Figure 6–9. The anterior commissure laryngoscope is displaced toward the patients feet as a unit. In this manner, force is borne by the muscular base of the tongue.

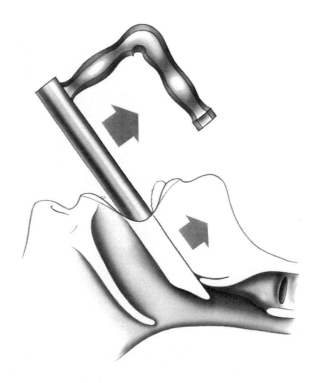

The tip of the laryngoscope is dropped just below the epiglottis and advanced slightly to engage it. The instrument is then advanced toward the patient's feet, *without changing its angulation*. This maneuver displaces the base of tongue and the epiglottis and exposes the arytenoids (Fig. 6–11). The laryngoscope is next advanced slightly further and elevated toward the ceiling to expose the remainder of the glottis (Fig. 6–12). Once the desired exposure has been achieved, the suspension arm can be attached and adjusted while the proper position is maintained by the examiner. If

Figure 6–10. Initial view of larynx with laryngoscope in place.

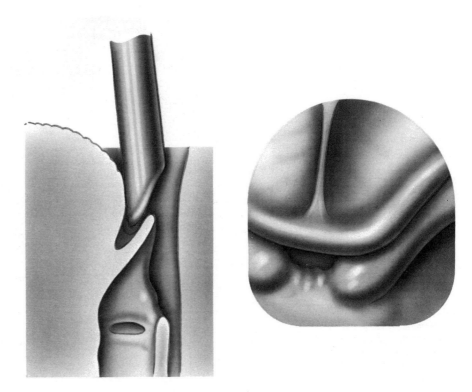

Figure 6–11. Laryngoscope is advanced into supraglottis to expose arytenoids.

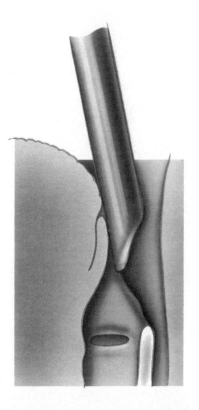
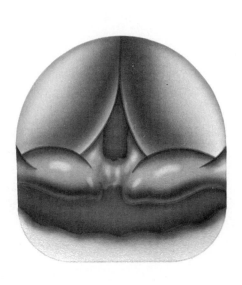

hand-held laryngoscopy is to be carried out, the surgeon supports his left arm holding the laryngoscope by bringing the elbow against his left iliac crest. When the proper position has been achieved, the right hand is no longer needed to protect the teeth and is free for other manipulations.

Instrumentation

Once the larynx has been properly exposed (and the laryngoscope suspended, if so desired), the entire structure can be inspected and decisions made regarding necessary instrumentation. The most commonly used in-

Figure 6–12. Glottis fully exposed.

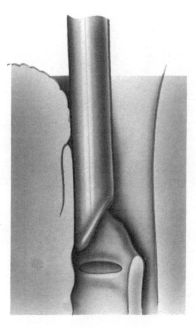
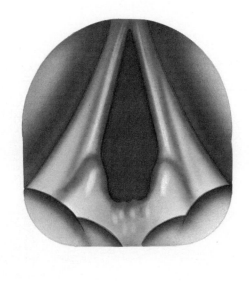

Figure 6–13.
Microlaryngoscopy instruments.

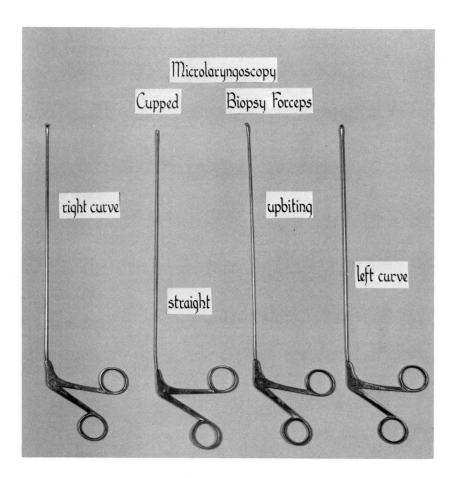

strument is the *suction tip*. Both open-ended and "velvet eye" types exist in various sizes and designs, including specialized ones to displace and protect one vocal fold during laser procedures. Assorted straight and angulated *cup forceps, alligator forceps,* and Belucci-type *scissors* are available in sizes suitable to either hand-held or microlaryngeal surgery (Fig. 6–13). Microsurgical *knives, probes, spatulas,* and *mirrors* can also be useful.

Technique of Laryngeal Surgery

Certain surgical concepts and techniques apply, whether laryngeal manipulation is carried out under hand-held, suspension or microscopic conditions. These include maintaining proper exposure, manipulation, and removal of tissues and hemostasis.

Necessary *exposure* is best achieved by proper placement of an appropriately chosen laryngoscope and fixing it in position, as already described. However, small maneuvers may be needed from time to time during the conduct of laryngoscopy to provide better visualization and access to various structures. Simple rotation of the tip of an anterior commissure laryngoscope can expose the ventricle, displace the false cord, and fix the true vocal fold in position for surgical manipulation (Fig. 6–14). Sometimes, it is difficult to see the anterior commissure, especially when using the suspension apparatus. Firm downward pressure on the thyroid cartilage by either the examiner or an assistant can bring the rest of the glottis and the petiole of the epiglottis into view. The undersurface of the vocal fold can be brought into view by light pressure on its upper surface at a point well into the ventricle. A suction tip or blunt probe can be used to displace

Figure 6–14. Tip of anterior commissure laryngoscope can be rotated just above the true vocal fold to displace the false cord and expose lesions deep in the ventrical.

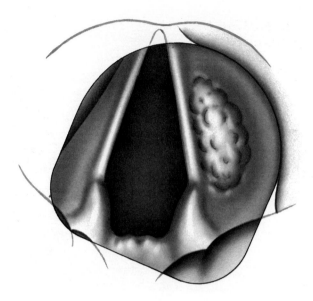

the false vocal fold and permit this maneuver. It is also quite possible to see the undersurface of the vocal folds and the upper trachea by simply advancing the tip of the laryngoscope slightly through the glottis or by using small mirrors or telescopes.

Tissue handling can be critical to successful diagnosis and management of laryngeal disease. Various microsurgical instruments permit grasping and cutting of lesions as necessary. It is essential that the surgeon develop ambidexterity in the use of any of these, since the proper placement of these instruments, often in reversed sequence from one side to the other, is essential to successful tissue manipulation.

Most mucosal lesions, such as polyps, nodules, and superficial leukoplakia can be avulsed cleanly and with minimal damage to adjacent tissues if the following technique is followed:

''The laryngoscope is rotated slightly so that the lip is towards the side of the lesion, thus fixing the vocal cord at its tip and minimizing any movement of the lesions. . . . A small up-biting cup forceps is introduced and the lesion is grasped gently, but not so firmly as to cut through its attachment. If the forceps is quickly and sharply advanced along the long axis of the trachea and then immediately drawn back in a single in and out motion, the mucosa at the point of attachment of the lesion will tear neatly away through Reinke's space, leaving a smooth, denuded vocal cord''[6] (Figs. 6–15 and 6–16).

Hemostasis is more often a problem in maintaining exposure than in prevention of blood loss or airway obstruction. Even a few drops of blood can obscure important findings and interfere with surgical manipulations. Most particularly, bloody lesions (i.e., papillomas) are treated today with the carbon dioxide laser (see later), with which it is possible to cauterize small bleeding vessels. This is done by slightly defocusing the laser and decreasing power to approximately 15 W before striking the bleeding point. Other ways to handle bleeding include suctioning, placement of cottonoids soaked in epinephrine 1:100,000, application of tannic acid powder, and electrocautery.

Laser Surgery

The development of the carbon dioxide laser for endoscopic use has, to a large extent, revolutionized modern laryngoscopic surgery. It permits precise destruction of tissues with much less damage to remaining struc-

Figure 6–15. Vocal fold is fixed
by rotation and inward pressure
of the laryngoscope. The lesion
is grasped gently in angulated
cup forceps.

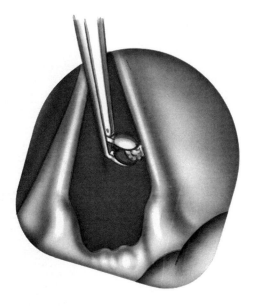

*Because of the wavelength of the
carbon dioxide laser, the distance
from total tissue vaporization to the
first intact, undamaged cells is
approximately 60 micra or the
width of eight red blood cells side
by side. The zone of tissue
distortion at the periphery of a
lesion excised with the laser is so
small that the pathologist can
usually interpret the margins of
such specimens without difficulty.*

tures than can usually be achieved even by the most meticulous mechanical
microsurgery.◁ Because the laser is a coherent light beam, it permits manipulation of the larynx under better visualization, reduces the number of
instruments that must take up available space in the laryngoscope, lessens
distortion of the structures, and often permits an almost bloodless field.
Nevertheless, it is not the answer to every problem in management of laryngeal lesions that some of its early proponents had hoped it would be.

Certain *precautions* must be observed in the use of the laser, especially regarding the possibility of ignition of flammable materials.

1.   The eyes of every person in the room should be protected against
stray contact with the laser beam. For the patient this can best be accomplished by taping the eyes shut in the usual manner and then placing sa-
line-moistened eye patches over them. With the possible exception of the
operator, who is protected by the microscope lenses, all personnel should
wear protective glasses or contact lenses.

2.   Endotracheal tubes used with the laser must be protected from
contact with the beam. Standard polyvinyl chloride and Silastic tubes can
be adequately protected by wrapping them with aluminized tape from the

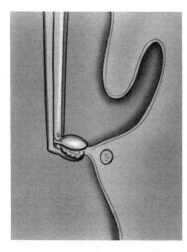
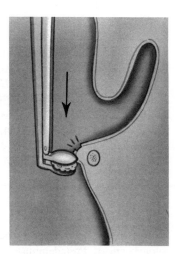
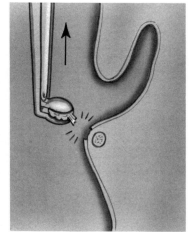

Figure 6–16. Proper technique for avulsion of mucosal lesions of the vocal fold.

Figure 6–17. Safety implements
and aluminum tape wrapped
endotracheal tube for laser
surgery.

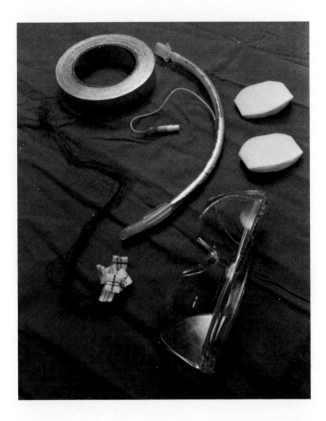

point of contact between the cuff and the body of the tube, up to the point
at which the filler tube leaves it. For most tubes of appropriate size for
endoscopic procedures, a single strip can be oriented along the long axis
of the endotracheal tube and wrapped around it lengthwise (Fig. 6–17). In
this manner, only a small gap is left along the the side of the tube that will
be away from the operative field and any gaps that might result from the
more traditional spiral wrapping technique are avoided. Metal endotracheal
tubes have been introduced for use with the laser, but, at least in my hands,
have been unsatisfactory because of leakage through the many joints. Metal
impregnated plastic laser tubes have also been made commercially available recently and, if they prove as safe as the manufacturer claims, may
be a useful substitute for metallic wrapping.

3.   Saline-soaked neurosurgical patties should be placed around the
cuff of the endotracheal tube to prevent inadvertent laser damage. Also,
the anesthetist must be constantly alert to a sudden change in compliance
or to air leakage that may signal that such loss of integrity of the cuff has
occurred, so that the operator can be warned. If this happens, *IT IS IM-
PERATIVE THAT ALL FURTHER LASER TREATMENT BE STOPPED
AND THE TUBE REPLACED.* Once the cuff is down, the risk of ignition
of the tube is very high, not only because of the exposure of the un-
wrapped distal portion of the tube, but also because of the high oxygen
atmosphere that can now flow proximally.

References

1.   Lejeune FE Jr: Laryngoscopy. In English GE
      (Ed): Otolaryngology, vol 3. Philadelphia,
      Harper & Row, 1983, p 1.

2.   Abelson TI, Tucker HM: Superior laryngeal
      nerve paralysis: A controversy. Otolaryngol
      Head Neck Surg, 89:463, 1981.

3. Clark WD: Diagnosis and staging of laryngeal disease. In Bailey BJ, Biller HF (Eds): Surgery of the Larynx, Philadelphia, WB Saunders, 1985, p 49.

4. Jackson C, Jackson CL: Bronchoscopy, esophagoscopy and gastroscopy: A manual of peroral fundoscopy and laryngeal surgery, 3rd ed. Philadelphia, WB Saunders, 1934.

5. Brunnett RE: The pharmacology of drugs used in otolaryngology. In English GE (Ed): Otolaryngology, vol 5. Philadelphia, Harper & Row, 1974.

6. Tucker HM: Surgery for Phonatory Disorders, New York, Churchill Livingstone, 1981, p 20.

7. Strong MS: Endoscopic surgery of the larynx. In Bailey BJ, Biller HF (Eds): Surgery of the Larynx. Philadelphia, WB Saunders, 1985, p 107.

8. Strong MS, et al: Cardiac complications of microsurgery of the larynx: Etiology, incidence, and prevention. Laryngoscope, 84:908–920, 1974.

9. Norton ML, et al: Endotracheal intubation and Venturi (jet) ventilation for microsurgery of the larynx. Ann Otolaryngol, 85:656, 1974.

10. Carden E, Crutchfield W: Anesthesia for microsurgery of the larynx. Can Anaesth Soc J, 20:378, 1973.

Chapter 7

Congenital Disorders
of the Larynx

See Chapter 1.

Congenital disorders of the larynx may result from genetic accidents, embryologic abnormalities,◁ or injuries sustained during delivery. Although present at birth, some of these disorders are not clinically apparent for months or even years afterward. Most of them, however, result in symptoms suggestive of a laryngeal problem at or shortly after delivery.

Diagnosis

Symptoms

Three symptoms occur in varying degree and combination in infants with congenital anomalies of the larynx: Respiratory obstruction, abnormal cry, and difficulty in swallowing. Although any of these may be due to nonlaryngeal causes, the simultaneous presence of all of them strongly suggests laryngeal origin.

Laryngeal obstruction usually results in *both* vigorous efforts at breathing and in cyanosis, whereas cyanosis alone suggests either a cardiac or central nervous system problem. When both are present, but disappear promptly if the infant cries, upper airway obstruction above the larynx (i.e., choanal atresia) is usually at fault.◁

Infants at birth are obligate nasal breathers. This has survival value, inasmuch as the newborn must be able to continue breathing while suckling and without aspiration (see Chapter 2). As a result, however, complete nasal obstruction can be life-threatening. Respiratory function will seem to be normal as long as the infant cries, but distress and cyanosis will ensue promptly when he becomes quiet. This will instigate a renewed bout of crying with clearing of the cyanosis, but eventually the infant becomes too tired to go on and will succumb unless the situation is recognized and remedied by placement of some kind of oral airway.—HMT

Abnormal cry may be characterized as muffled (suggesting supraglottic swelling or mass), stridorous (laryngeal obstruction), weak, hoarse, or absent. Careful observation and experience in relating the type of voice change to potential diagnosis can be helpful in directing attempts at evaluation of laryngeal problems in the newborn. For example, the presence of inspiratory and expiratory stridor coupled with a weak cry suggests a web. The same pattern of stridor, when associated with an essentially normal voice, on the other hand, may be due to subglottic stenosis. Although it is possible to gain a great deal of information by observing the pattern and combination of symptoms, a presumptive diagnosis is provided at best, which *must* be confirmed by other means.

Dysphagia or aspiration often result from laryngeal anomalies. However, any lesion of the esophagus itself (i.e., atresia) and several neurologic causes can produce similar difficulty in swallowing. When this symptom is seen in conjunction with one or more of the other findings already mentioned, laryngeal anomaly is more strongly suggested.

Evaluation

After a thorough physical examination has been carried out and if immediate intervention is not required, several other studies may be considered, which can be very helpful not only in establishing a diagnosis, but also in determining what to do next.◁ *Lateral soft tissue radiographs* can identify masses impinging on the hypopharynx or trachea. These and *xeroradiograms* may be very helpful in delineating the cartilaginous structures or stenoses. *Cine barium swallow* may demonstrate a small upper esophageal stenosis or fistula. *Computed tomography (CT)* has offered little or no advantage over some appropriate combination of the studies mentioned, at least in my hands, and is both difficult to carry out in infants and quite expensive. On rare occasions *vascular studies* may be useful, if other observations suggest such a lesion.

Direct laryngoscopy, with or without the addition of *bronchoscopy* and *esophagoscopy,* remains the definitive means of establishing a diagnosis. Because of the difficulties inherent in intubation of infants, even when the airway is *not* compromised, this is best carried out without anesthesia. Moreover, it is necessary to establish whether or not there is paralysis or fixation of one or both of the vocal folds, which cannot be determined if the infant is deeply anesthetized.◁

Classification

Table 7–1 provides a classification of these lesions.[1] Unless the physician has a mental list of potential diagnoses that will allow him to *think* of the correct one while evaluating an infant with symptoms suggestive of a congenital laryngeal problem, it is unlikely that the appropriate diagnosis will be made.

Management

Anomalies of Cartilaginous Support

Laryngomalacia

At birth, the supporting structures of the laryngotracheal complex are soft and flaccid. They do not usually collapse during respiration only because the resting tissue turgor is sufficiently stiff to prevent collapse in response to Bernoulli's effect.◁ In some infants at birth, but more often a few weeks thereafter, soft tissue support proves insufficient for this purpose and the syndrome of congenital laryngeal stridor (as Laryngomalacia is also called) ensues. Typically, the infant thus affected begins to manifest inspiratory stridor and suprasternal retractions. Pectus excavatum is often seen in these patients, but whether this is a cause or a result of the laryngomalacia is not entirely clear. Laryngomalacia is the single-most common congenital laryngeal anomaly (75 percent). The *diagnosis* is made primarily by excluding other lesions.◁ At laryngoscopy, one commonly observes an omega-shaped or scrolled epiglottis, which, along with the other supraglottic structures, collapses inward during inspiration (Fig. 7–1) and opens passively in response to expiratory airflow. Since the condition is almost always self-limited, *treatment* is expectant. The parents can be reassured that with further growth and calcium deposition into the supporting cartilages, stridor will diminish and eventually disappear. In rare cases, trache-

See Chapter 4.

"Visualization of the mobility of the true cords may be accomplished best by inserting the tip of the laryngoscope into the vallecula. . . . Care must be taken to avoid limiting vocal cord mobility with the laryngoscope. General anesthesia gives a false impression of decreased vocal cord mobility and should be avoided." —P Holinger[1]

See Chapter 2.

"Early intubation of the dyspneic child" (without first examining the airway endoscopically—HMT) "may obscure forever whether a later [stenosis] was congenital, acquired, or mixed. The tracheotomy required by acquired stenosis may, indeed, be thought of as a complication of intubation."— GF Tucker[15]

Table 7–1   Classification of Congenital Disorders of the Larynx

Cartilaginous anomalies
   Laryngomalacia (congenital laryngeal stridor)
   Epiglottic anomalies
      Absent
      Bifid
      Tubular
   Thyroid cartilage anomalies
      Nonfusion of ala
      Absence of superior or inferior horns
   Arytenoid anomalies
      Atavistic
   Cricoid cartilage anomalies
      Subglottic stenosis
      Fusion of entire ring
      Failure of dorsal fusion (cleft)
Soft tissue anomalies
   Cysts and laryngoceles
      Internal: ventricular; aryepiglottic fold and arytenoid
      External
      Combined
   Webs, stenoses, and atresias
      Supraglottic
      Glottic
      Subglottic
   Cri du chat syndrome
Neurologic lesions
   Unilateral vocal cord paralysis
   Bilateral vocal cord paralysis
Vascular anomalies
   Hemangiomas
   Lymphangiomas

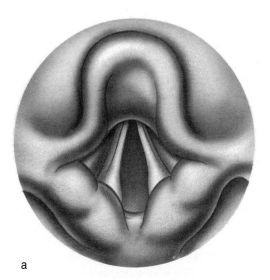
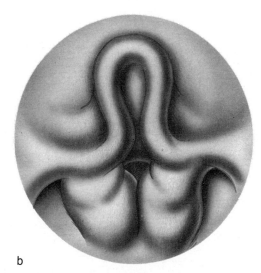

a   b

Figure 7–1. **a,** Omega-shaped epiglottis of pediatic larynx at rest. **b,** Inward collapse of epiglottis, false vocal cords, and arytenoids seen in laryngomalacia.

ostomy may be necessary if respiratory effort is so difficult that it results in failure to thrive or severe sleep disruption.

Epiglottic Anomalies

The epiglottis may be absent, bifid, or tubular. With the exception of the last, these abnormalities are rarely recognized in infancy, since they generally produce no symptoms that would lead to laryngoscopy. Bifid epiglottis is sometimes associated with polydactyly. Tubular epiglottis is occasionally seen in laryngomalacia or *cri du chat* syndrome.

Thyroid Cartilage Anomalies

Although not unusual, failure of fusion of the thyroid alae and absence or deformities of the superior or inferior cornua are rarely of clinical significance.

Anomalies of the Arytenoid Cartilage

"Probably the most frequently encountered [anomaly] is an atavistic ("throwback") appearance. . . . The cartilage and aryepiglottic folds have an anteroposterior configuration rather than a midline to lateral position similar to that seen in the canine larynx."—Holinger and Holinger[1]

Ankylosis or fixation of the cricoarytenoid joint is difficult to distinguish from paralysis in adults; it may be almost impossible in small children. This differentiation requires both observation of the vocal folds at direct laryngoscopy without anesthesia and palpation of the arytenoids while the infant is paralyzed (see Chapter 11). It is imperative that the tip of the laryngoscope be placed so as not to limit motion, that the tip of the palpating spatula be as far posterior as possible, and that the spatula not be inserted to the point where it will impact on the cricoid cartilage, thus giving a false impression of fixation.—HMT

See Chapter 11.

Various deformities of the arytenoids are encountered but are seldom of clinical significance. Fusion of the arytenoid, cuneiform, and corniculate cartilages is sometimes seen but is rarely discovered unless surgery is required for other causes.◁

Uni- or bilateral fixation of the cricoarytenoid joints can occur. This condition, even when it is only unilateral, usually results in severe respiratory distress and may even be incompatible with life unless immediately recognized and the airway secured. It is often unclear whether this is due to a developmental anomaly or to perinatal trauma with subsequent ankylosis in unilateral cases, especially if respiratory distress is sufficiently mild that the diagnosis is not made for several weeks or months.◁

The *diagnosis* is made at direct laryngoscopy by palpation of the arytenoids under paralytic anesthesia, after first having observed nonmovement of the vocal folds without anesthesia. *Treatment* depends on the severity of the airway compromise, but tracheotomy (or anterior cricoid cartilage split) will always be required in bilateral fixation and frequently in unilateral fixation (see Vocal Fold Paralysis). After securing a long-term airway, consideration can be given to definitive management. In unilateral cases, tracheotomy can simply be maintained until laryngeal growth is sufficient that the child can tolerate immobility of one vocal fold without significant airway compromise. This may be as early as 1 year of age, but is more likely to be at 3 or 4 years. Voice development is usually very good due to the ability of such a young and growing larynx to compensate. After extubation has been accomplished, further intervention for voice improvement is rarely necessary. Since the vocal fold is fixed rather than simply paralyzed, Teflon injection is not likely to be helpful in those cases in which voice is unsatisfactory. Such patients should be managed by surgical medialization of the vocal fold.◁ In bilateral fixation, some form of vocal fold lateralization will be required if the tracheotomy tube is to be dispensed with. Since this approach will always result in a poor voice, I believe that it is better for the child to be managed by long-term tracheotomy. In this manner, voice is preserved until the child is old enough to take part in the decision whether or not to lateralize a vocal fold at a later date. Moreover, vocal fold lateralization is essentially irreversible, whereas tracheotomy can always be undone.

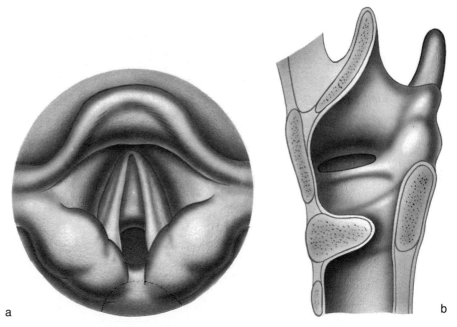

Figure 7–2. Cartilagenous subglottic stenosis. **a,** Laryngoscopic view from above. **b,** Sagittal section reveals cartilagenous component.

Cricoid Cartilage Anomalies

These may include deformities resulting in cartilaginous subglottic stenosis and laryngotracheal clefts.

Cartilaginous subglottic stenosis results from a platelike shelf extending posteriorly from the anterior cricoid ring (Fig. 7–2). The child will have both inspiratory and expiratory stridor. *Diagnosis* is made by palpation of the stenosis at laryngoscopy. Xeroradiography may assist in determining the vertical extent of the lesion, and this knowledge may be important in deciding the best management.

Treatment will include tracheotomy in severe cases (about 45 percent of all subglottic stenoses in children[2]). If tracheotomy can be avoided safely, every effort should be made to do so. Unlike the situation in soft tissue stenoses (see later), dilation is of no value. If the cartilage plate is thin enough, it may be possible to remove it with a laser, although this approach will sometimes substitute a fibrous acquired stenosis for the cartilaginous one originally present. In a small number of cases, simply waiting for differential growth of the larynx to take place will result in successful extubation.◁ If, after several months of observation, there does not appear to be appreciable increase in relative subglottic airway, or if it is apparent at the outset that the stenosis is so severe that there is no hope of spontaneous improvement, further surgical intervention will be the only recourse. In my hands, thyrotomy with excision of the stenosis and placement of an anterior rib cartilage graft has been most useful.[3]◁ There is really no reason to delay repair beyond the time when the infant has regained its birth weight and the diagnosis has been confirmed. However, surgical intervention is often put off until about 6 months to 1 year have elapsed to allow for spontaneous improvement and to take advantage of the larger size of the larynx in a 1-year-old. Moreover, even if early repair is successful, it is notoriously difficult to remove tracheotomy tubes in small infants and children up to approximately 2 years of age.

When there is stenosis of the airway, whether acquired or congenital, there are three possible outcomes if one awaits further laryngeal growth: (1) The larynx may enlarge and the stenosis remain the same. This effectively results in worsening of the stenosis; (2) the larynx may enlarge and the stenosis may grow with it at about the same rate. In this case, although the stenosis remains the same relative to the rest of the airway, it may grow beyond a critical minimum and, thus, become adequate without further intervention; (3) the stenosis may actually enlarge faster than the rest of the airway, in which situation respiratory restriction may also resolve itself.—HMT

See Chapter 8 for a general discussion of this approach.

Figure 7–3. Posterior laryngeal clefts, seen from behind.

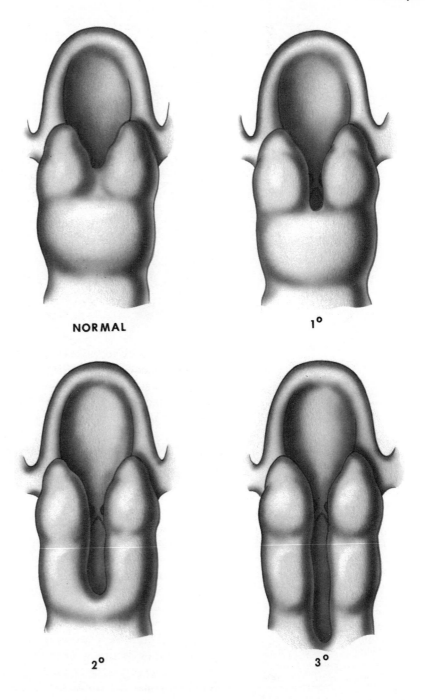

NORMAL

1°

2°

3°

See Chapter 1.

Laryngotracheal cleft results from varying degrees of failure of complete fusion of the posterior cricoid lamina.[4,5]◁ It may be classified as first, second, or third degree, depending on the extent of the cleft (Fig. 7–3). First-degree cleft is limited to the interarytenoid muscles and mucosal septum, not involving the cartilage. Second degree implies any subtotal defect of the posterior cricoid lamina. Third degree refers to a complete cleft of the entire vertical dimension of the cricoid cartilage. In rare cases, the cleft may extend down the posterior tracheal wall as far as the carina. Symptoms include aspiration, weak or absent cry, and respiratory distress. *Diagnosis* is made by oral panendoscopy. Gastrografin swallow may be helpful in diagnosis, but can be dangerous in the newborn. In first-degree cleft the findings may be subtle. It is necessary to observe the typical failure of closure of the posterior commissure during phonatory effort and without

Figure 7–4. Repair of posterior laryngeal cleft.

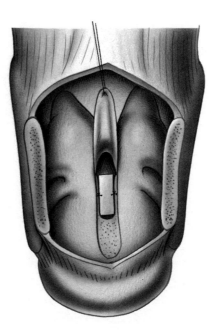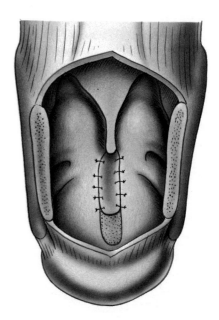

anesthesia, as well as to demonstrate the defect by gently separating the arytenoids under paralytic anesthesia. In second- and third-degree clefts the findings are similar but more dramatic. There is usually little difficulty in observing the cartilaginous defect in these more advanced cases.

Treatment depends on the severity of the cleft. Most first-degree clefts require only parental awareness and counseling, so that feeding difficulties can be minimized. Upright nursing and early addition of semisolid foods can be helpful. Second- and third-degree clefts usually necessitate tracheostomy for airway control and toilette, followed promptly by surgical repair. This is usually carried out via thyrotomy (Fig. 7–4). A posterior mucosal flap is raised and a cartilage graft obtained from the ear, the nasal septum, the thyroid lamina, or from rib cartilage is inserted into the defect. It is also helpful to interpose a muscle flap between the trachea and esophagus in larger clefts.[6,7]

Soft Tissue Anomalies

Cystic Lesions

Simple *cysts* are probably the result of obstruction of the ducts of mucous, serous, or minor salivary glands. They can occur anywhere in the larynx, but usually become symptomatic only if they are large enough to produce obstruction.

Laryngoceles, on the other hand, are due to the entrapment of air or secretions in the anterior recess (saccule, appendix) of the ventricle. They may become distended only during Valsalva maneuvers, such as crying or straining at stool. The symptoms of any cystic lesion include a muffled cry and varying degrees of airway obstruction, depending on location. Laryngoceles, on the other hand, may break through the thyrohyoid membrane (Fig. 7–5) and present as a neck mass.

Diagnosis can be made by soft tissue or xeroradiography. It is confirmed by laryngoscopy. *Treatment* of simple cysts and internal laryngoceles is by aspiration using a large-bore needle. If necessary, this can be repeated, but recurrent cysts generally should be marsupialized microlaryngoscopically or removed with the laser. External laryngoceles must be removed by a lateral neck approach.[8] The larynx is reached through a lat-

Figure 7–5. Laryngocele. **a,** Laryngoscopic view. **b,** Coronal view showing combined internal and external laryngocele breaking through thyrohyoid membrane and presenting as a mass in the neck.

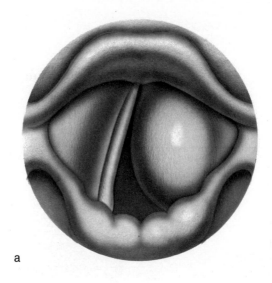

a

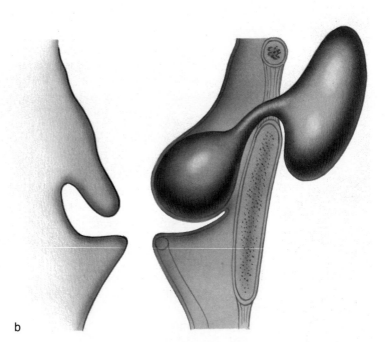

b

eral neck incision (Fig. 7–6). If the laryngocele has penetrated through the thyrohyoid membrane, it will be encountered or identified in the neck. The upper border of the thyroid lamina is incised through the perichondrium, the external and internal perichondrium are elevated, and the upper third of the thyroid cartilage is removed for exposure. The internal portion of the laryngocele is traced to its attachment to the ventricle and suture ligated.

Glottic Webs

These result from incomplete recanalization of the larynx during fetal development.◁ As a result, they may occupy any part of the glottis, but usually extend from anterior to posterior. They may vary from a thin, diaphenous membrane involving only the anterior third of the vocal folds to a thick fusion of the entire membranous portion of the glottis. In rare cases,

See Chapter 1.

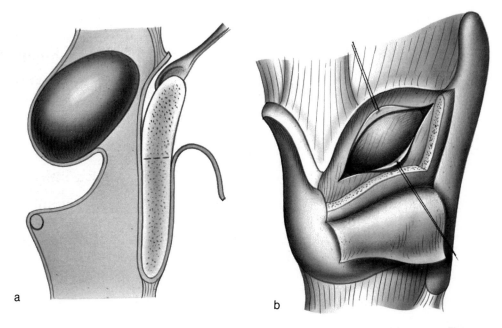

a   b

Figure 7–6. Surgical approach to internal laryngocele. **a,** Subperichondrial dissection and removal of upper portion of thyroid ala. **b,** Inner perichondrium is opened to expose mass in substance of false vocal cord.

the fusion of the vocal folds is complete and is referred to as *laryngeal atresia*. This degree of fusion is incompatible with life unless it is recognized immediately and an emergency tracheotomy carried out.

Diagnosis is made by direct laryngoscopy in an infant who manifests little or no voice when it attempts to cry, associated with inspiratory and expiratory stridor of varying degree. Treatment depends on severity. If tracheotomy is not necessary, endoscopic dilation is often quite successful, especially in thin anterior webs. The thicker ones and those that do not respond to dilation can best be managed by anterior thyrotomy and placement of a keel.[8] (Fig. 7–7)

Figure 7–7. Anterior thyrotomy and placement of tantalum keel.

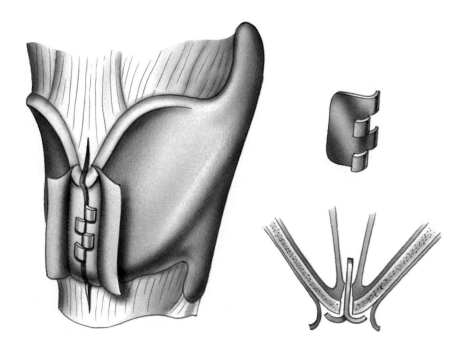

See Chapter 9.

"The least laryngeal inflammation may precipitate the need for intubation or tracheotomy since the limiting cricoid cartilage does not permit swelling of tissues in any direction other than inward at the expense of the airway."—Holinger and Holinger[1]

"One mm of edema in the subglottic region of the normal newborn reduces the airway to thirty-two percent of. . . . normal."—Holinger and Holinger[1]

Subglottic Stenosis

This is due to a thickening of the soft tissues lining the cricoid cartilage. It may be difficult to distinguish from cartilaginous subglottic stenosis (see before) and, particularly, from subglottic hemangioma. Symptoms suggestive of croup[2]◁ but of insidious onset and which are persistent should alert the physician to this possibility. The *diagnosis* is made at direct laryngoscopy. The usual site of stenosis is 2 to 3 mm below the glottis.◁

Treatment depends on severity of obstruction. Very mild degrees of subglottic stenosis tend to diminish as the child grows and thus may require only careful observation. More severe stenosis will usually respond to gentle dilation, but this approach almost always mandates a tracheotomy because of the threat of postdilation edema.◁ This can sometimes be avoided by supramaximal doses of dexamethasone given intravenously 20 minutes before laryngeal manipulation. Approximately two-thirds of infants with congenital subglottic stenosis will respond satisfactorily to a single such dilatation.[2] Anterior cricoid split has been advocated as a means of avoiding tracheotomy, especially in premature infants.[3,16]

Cri du Chat Syndrome

This is characterized by inspiratory stridor and a peculiar, mewling cry that has been likened to the sound of a kitten. It is thought to be due to a defect in the short arm of chromosome 5 in the B group. The condition presents with a flaccid, tubular epiglottis, which is sucked down over the glottis during inspiratory efforts. There is usually also paralysis of the interarytenoideus muscle.[9] As a result, the posterior glottis does not close completely. Air escapes during phonation, which, coupled with the adduction of the membranous vocal folds, produces the characteristic cry. The condition may be associated with other anomalies, including hypertelorism, low-set ears, microcephaly, and mental retardation.

Diagnosis is suspected from the characteristic cry, associated findings, and by direct laryngoscopy. It must be confirmed by chromosomal analysis. *Treatment* is not often necessary, since airway obstruction is usually mild. Tracheotomy may be needed in occasional cases. Parental counseling is obviously very important.

Vascular Anomalies

Hemangiomas

"Conversely, the clinical presentation may be a protracted episode of laryngotracheobronchitis."—T McGill[10]

Although hemagiomas occur frequently about the head and neck, they have a peculiar propensity for the subglottic area. They may be *cavernous* or *capillary* in histologic type. The capillary type is considerably more frequently encountered. They are five times more common in females than in males. In approximately 50 percent of cases, subglottic lesions are associated with cutaneous hemangiomas. The usual presentation is a pattern of progressive biphasic stridor appearing within a few weeks of birth.◁

Diagnosis is suspected from the presentation of inspiratory and expiratory stridor in association with other hemangiomas. Xeroradiography may show a subglottic soft tissue shadow. Confirmation of diagnosis is made at direct laryngoscopy. A smooth, sometimes bluish, mucosal covered mass is encountered in the cricoid area. Biopsy is rarely necessary, but, in any event, ought not to be carried out unless a tracheotomy has been performed, because of the threat of serious bleeding.

Treatment is aimed at securing the airway, since most of these lesions undergo spontaneous involution between 18 months and 3 years of age. Tracheotomy is frequently necessary, but can occasionally be avoided by use of systemic steroids.◁ Some success has been reported in avoiding or shortening the period during which tracheotomy is needed by use of the carbon dioxide laser.[11]

Lymphangiomas

These lesions are most often part of a larger cystic hygroma involving the larynx as well as the neck. They are usually present at birth and are soft, compressible and have a tendency to worsen gradually without treatment.

I have been able to manage two of these lymphangiomas without tracheotomy by judicious use of the carbon dioxide laser. One must be very cautious about serious bleeding, at least at the first attempt at laser surgery, because some of these lesions are mixed hemangioma-lymphangiomas.—HMT

Diagnosis is made at direct laryngoscopy in an infant with a soft mass that feels like a "bag of worms" on palpation of the neck. The mass becomes tense and may enlarge dramatically during crying. Tracheotomy is usually necessary, not only to secure the airway, but because definitive excision of the entire mass in the neck is the proper *treatment*, when possible.◁

Neurological Anomalies

After laryngomalacia, neurologic lesions are the most common congenital anomalies of the larynx, comprising about 10 percent of all such cases.

Vocal Fold Paralysis

Paralysis of the vocal folds at birth may be unilateral or bilateral. Approximately 20 percent of these are associated with traumatic delivery, probably due to stretching of the recurrent laryngeal nerve or, in forceps deliveries, perhaps due to direct trauma. Most of the rest are associated with other central nervous system anomalies, such as the Arnold-Chiari malformation,[12] or with other congenital defects.[13]

The 40 to 50 percent reduction in the diameter of the infant airway that results from unilateral vocal fold paralysis, coupled with the relative softness and collapsibility of the supporting tissues, frequently produces almost as severe compromise as does bilateral paralysis in adults.—HMT

Newborn infants with bilateral paralysis manifest severe respiratory distress, which will require intubation and eventual tracheotomy once the *diagnosis* is established by laryngoscopy. Even unilateral paralysis is not as well tolerated in the infant as in adults and may require similar intervention.◁

A possible exception to this is in Arnold-Chiari malformation with meningomyelocele, in which case "tracheotomy should be delayed until a shunt has been performed. Following the shunt procedure the child should be left intubated for 48 hours; then a trial of extubation can be carried out."—T McGill[10]

See Chapter 11.

Treatment requires tracheotomy for stabilization of the airway in bilateral paralysis and even in some cases of unilateral paralysis.◁ Once the airway has been established, thorough assessment of the problem can be carried out under nonemergent conditions.

In *unilateral* paralysis, no intervention is generally indicated in small children. If the airway is not significantly compromised, the only resultant deficit is a somewhat weak and breathy voice, which is usually not a serious problem. In most such cases, spontaneous recovery or compensation can be expected, especially if speech therapy is added to the regimen beginning at about 1 year of age. Teflon injection or reinnervation can be considered if there is no recovery or adequate compensation◁ after 1 or 2 years but these should rarely be necessary.

Bilateral paralysis, on the other hand, almost always requires some kind of surgical rehabilitation, since most of these do not recover spontaneously. After tracheotomy has been established, further intervention should be delayed until the child is 1 or 2 years of age. If return of function of at least one vocal fold has not taken place by then, consideration should be given to reinnervation.[13,14] When successful, (80 percent of attempted cases) sufficient vocal fold motion can be achieved to allow safe extubation without further compromise of voice. If reinnervation cannot be carried out or fails, long-term tracheotomy seems to be the best solution, since it is generally well tolerated and does not lessen the voice. Although arytenoid lateralization procedures can be performed successfully in children, I believe that they should be delayed in most cases until the child is sufficiently mature to take part in the decision whether or not to sacrifice voice for airway.

References

1. Holinger PH, Holinger LD: Congenital anomalies of the larynx. In English GE (Ed): Otolaryngology. Philadelphia, Harper & Row, 1984.
2. Holinger PH, Kutnick SL, Schild JL, Holinger LD: Subglottic stenosis in infants and children. Ann Otol Rhinol Laryngol, 85:591–599, 1976.
3. Cotton R: Management of subglottic stenosis in infancy and childhood. Ann Otol Rhinol Laryngol, 87:649–657, 1978.
4. Doyle PJ, Imbrie D: Laryngotracheoesophageal cleft. In Bergsma D (Ed): Birth Defects Atlas and Compendium. New York, Alan R. Liss, 1979.
5. Lim TA, Spanier SS, Kohut RI: Laryngeal clefts. Ann Otol Rhinol Laryngol, 88:837, 1979.
6. Bell DW, Christiansen TA, Smith TE Jr, Stucker FJ: Laryngotracheoesophageal cleft: The anterior approach. Ann Otol Rhinol Laryngol, 86:616, 1977.
7. Cotton RT, Schreiber JT: Management of laryngotracheoesophageal cleft. Ann Otol Rhinol Laryngol, 90:401, 1981.
8. Tucker HM: Surgery for Phonatory Disorders. New York, Churchill Livingstone, 1981, p 54.
9. Ferguson CF: Congenital malformations. In Ferguson CF, Kendig EL (Eds): Pediatric Otolaryngology. Philadelphia, WB Saunders, 1972, pp 1166–1175.
10. McGill T: Congenital diseases of the larynx. Otol Clin North Am, 17:61, 1984.
11. Healy GB, Fearon B, French R, McGill T: Treatment of subglottic hemangioma with the carbon dioxide laser. Laryngoscope, 90:809–813, 1980.
12. Cohen S, Geller K, Birns J, Thompson J: Laryngeal paralysis in children: A long-term retrospective study. Ann Otol Rhinol Laryngol, 91:4, 1982.
13. Tucker HM: Congenital bilateral recurrent nerve paralysis and ptosis: A new syndrome. Laryngoscope, 93:1405–1407, 1983.
14. Tucker HM: Vocal Cord Paralysis in Children: Principles in Management. Ann Otol Rhinol Laryngol, 95:618–621, 1986.
15. Tucker GF: Congenital (and acquired) laryngeal disease. Presented at the Albert Einstein College of Medicine Symposium on Benign Laryngeal Disease, New York, March 4–5, 1983.
16. Cotton RT, Seid AB: Management of the extubation problem in the premature child. Ann Otol Rhinol Laryngol, 89:508, 1980.

Chapter 8

Laryngeal Trauma

Mechanism of Injury

Blunt Trauma

The larynx enjoys a relatively well-protected position in the neck. It is shielded from lateral impact by the bulk of the sternocleidomastoid muscles, from behind by the cervical vertebrae and the other muscles of the neck, and from above by the overhanging mandible. When the individual is in normal anatomic position, it is even shielded from the front by the mandible, especially since the normal reflexive reaction to impending anterior trauma is to simultaneously withdraw the head and to lower the jaw. (Fig. 8–1).◁ Increasing incidence of automobile accidents, however, frequently places the head and neck in a fully extended position (Fig. 8–2), especially if shoulder restraints are not in use. This not only withdraws the anterior (mandible) and lateral (sternocleidomastoid) protections, but pulls the larynx forward and fixes it in an exposed position. The steering wheel, dashboard, and backs of the front seats are then ideally positioned for direct crushing impact, sandwiching the larynx between themselves and the vertebral column. Similar trauma may result from karate chops, "clothesline" injuries (often sustained while riding bicycles or in snowmobiles at night), and sports injuries (elbows, hockey sticks, etc.)

Such a blow may do relatively little damage in young, flexible larynges whose cartilages can absorb the impact and spring back into position without fracturing. In such cases, only submucosal *edema* or minor *hemorrhage* may ensue, but even this degree of injury can result in airway compromise. Indeed, flexible laryngeal cartilages may potentiate the mechanism of *dislocation of the arytenoids* and *rupture of the membranous vocal folds*. (Fig. 8–3) The thyroid cartilage is driven back against the vertebral bodies, whose convex anterior shape acts like a wedge to force the posterior thyroid alae apart. The posterior cricoid lamina is driven anteriorly, in turn, releasing all tension on the vocal ligaments and simultaneously displacing the arytenoid cartilages anteriorly. At this moment, if the anterior force is suddenly withdrawn, the larynx springs back, instantaneously increasing the tension in the vocal ligaments. This may result in rupture of the membranous vocal folds or *dislocation of the arytenoids* anterior to the cricoid lamina.

When a glancing blow is struck from the front, it may bounce off the mandible and be redirected downward to strike the sternum. Therefore, all unconscious patients who have sustained such mandibular injuries should be suspected of sternal or upper thoracic injuries, as well. Moreover, if an unconscious patient has had mandibular and thoracic trauma, intubation or tracheotomy are often undertaken as an emergency procedure, sometimes without having adequately assessed possible laryngeal injuries. The larynx should be examined in all such patients as soon as stabilization of other injuries will permit.—HMT

Figure 8–1. The mandible tends to protect the larynx from blows from the front.

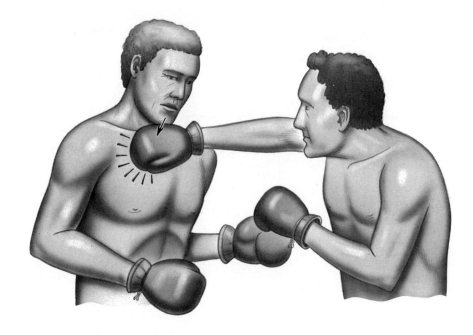

When a blow has been sustained of sufficient magnitude to produce severe laryngeal trauma, the possibility of associated injuries, such as cervical fracture or dislocation, pharyngeal or esophageal rupture or pneumothorax without direct chest trauma must be considered.—HMT

Fracture of any or all of the cartilaginous structures can and does occur by the same mechanism, especially in patients whose larynges are calcified. These fractures tend to occur in patterns corresponding to the point of impact. Midline or paramedian fractures are most common, but comminution and complex fractures often occur. *Laryngotracheal separation* is the most serious type of injury because it can result in severe airway compromise, which may be precipitated by attempts at intubation, (see later). ◁

Figure 8–2. When the head and neck are extended, the larynx is brought forward into an unprotected position.

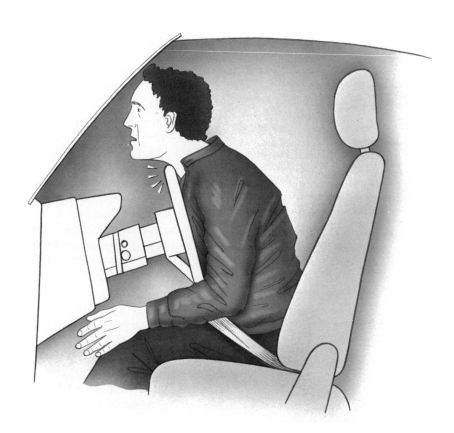

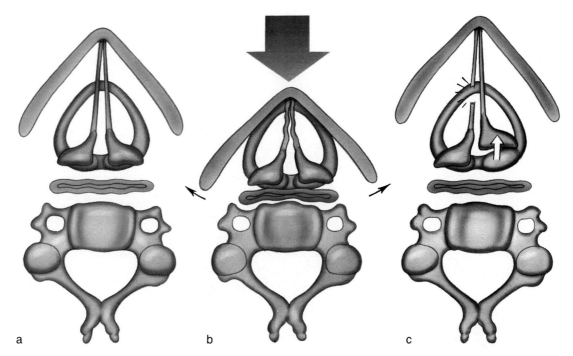

Figure 8–3. Mechanism of rupture of vocal folds and/or anterior dislocation of the arytenoid cartilage. **a,** Larynx at rest. **b,** Anterior blow displaces larynx posteriorly toward vertebral bodies, which splays the thyroid cartilage and releases all tension on the vocal ligaments. **c,** With the anterior pressure removed, the thyroid cartilage springs forward, either avulsing the vocal fold or dislocating the arytenoid forward, where it impacts against the cricoid lamina and is trapped.

Penetrating Trauma

Although vascular injuries are the most common cause of death after penetrating trauma of the neck,[1] damage to the airway is also quite common and can be life-threatening. Unless it is fixed in the neck at the moment of impact, the larynx is often displaced without serious injury by knife thrusts and low-velocity civilian type bullets, whereas shotgun blasts tend to destroy rather than displace such rigid structures. Depending on the type of instrument, penetrating injuries can result in any of the problems just outlined or discrete *perforation* of the laryngeal membranes.

Intubation Trauma

Even when performed under optimal conditions, intubation carries the risk of transient or permanent laryngeal injury. *Mucosal ulceration,* at least at a microscopic level, probably occurs after most intubations, but is apparently not often clinically significant.[2] Factors that have been incriminated in intubation trauma are listed in Table 8–1.[3]

The late injuries most commonly encountered as a result of intubation are *intubation granuloma,* ◁ *cricoarytenoid ankylosis (fibrosis),* and *acquired subglottic stenosis.* With the possible exception of cricoarytenoid ankylosis, which may also result from subluxation of the arytenoid during traumatic intubation, the pathophysiology of all of these is related to secondary infection and chondritis. Such injuries are best prevented (See Management of Intubation Trauma).

See Chapter 10.

Table 8–1   Factors in Intubation as a Cause of Subglottic Stenosis*

Duration of intubation: likelihood of damage increases after 72 hours

Tube size: the smallest tube that will adequately ventilate the patient for the anticipated duration of intubation should be used

Infection: mucosal ulceration in a potentially infected area predisposes to chondritis and stenosis

Movement: the in and out pistonlike movement of an improperly immobilized endotracheal tube results in subglottic injury, especially during mechanically assisted ventilation

Cuff pressure: pressures greater than 5 mmHg completely obstruct venous return and can produce local necrosis

Nasogastric intubation: Cricoid chondritis secondary to gastroesophageal reflex has been implicated in subglottic stenosis.

Systemic factors: Such factors as anemia, toxicity, avitaminosis, and dehydration may all play a part in development of subglottic stenosis.

*Modified with permission from Toohill and Duncavage.[3]

Thermal and Chemical Trauma

Inhalation of hot gases, whether caustic or not, can result in both short- and long-term laryngeal damage. Initial problems all relate to stabilization of the airway, which may respond to such injury with severe and rather sudden *edema*.◁ Long-term injuries are associated with *loss of mucosal integrity*, *infection*, *chondritis*, and *fibrosis*. They are in many ways similar to those seen as a result of prolonged intubation (since endotracheal respiratory support is usually needed), but are often much more severe.

Diagnosis

Signs and Symptoms

Symptoms of laryngeal trauma include stridor, voice change, hemoptysis, pain (especially on swallowing), and swelling of the neck. Associated clinical findings that suggest laryngeal trauma are respiratory distress, hoarseness or aphonia, subcutaneous emphysema and ecchymosis, and blood-tinged sputum. When coupled with a history of neck trauma, any or all of these findings strongly suggest laryngeal injury until proved otherwise.

History and Physical Examination

If stabilization of the airway and other injuries do not demand immediate attention, physical examination should be carried out.◁ IT IS IMPERATIVE, HOWEVER, THAT THE NECK NOT BE MOVED UNTIL ASSOCIATED CERVICAL FRACTURE HAS BEEN RULED OUT. After the history has been obtained, a thorough head and neck examination should be undertaken, with special attention to the larynx. (Sufficient general physical examination must be done to identify other significant injuries.) In most laryngeal trauma, *indirect mirror examination* will either identify it, or at least provide strong suspicion of the location and severity. Edema, submucosal hemorrhage, lacerations, dislocation of the arytenoid, and immobility of one or both vocal folds can usually be observed, providing the patient can cooperate and secretions can be cleared. *Palpation* and *auscultation* of the neck will reveal cervical emphysema (a strong suggestion of perforation of a viscus),◁ edema of the overlying soft tissues (suggestive

Chemical and thermal trauma produce laryngeal damage that often results in delayed edema and obstruction. Moreover, the onset of airway compromise is usually abrupt. Therefore, it is important that the means of intubation and the personnel able to do it be immediately available in the management of such patients until it has been determined that all danger of obstruction is past.—HMT

In any severe neck injury, the neck should be braced to prevent movement of the head because of the danger of cervical fracture or dislocation, the further disturbance of which might result in injury to the spinal cord. Appropriate radiographs should be obtained in all such cases before any manipulation of the head is permitted. The radiology technician should be alerted to this concern— HMT

Nonpenetrating trauma of the neck can result in pharyngeal or esophageal rupture with subsequent subcutaneous or mediastinal emphysema. If the vocal folds are closed, subglottic pressure is elevated and the cricopharyngeus and velopharyngeal port are closed at the moment of impact, the sudden increase in intrapharyngeal pressure can rupture the wall. —Tucker and Padula.[4]

of hemorrhage), loss of normal laryngeal prominance, and even palpable fragmentation of the laryngeal cartilages.

Radiologic Evaluation

See Chapter 4.

An important finding on radiographs that may alert the physician to trauma in the absence of obvious fracture is loss of the normal lordotic curve of the cervical spine.—HMT

If the patient's condition permits and the airway has been assured, appropriate radiographic studies can be obtained.◁ These should include a *chest radiograph* (to rule out associated chest trauma or pneumothorax), *cervical spine films* (to rule out fracture or dislocation),◁ and *xeroradiograms* (to identify cervical emphysema, cartilage fragmentation, or widening of the prevertebral space). *Tomography* has been used in the past to assess actual fractures of the larynx, but I feel that xeroradiography (or, in certain cases, *computed tomography (CAT scanning)* is more effective and less expensive. *Gastrografin swallow* has been recommended to identify associated esophageal tears, and is felt to be more sensitive than esophagoscopy.[5]

Laboratory Studies

Appropriate studies to permit safe general anesthesia and to identify present status of such intercurrent conditions as diabetes, use of anticoagulants, or electrolyte imbalance should be carried out if time and the patient's condition permit. An electrocardiogram is also useful as a baseline. Type and cross-match of several units of blood is frequently advisable, especially when other injuries are evident. Blood alcohol levels may have both medical and legal significance.

Endoscopic Evaluation

Unless noninvasive studies have identified the full extent of the trauma and the physician is satisfied that no immediate intervention is necessary, *direct laryngoscopy, esophagoscopy,* and *bronchoscopy* are indicated. However, since they are usually carried out in the operating room and only when prepared to proceed with surgical management if endoscopic findings confirm the need, these evaluations will be considered under Management.

Management

Closed neck injury can result in transection of the trachea. If the patient survives the initial injury, he may maintain a precarious airway until he reaches the emergency room, providing his head is stabilized and he is not forced to lie down. When such an injury is suspected, it is imperative that all preparations for emergency tracheotomy be made, including preparing and anesthetizing the neck, before the patient is made to lie down or intubation is attempted. Indeed, attempts at intubation, even with a bronchoscope, are likely to precipitate an immediate respiratory emergency that can be resolved only by prompt tracheotomy.—HMT

Airway

In cases of acute laryngeal trauma, assessment and stabilization of the airway is of paramount importance and should take precedence over virtually all other issues (with the possible exception of massive bleeding or cardiac arrest). In any situation that requires control of the airway, peroral intubation is the most common approach. Although this is also true in most cases of laryngeal trauma, it is essential that *no attempt at intubation* be made until: (1) the neck has been stabilized or cervical fracture has been ruled out; (2) the larynx has been visualized (if possible); (3) the necessary equipment for rigid intubation (bronchoscope) and the personnel necessary for emergency tracheotomy are immediately available. Therefore, except under dire conditions, an otolaryngologist-head and neck surgeon or other specialist equally qualified to carry out *all* of the steps just outlined is the appropriate person to manage such cases.◁ In addition to other advantages, this approach may permit certain vital observations before intubation obscures the field or complicates the situation.

Once the airway has been stabilized by intubation or bronchoscopy performed, *orderly tracheotomy* is usually indicated. If intubation was necessary, it is not likely that the patient can be safely extubated in a short time; thus, the presence of the endotracheal tube will both interfere with subsequent evaluation and therapy for the damaged larynx and further traumatize lacerated tissues. If circumstances permit, the intubated patient should be transported to the operating room so that endoscopic evaluation or further surgical intervention can be carried out at the same time as the tracheotomy, which can then be planned to take advantage of the incisions necessary for exploration.

When *emergency tracheotomy* is necessary, it should be carried out through a vertical midline incision. This allows extension for additional exposure that may be needed, as well as permitting the tracheostoma to be established at the usual level, rather than forcing the use of a *cricothyroidotomy*. Cricothyroidotomy is advantageous as a means of obtaining an emergency airway only under circumstances that do not permit intubation or a normal tracheotomy. Its several disadvantages include: (1) Risk of damage to the vocal cords and cricoid cartilage, especially if left in place for more than a few hours; (2) need for prompt revision to a position below the second tracheal ring; and (3) interference with ability to speak while the cannula is in place. In my opinion, because of proximity to the only complete tracheal ring (cricoid cartilage), cricothyroidotomy should *always* be removed or replaced by a proper tracheotomy as soon as possible. This approach is particularly important, inasmuch as there may have been a tracheolaryngeal transection with distraction of the tracheal segment. In such a situation, cricothyroidotomy not only would fail to demonstrate the injury, but would not establish an adequate airway, either. ◁

". . . The reason for the need of tracheotomy is forgotten during the management of thoracic and abdominal or perhaps intracranial injuries. The laryngeal trauma is rediscovered 10 or so days later when it appears that it would be appropriate to remove the tracheotomy tube. Evaluation of the larynx should be carried out as soon as possible"—JB Snow, Jr.[5] p 103

Blunt Trauma

Aims of management of blunt laryngeal trauma are outlined in Table 8–2.

Immediate

After endoscopic evaluation, a decision must be made regarding the need for tracheotomy. If the findings are limited to minimal edema, submucosal hemorrhage (mucous membrane intact), and either no evidence of laryngeal fracture or simple, undisplaced fracture, tracheotomy may not be necessary. Such cases can be managed by careful observation (since tracheotomy *may* become necessary later), cool mist inhalation, broad-spectrum antibiotics, intravenous fluids, and, if necessary to reduce edema, judicious use of steroids. ◁

If endoscopic findings exceed those just outlined, tracheotomy should

Only one or two intravenous boluses should be needed. I prefer intravenous dexamethasone, 12 mg (in an adult male), which is a supramaximal dose. Prolonged use of steroids should be avoided, since they may potentiate infection.— HMT

Table 8–2   Management of Blunt Laryngeal Trauma
Immediate aims
Recognition of the extent of injury
Stabilization of the airway
Restoration of an intact cartilaginous framework
Reestablishment of internal mucosal integrity
Prevention of infection
Long-term aims
Prevent laryngeal stenosis
Restore normal phonatory functions

be carried out. Depending on the reliability of preoperative evaluation, the surgeon may decide to do nothing more for 2 to 3 days and then reassess the degree of injury when obscuring edema and secretions have been allowed to subside, or he may proceed directly to exploration of the larynx.

I find that an apron flap incision is best for exposure and cosmesis. The tracheotomy may be performed after the flap is raised and be placed in the incision, if it has not been previously carried out. After adequate exposure has been obtained, the strap muscles are separated in the midline and the laryngeal cartilages and hyoid bone are explored. The larynx is entered either through an appropriately placed fracture line or via a purposeful midline thyrotomy. The interior of the larynx is inspected and *repair of all mucosal tears* is carried out, under microscopic control, if necessary. Debridement of tissue should be avoided if at all possible. When there has been significant mucosal loss, flaps obtained from the pyriform sinus or free grafts should be used to reestablish mucosal integrity. Fine absorbable sutures should be used throughout. It is imperative that the vocal ligaments and particularly their *anterior commissure attachment* be *reestablished. Dislocation of the arytenoid cartilages* can be *reduced,* but if one cartilage is missing, the *vocal cord remnant* should be *fixed to the cricoid cartilage at the midline* in order to allow good apposition of the remaining mobile cord and avoid later aspiration. In the unlikely event that both arytenoids are lost, the vocal cord remnants should be fixed to the cricoid with sufficient separation to permit eventual extubation. If the *epiglottis* has been avulsed, it may be *repaired,* but probably it is better to amputate it.[6]

All cartilaginous and bony *fractures should be reduced* and directly wired, although nonabsorbable sutures can often be used instead if there is little calcification. In some cases, simple suture repair of the outer perichondrium is sufficient to stabilize small fragments. Although all cartilage fragments should be preserved when possible, the critical elements are reestablishment of the cricoid ring, stabilization of the anterior commissure, and reestablishment of the cornua and posterior edges of the thyroid alae, including their relationship to the hyoid bone via the thyrohyoid ligaments.

Stenting should be avoided whenever possible and, if it *is* necessary, should be maintained only for 3 to 5 days, beyond which time it becomes a source of significant trauma, itself. A variety of stents have been employed, each having its relative advantages. A simple, soft stent for short-term use may be made at the table from a condom packed with gauze.

If a stent can be avoided, it is often wise to use an *anterior keel* (Fig. 8–4), usually made of tantalum plate. This will avoid webbing at the anterior commissure and, if extended far enough posteriorly in the larynx, prevents adherence of the vocal cords if they are denuded of mucosa on opposing surfaces. Such a keel can be removed under local anesthesia in 10 days to 2 weeks.

Long-Term

Long-term management of blunt laryngeal trauma is concerned mainly with prevention or correction of stenosis and preservation or restoration of normal vocal cord mobility. Despite strict adherence to the principles of immediate management just outlined, stenosis or paralysis or fixation of the glottis often occurs. This may be due to infection, chondronecrosis, or failure to assess adequately the extent of the initial injury because of other pressing concerns. In addition, the tracheotomy that is so often necessary in management of laryngeal injuries carries with it a significant incidence of complications, although most of these are localized below the larynx.

Figure 8–4. Placement of tantlum keel via thyrotomy for anterior web.

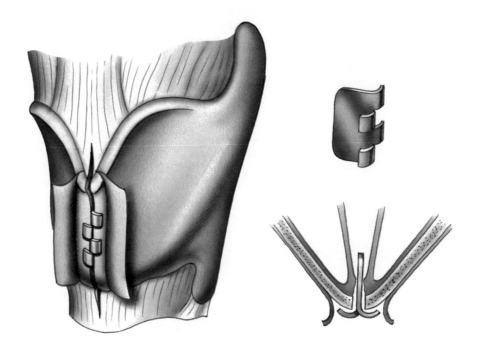

CT scanning or laminograms may be used to determine if stenosis is due to skeletal collapse or only because of soft tissue scarring. It is extremely important to make this distinction, since nothing short of open surgical correction will suffice if the cartilage framework has collapsed.—HMT

Rethi[7] pointed out that no scar tissue should be removed that is not essential to enlarge the lumen, since the resultant denudation of submucosal soft tissue, coupled with the stimulus to more scar formation during healing, are the factors that lead to recurrent stenosis.—HMT

Acquired *laryngotracheal stenosis* is best prevented, inasmuch as its management is difficult and often not completely successful. It may result from the injury itself, associated tracheotomy, or secondary to intubation. Depending on the extent and severity of stenosis, appropriate management may consist of dilation, laser surgery, with or without stenting, and surgical correction via anterior or posterior laryngotracheoplasty.

Dilations may be successful, providing the stenosis is not too severe and there is no loss of cartilaginous support. ◁ If the stenosis is more severe, but is still limited to the soft tissue, *laser surgery* can be used to "core out" the stenosis, on a repeated basis, if necessary. This is often successful, providing that wedges of soft tissue are removed from three or four quadrants (Fig. 8–5) rather than attempting circumferential excision. ◁ Stenting with a soft Silastic T-tube[8] has been most useful in my hands, although other stents have been reported to be successful, as well.[9]

The decision to intervene surgically in laryngotracheal stenosis is not difficult if cartilaginous collapse has been identified, but is often troublesome when the stenosis is limited to soft tissue. Useful guidelines[3] in making this decision include:

1. Tracheostomy care cannot be managed safely on an outpatient basis.

Figure 8–5. Laser surgery for soft tracheal stenosis. Removal of limited amounts of tissue at each quadrant tends to prevent restenosis.

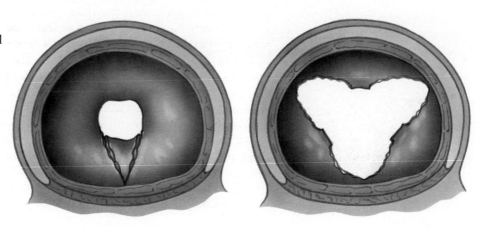

Figure 8–6. Management of tracheal stenosis. **a,** Simple incision through stenosis and stenting. **b,** Crenellated incision.

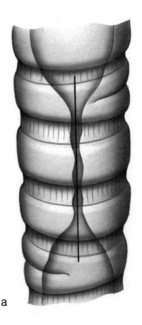

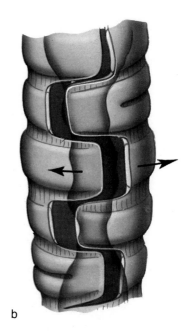

a   b

I prefer costal cartilage for this purpose, because it is available in ample supply and can be carved to almost any thickness or shape desired. Montgomery[13] prefers autogenous thyroid cartilage.— HMT

2. There is no improvement after several conservative procedures, such as dilations or laser surgery.
3. The "wait and see" approach is not accompanied by progressive improvement of the airway.

Laryngotracheoplasty can be accomplished in many ways. Rethi[7] and Evans and Todd[10] (Fig. 8–6 a and b) have recommended simple anterior incision of the stenotic area along its vertical axis, with internal stenting to hold the new lumen until healing takes place. Such an approach has the advantage that it enlarges the lumen with little additional damage to the interior. However, prolonged stenting is in itself a source of granulation tissue formation and subsequent restenosis. Therefore, I prefer the technique of cartilage interposition,[11,12] which permits significant widening of the lumen without the need for long-term stenting, in most cases. In my opinion, most subglottic stenoses requiring surgical intervention benefit from interposition of cartilage both anteriorly and posteriorly (Fig. 8–7 a and b). ◁ The larynx is exposed via an anterior approach and a median thyrotomy, including the anterior cricoid ring, is carried out through the stenosis. A superiorly based flap of mucosa is raised in the posterior commissure, leaving it attached to its reflection on the posterior aspect of the cricoid lamina. The interarytenoideus muscle is resected if it is fibrotic and the posterior cricoid lamina is split vertically in the midline, too, but not through the mucosa on its posterior surface. An appropriately sized piece of cartilage with perichondrium intact on at least one surface is fashioned and sutured in place to hold the laminae apart, using fine, nonabsorbable sutures placed entirely within the cartilage itself. The posterior mucosal flap is mobilized onto the posterior surface of the cricoid to gain additional length and repositioned to cover the cartilage graft. A suitable piece of cartilage is likewise sutured to the anterior cricotracheal defect, perichondrium toward the lumen. The intact perichondrium both increases the chance for establishment of good blood supply and serves as a mucosal substitute. Most of these patients do not require stenting. The rotary door flap has also been described recently for such defects (Fig. 8–8).

Nonmovement of the vocal cords may result from paralysis, fixation of the cricoarytenoid joints, or both. Therefore, when this situation is dis-

Figure 8–7. Cartilage interposition laryngotracheoplasty.
a, Anterior placement.
b, Posterior commissuroplasty.

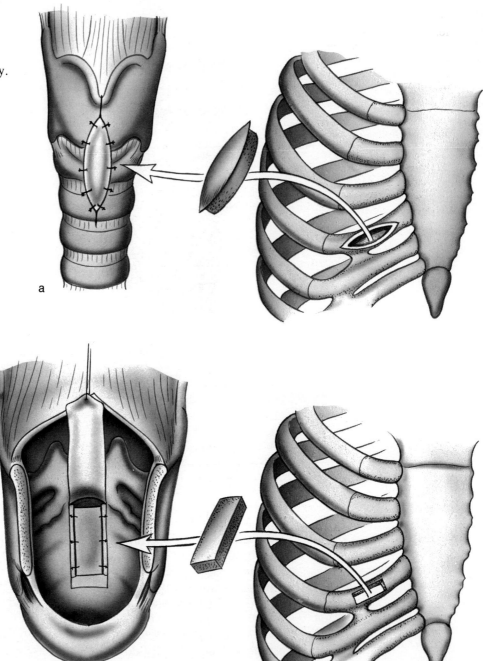

a

b

In those few cases in which anastomosis has been attempted,[14,15] if anything has been achieved it has been limited to adduction. Since there are at least three times as many adductor as abductor fibers in the recurrent laryngeal nerve, it is not surprising that this is so. Miglets[16] was able selectively to reimplant the avulsed end of the recurrent laryngeal nerves into the posterior cricoarytenoid muscle. There was return of abductor function several months later on one side.—HMT

covered late, it is imperative to determine whether the vocal folds are passively mobile, inasmuch as this finding will be important in determining best management. Discussion of surgical intervention for vocal cord paralysis and/or fixation can be found in Chapter 11.

If there has been severe trauma to the neck and the vocal cords do not move immediately after the injury, should the recurrent laryngeal nerves be explored and repaired? In my opinion, such exploration is both pointless and may even worsen the situation. If the vocal cords do not move, either they are permanently paralyzed or they will recover without intervention. Since repair of severed recurrent laryngeal nerves has been generally unsuccessful,◁ there is little point in trying to explore them, espe-

Figure 8–8. Rotary door flap repair for laryngotracheal stenosis. A myocutaneous flap of the sternothyroid muscle and its overlying skin can be rotated with intact nerve and blood supply to fill such a defect. (Courtesy Isaac Eliachar, MD, Department of Otolaryngology, Cleveland Clinic Foundation, Cleveland, OH.)

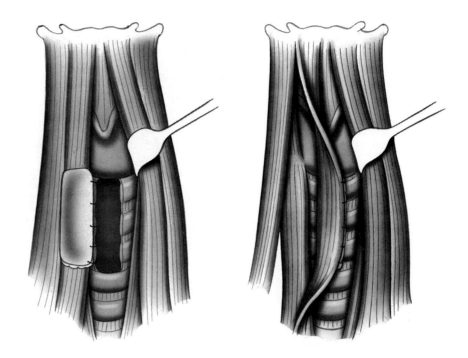

cially since additional trauma may ensue during the attempt to find the nerves in a bloody and anatomically disrupted field. Since nerve-muscle pedicle reinnervation[17] does not require manipulation of the recurrent laryngeal nerve and does not interfere with spontaneous recovery if it is destined to take place, this technique can be applied without waiting for spontaneous recovery. Although the surgeon could consider immediate nerve-muscle pedicle reinnervation under these circumstances, in practice one usually waits from 3 months to 1 year for spontaneous recovery, before intervening.

Intubation Trauma

No matter how skillfully or carefully done, intubation of the larynx carries with it the risk of acute and long-term complications. It is a tribute to the competence of most of the anesthesiologists and nurse anesthetists who perform the enormous number of intubations that now take place daily around the world that there is not an even higher incidence of unwanted side effects from this procedure.

Immediate laryngeal complications of intubation include glottic or subglottic edema, mucosal laceration, dislocation of the arytenoid, avulsion of the epiglottis, and vocal cord paralysis. These injuries are more likely to occur under emergency conditions than after orderly intubation. Since patients often complain of throat discomfort or slight voice change after even ''atraumatic'' intubation, these injuries can remain undiagnosed for some period of time after the injury. It is imperative, therefore, that *any* significant voice change, stridor, dysphagia, or persistent laryngeal discomfort be evaluated by indirect laryngoscopy. *Laryngeal edema* can often be prevented by administering a bolus of dexamethasone (in supramaximal dose) about 20 minutes before intubation in patients at high risk because of local laryngeal problems. Once significant edema has occurred, however, reintubation and treatment with steroids and antibiotics may be needed for 1 or 2 days. Tracheotomy should only rarely be necessary. The other three immediate complications, when recognized, will often require prompt endoscopic or surgical intervention. *Mucosal lacerations,* if severe enough, should be managed as described for blunt trauma. *Arytenoid dis-*

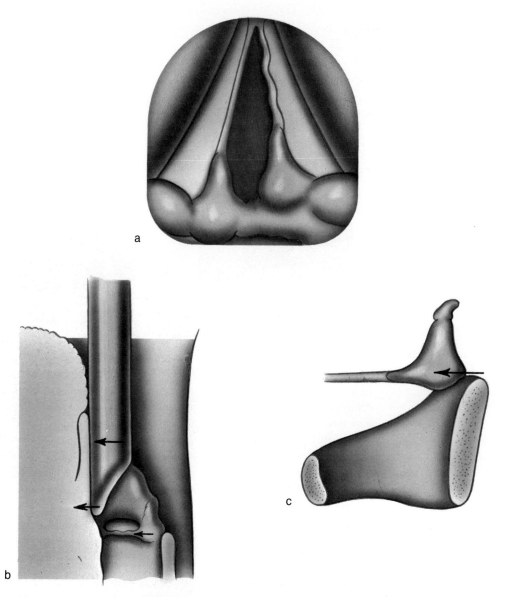

Figure 8–9. **a,** Appearance of dislocated arytenoid cartilage. **b,c,** Simple anterior pressure on the petiole of the epiglottis at laryngoscopy may be sufficient to disimpact the arytenoid and to permit it to return to normal position.

Although unproved, I believe that the mechanism of injury in these cases is due to entrapment of a recurrent laryngeal nerve that passes anterior (rather than posterior, as is usually the case,) to the lesser cornu of the thyroid cartilage (see Chapter 1). This variant exists in perhaps 5 percent of normal adults. Both the forceful elevation of the thyroid cartilage relative to the cricoid cartilage that takes place during laryngoscopy and the posterior displacement of the cricoid lamina relative to the thyroid cartilage because of position of the endotracheal tube offer opportunities for such an injury. —HMT

location should be reduced as soon as possible, since after 24 to 48 hours, reduction usually will not prevent long-term ankylosis. The simple act of elevating the larynx during endoscopy is usually sufficient to disimpact the arytenoid and to allow it to reposition itself. (Fig. 8–9) *Avulsion of the epiglottis* requires open repair or laser excision. *Vocal cord paralysis* as a result of otherwise uncomplicated intubation is an unusual, but not unheard of, complication. Most of these recover, except in the cases where the paralysis existed undetected before intubation.[18]◁

Delayed complications of intubation include intubation granuloma, cricoarytenoid ankylosis or fibrosis, glottic webs, and subglottic stenosis. Most of these can be prevented or minimized by limiting intubation time whenever possible, selection of the smallest tube that will permit adequate respiratory support, use of low-pressure cuffs, careful fixation of the tube to limit movement during assisted ventilation, use of steroids and antibiot-

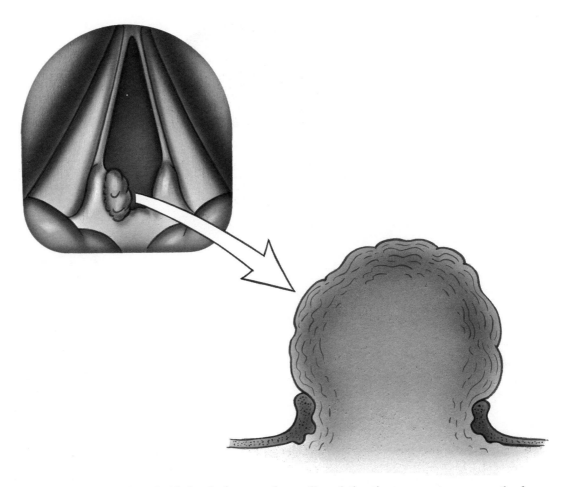

Figure 8–10. Intubation granuloma. Granulation tissue prevents overgrowth of epithelium.

ics in high-risk cases, and early recognition and treatment of such laryngeal injuries.

   Intubation granuloma (Fig. 8–10) results from denudation of the mucosa overlying the bodies or vocal processes of the arytenoid cartilages. Because there is no submucosa, the blood supply is rather poor, and the area is always exposed to potential contamination, the circumstances that favor chronic infection and formation of granulation tissue are all present. Heaping up of the granulation tissue prevents remucosalization. These can sometimes be resolved by a course of steroids (prednisone, 10 mg orally four times daily for 10 days, with tapering doses thereafter) antibiotics (penicillin V or cephalexin, 250 mg orally four times daily for 30 days) and zinc sulfate (220 mg, three times daily after meals for 30 to 60 days). The steroids are intended to suppress the formation of granulation tissue, the antibiotics control the infection, and the zinc has been suggested empirically as an adjunct to wound healing.[19] The assistance of a speech therapist is also strongly advised. If a reasonable course of such medical therapy is unsuccessful, removal via laser surgery is indicated. If followed by a repeated course of medical therapy, approximately 50 percent will be cured. Of the remainder, about half can be cured by a second attempt at surgical removal. This lesion, however, is sometimes refractory to any means of therapy, so that the best that can be achieved in some cases is a stable but persistent small granuloma.

   Glottic web has been considered in Chapter 7 when of congenital or-

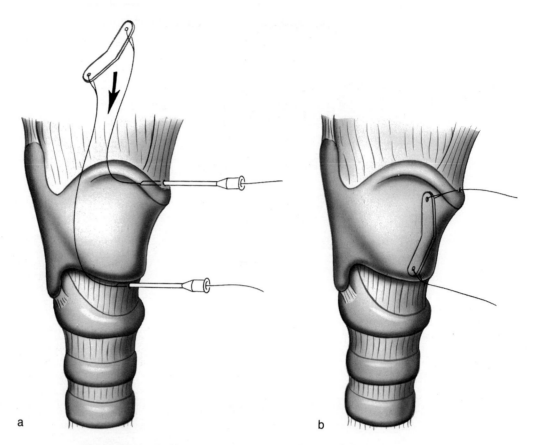

Figure 8–11. Endoscopic placement of a Teflon keel.

See Chapter 6.

igin. It can occur as a result of simultaneous denudation of both vocal folds near the anterior commissure, which, when they heal together, produce a web. Webs probably result from improper laryngeal surgery◁ more often than from intubation. In addition to the technique described for placement of an anterior tantalum keel (see before), they can be managed endoscopically by laser or mechanical lysis, followed by placement of an internal Teflon keel (Fig. 8–11) held in place by wires passed through the skin.[20] The keel is removed endoscopically, as well, after about 10 days to 2 weeks.

Cricoarytenoid ankylosis is considered in Chapter 9 and *acquired subglottic stenosis* has been discussed before.

Thermal and Chemical Injuries

Immediate management of suspected inhalation of hot or caustic gases must include anticipation of delayed, but often of sudden onset, severe upper airway obstruction. It is common for such a patient to demonstrate few symptoms when first seen and then to be in severe distress a few minutes later. Burns of the lower respiratory tract are relatively uncommon, since inhalation of gases hot enough to produce them would result in laryngeal edema and obstruction before pulmonary injuries could occur.[21] Thus, it is more often the irritants contained within the smoke than its temperature that are responsible for laryngeal burns. Moreover, the absence of visible external burns does not preclude the possibility of life-threatening injury to the airway.

Such *signs* and *symptoms* as cough, carbon particles, or blood in the sputum, voice change, stridor, or dyspnea should alert the physician to the

"A cherry-red color is a manifestation of carbon monoxyhemoglobin and may mask a coexistent cyanosis."—Cohen and Peppard[22]

possibility of impending severe obstruction or pulmonary edema. If in doubt, the patient should be admitted for observation, an intravenous line started, and the necessary instruments for prompt intubation kept at hand.◁ Cultures should be obtained of both sputum and blood. If there is any doubt about the patient's respiratory competency, he should be intubated and placed on assisted positive-pressure breathing support. In addition to anticipating and preventing laryngeal obstruction, positive-pressure breathing can help minimize pulmonary edema. Arterial blood gas monitoring can be very useful in assessing the effectiveness of the patient's own respiratory efforts, as well as in artificial control of ventilation.

The decision whether or not to perform a *tracheotomy in patients with upper airway burns* is a difficult one. Tracheotomy can reduce dead space, greatly simplify bronchopulmonary toilette, is more comfortable for the patient (thus reducing the need for sedation), may permit peroral rather than nasogastric tube feeding, and reduces the chance for further injuring an already traumatized larynx by removing the endotracheal tube from between the vocal cords.◁ On the other hand, especially since we have greatly improved the ability to maintain long-term endotracheal intubation in recent years, airway management by the peroral route can avoid certain uncommon, but potentially devastating, complications of tracheotomy. Paramount among these is secondary infection. *All* tracheotomy tracts become at least superficially infected. A burned airway, especially in a patient who must be treated with steroids, is a prime candidate for secondary infection, often with *Pseudomonas*. Therefore, *if* tracheotomy is undertaken, local wound care must be meticulous and a careful watch for signs of infection, followed by prompt antibiotic treatment, is mandatory.

Long-term management of laryngeal burns depends on the success of initial treatment in preventing such complications as stenosis and ankylosis of the cricoarytenoid joints. Specific measures to deal with these problems have been discussed.

"The indication for tracheostomy is determined by the degree of pulmonary toilet required and the anticipated time of intubation."—Cohen and Peppard[22]

References

1. May M, Tucker HM, Dillard BM: Penetrating wounds of the neck in civilians. Otol Clin North Am, 9:361–391, 1976.

2. Hilding AC: Laryngotracheal damage during intratracheal anesthesia. Ann Otol Rhinol Laryngol, 80:565, 1971.

3. Toohill RJ, Duncavage JA, Grossman TW, Lehman RH: Treatment of acquired and congenital subglottic stenosis. In English GE (Ed): Otolaryngology, vol 3. Philadelphia, Harper & Row, 1984, pp 3–4.

4. Tucker HM, Padula R: Nonpenetrating traumatic perforation of the pharynx. Arch Otol, 97:1, 1968.

5. Snow JB Jr: Diagnosis and therapy for acute laryngeal and tracheal injuries. Otol Clin North Am, 17:101–106, 1984.

6. Ogura JH, Biller HF: Reconstruction of the larynx after blunt trauma. Ann Otol Rhinol Laryngol, 80:492, 1971.

7. Rethi A: Operation for cicatricial stenosis of the larynx. Otolaryngol Head Neck Surg, 70:283–293, 1956.

8. Montgomery WW: Manual for care of the Montgomery silicone tracheal T-tube. Ann Otol Rhinol Laryngol, 89:(Suppl 73, pt 5):1–8, 1980.

9. Schaefer SD, Carder HM: How I do it-head and neck: Fabrication of a simple laryngeal stent. Laryngoscope, 90:1561–1563, 1980.

10. Evans JNR, Todd GB: Laryngotracheoplasty. J Laryngol Otol, 88:589–597, 1974.

11. Meyer R: New concepts in laryngotracheal reconstruction. Trans Am Acad Ophthalmol Otol, 76:758–766, 1972.

12. Cotton R: Management of subglottic stenosis in infancy and childhood. Ann Otol Rhinol Laryngol, 87:649–657, 1978.

13. Montgomery WW: Chronic subglottic stenosis. Otol Clin North Am 17:107–113, 1984.

14. Iwamura S: Functioning remobilization of the paralyzed vocal cord in dogs. Arch Otol, 199:122–129, 1974.

15. Doyle PJ, Brummett RE, Everts EC: Results of surgical section and repair of the recurrent

laryngeal nerve. Laryngoscope, 77:1245–1254, 1967.

16. Miglets AW: Functional laryngeal abduction following reimplantation of the recurrent laryngeal nerves. Laryngoscope, 84:1996–2005, 1974.

17. Tucker HM: Laryngeal reinnervation: A review. Head Neck Surg, 2:1, 1979.

18. Astor FC, Santilli P, Tucker HM: Incidence of cranial nerve dysfunction following carotid endarterectomy. Head Neck Surg, 6:660, 1983.

19. Levine H: Medical and surgical management of voice disorders. In English GM (Ed): Otolaryngology, vol 3. Philadelphia, Harper & Row, 1984.

20. Tucker HM: *Surgery for Phonatory Disorders.* New York, Churchill Livingstone, 1981, pp 47–51.

21. Stone HH, Rhame DW, Corbitt JD, et al: Respiratory burns: A correlation of clinical and laboratory results. Ann Surg, 165:157, 1967.

22. Cohen AM, Peppard SB: Laryngeal trauma. In English GE (Ed): Otolaryngology, vol 3. Philadelphia, Harper & Row, 1984.

Chapter 9

Degenerative Disorders of the Larynx

See Chapters 7 and 10.

It is sometimes difficult to distinguish degenerative conditions of the larynx from those that are the result of inflammation or infection or that are of congenital origin.◁ Indeed, in some instances, the ultimate degenerative changes are either initiated by infectious or inflammatory conditions or are exacerbated by concurrent ones. Nevertheless, it is useful to classify certain laryngeal conditions as degenerative, in some cases because they do not fit into any other classification and in others because they are clearly related to the aging process, physical abuse, or "wear and tear."

A list of such degenerative conditions of the larynx is included in Table 9–1.

Cystic Lesions

Pharyngoceles

Pharyngoceles are due to pathologic enlargement of the pyriform fossae or hypopharynx, or both. There are two potential natural defects in this area: between the superior and middle constrictor muscles, through which passes the glossopharyngeal nerve (Fig. 9–1a), and at the upper aspect of the pyriform fossa, via the thyrohyoid membrane at the point of passage of the superior laryngeal nerve, artery, and vein (Fig. 9–1b). The pharyngoepiglottic fold separates these two areas from each other, the tonsillar fossa above arising from the second pharyngeal pouch and the pyriform fossa below having been derived from the third and fourth pharyngeal pouches.◁ The term "pharyngocele" was first used by Atkinson[1] to distinguish these lateral enlargements from the midline posterior Zenker's diverticulum. Those that arise above the pharyngoepiglottic fold may be of *congenital* origin, in which case they are probably second branchial pouch remnants. This type usually has a long, slender neck, which may expand laterally in the neck and will demonstrate the histologic characteristics of a branchial cleft remnant.◁ The *acquired* variety tends to appear in old age and is often asymptomatic. Pharyngoceles that arise from the pyriform fossae usually occur in younger patients, in whom they are sometimes related to chronic dilation of the pharynx, as, for example, in brass musicians (Fig. 9–2).

Signs and *symptoms* include a visible mass, often brought on by the

See Chapter 1.

The criteria for pathologic diagnosis of branchial cleft remnant are lining of squamous or respiratory epithelium, or both, and containing foci of normal lymphoid follicles in the walls.—HMT

Table 9–1   Degenerative Conditions of the Larynx

Cystic lesions
   1. Pharyngoceles
   2. Laryngoceles
   3. Saccular cysts
   4. Ductal or inclusion cysts
Due to misuse
   1. Polypoid change and vocal polyps
   2. Nodules
   3. Contact ulcers
   4. Dysphonia plica ventricularis
Due to Aging and Systemic Disorders
   1. Cricoarytenoid arthritis
   2. Flaccid vocal folds

"A Valsalva maneuver with the airway closed at the laryngeal level will not inflate the pharyngocele."—LD Hollinger[2]

Certain Indian criminals were known to dilate their pharynges digitally to enlarge the pouches, into which they might place small stolen objects and thus avoid detection when searched. The dilation generally disappeared when the digital manipulation ceased.[1,3]

Valsalva maneuver, increasing collar size, and dysphagia, which is the most common complaint. Food tends to stick and even to be regurgitated some time after eating. Patients will occasionally experience cough or aspiration in severe cases. *Diagnosis* is made by physical examination and confirmed by xeroradiography with and without modified Valsalva maneuver.◁

If local measures, such as elimination of wind instrument playing and careful oropharyngeal hygiene to empty the sac, do not suffice,◁ *surgical management* becomes necessary. The sac is approached via a lateral neck incision appropriate to its level. If it has protruded through the constrictor

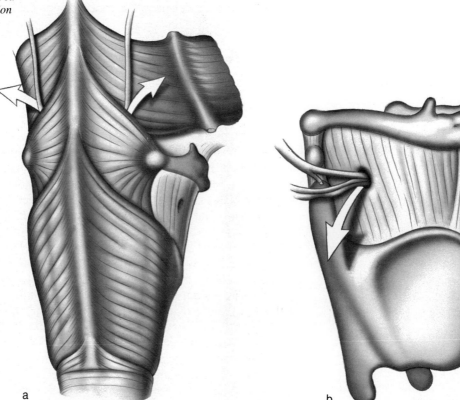

a   b

Figure 9–1. Potential anatomic weakpoints for egress of laryngocele from the larynx. **a,** junction of middle and superior constrictor muscles. **b,** Hiatus of the cricothyroid membrane for passage of the superior laryngeal vessels and nerves.

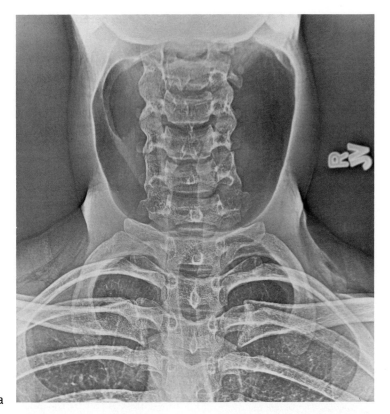

a

b

Figure 9–2. Massive dilatation of pyriform sinuses in a wind instrument player. **a,** Anteroposterior view. **b,** Lateral view (courtesy Howard Levine, MD, with permission of *Cleveland Clinic Quarterly*)

muscle, it is identified and traced to its origin, taking care not to injure the superior laryngeal nerve in the process. To this end, it may be helpful to distend the sac with a vaginal pack or inflated Foley catheter placed endoscopically.[4] It is important to delineate the sac carefully so that excess pharyngeal mucosa is not resected with it. A suction catheter drain should be used. The patient should be fed via a nasogastric tube for 5 to 7 days, by which time the wound ought to be sufficiently healed to permit oral alimentation.

Laryngoceles and Saccular Cysts

Diplophonia results (rather than hoarseness) if the saccular cyst is of sufficient size to distort the position of the vocal fold, but not large enough to interfere with apposition of the free margins. The weight of the cyst resting on the vocal fold changes its mass characteristics and, thus, its vibratory pattern.—HMT

The saccule of the ventricle is a blind pouch, directed superiorly between the substance of the ventricular band (false cord) and the medial aspect of the thyroid lamina. It contains a concentration of mucous glands and has small muscles in its wall to express its secretions onto the surface of the vocal folds.[5] If its neck or one of its glands becomes occluded, a *saccular cyst* can result (Fig. 9–3). They can be *congenital* or *acquired*, the former due to developmental anomaly of the sac itself and the latter due to obstruction secondary to trauma, foreign body, infection, or neoplasm. The most common *symptom* is voice change, often manifested as a muffled cry and inspiratory stridor in infants and diplophonia in adults.◁ The *diagnosis* is made by direct or indirect laryngoscopy. Such preoperative studies as xeroradiography and computed tomography (CT) scan can be helpful. *Treatment* is by needle aspiration in infants. This approach provides immediate relief of the airway at minimal risk and is often all that is necessary. In adults (and in recurrent cysts in children) endoscopic removal or marsupialization is appropriate. Although this has been accomplished with cup forceps for many years, the laser has allowed complete and essentially atraumatic removal in recent times. With this approach, tracheotomy should only occasionally be needed, even in small children.

Laryngocele is defined as "an abnormal dilatation or herniation of the saccule."[2] Classically, these lesions are filled with air, but may also contain mucus or other inspissated material. They may be *internal* (confined to the false cord), *external* (having escaped from the larynx via the thyrohyoid membrane), or *combined*. (Fig. 9–4) Internal laryngocele and saccular or even ductal cysts (see later) may be clinically and histologically

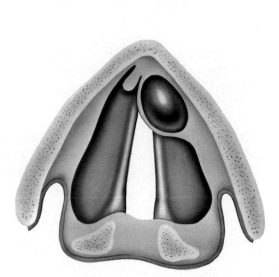
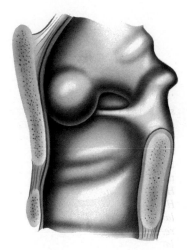

Figure 9–3. Saccular cyst. Note origin from appendix or saccule of the ventricle.

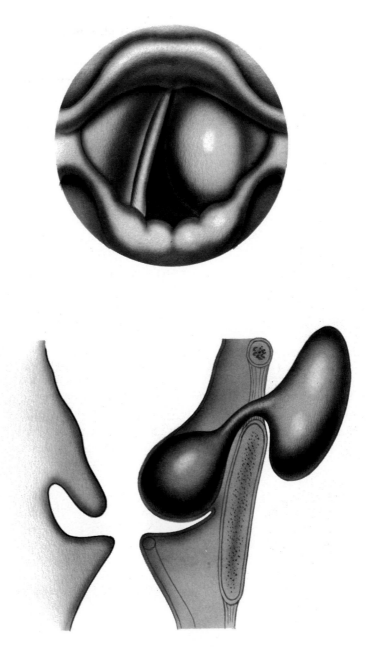

Figure 9–4. Combined internal-external laryngocele. It is not sufficient to remove only the cervical portion of such a lesion, since the internal component will continue to enlarge.

"The occurrence of a laryngocele, saccular cyst, or even a laryngopyocele in an adult should raise the suspicion of an associated laryngeal neoplasm. The literature is resplendent with case reports of this occurrence. The experience of Harrison[7] is typical in this regard: He reports a case in which a laryngocele or saccular cyst was resected only to have a large laryngeal tumor become apparent a short time later."—D Holinger[2]

indistinguishable from each other, especially if the laryngocele is filled with fluid. If any of these cystic intralaryngeal lesions becomes infected, it is referred to as a *laryngopyocele*.[6] Laryngocele is relatively uncommon in the newborn, in whom, however, it is clearly of *congenital* origin. In adults, on the other hand, most laryngoceles are thought to be *acquired*. Classic descriptions have led to such appellations as "glass-blowers' disease" which, coupled with the higher incidence of the problem in wind instrument players and in patients with partial laryngeal obstruction, ◁ suggests chronic increase in intralaryngeal pressure as a predisposing cause. Since most people included in the groups just described do not develop a laryngocele, it follows that there must be some preexisting weakness or congenital propensity in those who do.[1,8,9] *Symptoms* include muffled voice, inspiratory stri-

See Chapter 4.

dor, dysphagia, and, in the external and combined varieties, a transient or permanent mass in the neck. *Diagnosis* can be difficult because of the sometimes evanescent nature of the findings. If there is a neck mass whose contents can be evacuated by external pressure, especially in a patient whose history suggests repeated increase in intralaryngeal pressure, the diagnosis may be obvious. On the other hand, one is more likely to encounter a patient with vague fullness in the neck, occasional minor voice change, and few findings to explain the symptoms. Therefore, the examiner must have a high index of suspicion if appropriate studies to confirm the diagnosis are to be obtained. Indirect examination often shows little more than slight fullness of the false cord on the affected side, unless examined immediately after a Valsalva maneuver. CT scanning and xeroradiography are useful confirmatory studies and are most likely to demonstrate an air- or fluid-filled cystic mass, if one is present.◁

Treatment of small internal laryngoceles is often by *endoscopic removal* or marsupialization, as with other cysts. Combined and external laryngoceles require *external surgical removal,* usually via lateral thyrotomy[10] (Fig. 9–5) The mass is approached through an appropriately placed, horizontal skin-crease incision at about the level of the thyrohyoid membrane. If there is a sac in the neck, it is identified and mobilized from the surrounding structures. It is then traced to its point of escape from the larynx just above the upper border of the thyroid ala. An incision is made in the perichondrium along the upper border of the thyroid cartilage and the internal and external perichondrial leaflets thus described are elevated. The intervening portion of the upper thyroid ala is removed. If further dissection is needed within the larynx to reach the neck of the sac at the level of the ventricle, it is carried out extraperichondrially. The perichondrium is then incised to expose the intralaryngeal portion of the sac, its neck is suture ligated, and it is excised. In this manner, it is often possible to remove

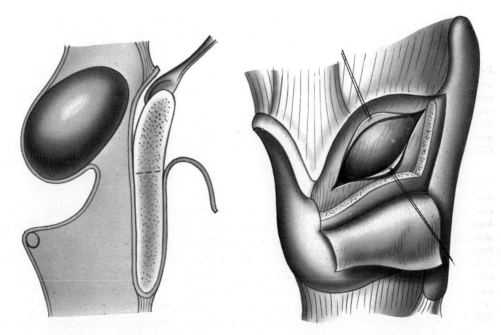

Figure 9–5. Surgical approach to internal laryngocele. Inner perichondrium is entered to expose the lesion only after it has been completely mobilized extralaryngeally. The neck of the sac is usually encountered anteriorly, since it arises from the saccule of the ventricle.

the entire laryngocele intact and to accomplish this without actually entering the mucosa-lined spaces of the larynx. Tracheotomy is generally advisable, at least for a few days after surgery. ◁

Ductal Cysts

The term "ductal cyst" is more appropriate than the commonly used *inclusion or retention cyst,* because these lesions are almost always lined by ductal epithelium. They are found anywhere in the larynx but, unlike saccular cysts and internal laryngoceles, they tend to be within the mucosa, rather than deep in the substance of the false cord. They are usually fairly small and are three times more common than sacular cysts.[6] Although aspiration is possible, it is probably best to remove them endoscopically.

Due to Misuse

The sequence of pathologic events that take place in the mucosa and underlying structures of the vocal folds in response to irritation or trauma of any kind can best be referred to as *polypoid change.* Although vocal abuse secondary to overuse or misuse of the voice is probably the most frequent cause of its earliest stages (Reinke's edema, see later), other factors, such as smoking, chronic sinusitis, allergy, and other inflammatory conditions, certainly are important contributors. Although many investigators tend to classify these lesions as *inflammatory,* it seems more appropriate to include them under *degenerative* conditions, inasmuch as degenerative changes are the common denominator in the pathophysiology of all of them, regardless of precipitating cause. In planning management, it is important to recognize that there is progressive deterioration of the vocal folds in response to continuing irritation; this "vicious cycle" can be broken and usually reversed by removing the source of injury. Only when the changes in the tissues have progressed to certain advanced levels does it become necessary to consider surgical intervention.

Polypoid Change and Vocal Polyps

The initial response of the vocal folds to irritation is the development of *Reinke's edema.* This is characterized by collection of fluid in the potential space that exists between the surface mucosa and underlying musculature. ◁ It is very common in heavy smokers, especially those older than 40 years of age, and often becomes chronic in this group. A less common and sometimes overlooked cause of Reinke's edema is *hypothyroidism.* ◁ It can be distinguished from polypoid changes in that the whole membranous portion of the vocal fold is uniformly involved, rather than in limited areas, as is usually the case with discrete polyps. *Symptoms* are usually limited to slight to moderate voice change. *Diagnosis* is confirmed by indirect laryngoscopy. The condition is *treated* by identifying and removing the source of irritation and will always benefit from the assistance of a speech pathologist. Indeed, since voice misuse is such a common underlying factor, failure to include *speech therapy* as part of the management plan is likely to result in failure. Such measures as stopping smoking, exogenous thyroid replacement where appropriate, humidification, and voice rest are obviously important, as well. In the occasional case that does not respond to these therapeutic efforts, surgical intervention via laryngoscopy and either cup forceps or *laser surgical removal* is necessary. Even then, if appro-

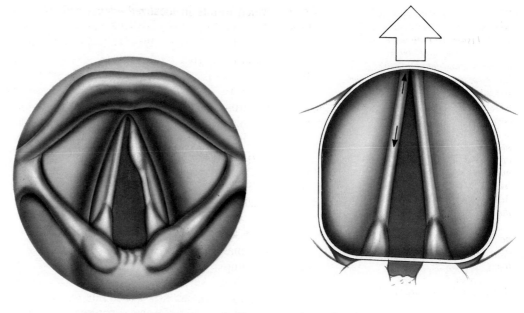

Figure 9–6. Mechanism of effacement of vocal polyp. **a,** Mirror view; note that image is reversed from direct view. **b,** Apparent disappearance of polyp because of tension on the vocal fold from the laryngoscope.

priate general measures as just outlined are not instituted postoperatively, the condition will probably return.

If the irritation producing Reinke's edema continues long enough, true *polypoid changes* will occur. The pathologic alterations that constitute the various types of polyps are reviewed in Chapter 3. Clinically, polyps may be classified as *pedunculated, fusiform, or generalized. Symptoms* include a foreign body sensation and voice change, which may wax and wane in severity, but usually does not return entirely to normal. Large, pedunculated polyps that hang below the free margin of the vocal folds can produce intermittent and rather abrupt aphonia or hoarseness. Voice change occurs only when the polyp flips up into the glottis and disappears just as quickly when it falls back to its dependent, subglottic position. *Diagnosis* is confirmed by indirect laryngoscopy, in most cases (Fig. 9–6).◁ *Treatment* is similar to that just described for Reinke's edema. Virtually every case should have a trial of removal of irritants and speech therapy before any consideration is given to surgical removal. The technique of laryngoscopic removal of polyps is discussed in Chapter 6.

Vocal Nodules

Vocal nodules are also called screamer's nodes or singer's nodes, and this terminology suggests the cause, which is invariably vocal abuse. It is important to distinguish between the otolaryngologist's use of the term "vocal nodule" and what is meant when the same term is used by the pathologist. To the clinician, a vocal nodule is a small, whitish or reddish elevation located at the junction of the anterior and middle thirds of the vocal fold. In the majority of such cases, the histologic findings are a deposition of scar or fibrous tissue, usually under the surface of intact but somewhat thickened mucous membrane. To the pathologist, however, this group of findings is only one of several that warrant the diagnosis of vocal polyp, a term that includes vocal nodules in most pathology classifications.

The probable *pathophysiology* of vocal nodules is trauma due to voice

Both small, fusiform polyps and large, pedunculated ones can be difficult to diagnose by mirror laryngoscopy. When the tongue is held in an extended position, the epiglottis is displaced anteriorly, which, in turn, puts the vocal folds under increased tension. Under these circumstances, a small, fusiform polyp may be effaced by the increased tension and, therefore, difficult to detect (Fig. 9–7). A similar situation may ensue during suspension laryngoscopy, making it difficult to identify a polyp seen previously on indirect examination. This problem can be avoided in appropriate cases by use of flexible, fiberoptic laryngoscopy with the larynx in normal position. Large, pedunculated polyps, on the other hand, may go unnoticed because they hang below the glottis, leaving only a slight change in contour at the point of origin from the free edge of the vocal fold.—HMT

"Children who develop vocal nodules differ in personality and family history from those who do not. . . . [They are] more aggressive and less mature and [have] more difficulty in managing stressful situations than children with normal voice. . . . The etiology and pathology of vocal nodules in adults are basically the same as in children. . . . Whereas the incidence . . . is higher in male children than in females, this trend is reversed in adults. . . . Adult(s) with nodules have some of the same personality characteristics . . . as children who develop nodules. They are talkative, . . . aggressive, and tense, and suffer from . . . interpersonal problems . . . , anxiety, anger, or depression."—AE Aronson[12]

This is especially true for singers and, to a lesser extent, other professional voice users. Whereas the speaking voice is usually quite satisfactory after careful removal of vocal nodules and a suitable recovery period, the ultimate singing voice is much more likely to be something less than what it was before the nodule developed. Therefore, SURGICAL INTERVENTION SHOULD BE AVOIDED if at all possible IN PROFESSIONAL VOICE PATIENTS. As a rule of thumb, I will not remove any obviously benign lesion in such individuals unless they are totally unable to perform. In this situation, the patient literally has nothing to lose, at least as far as his professional career is concerned. (See also Shechter and Coleman[13])—HMT

abuse, which results in localized edema and submucosal hemorrhage. These lesions form preferentially at the junction of the anterior and middle thirds of the vocal folds because this is the point of maximum amplitude during phonation at the higher pitch levels that occur during singing or screaming. If the trauma is of short duration and not repeated frequently, there is time for complete resolution of these changes. If, however, voice abuse is frequent or chronic, the changes persist and an *incipient nodule* results. At this point, histologic changes are limited to edema, mucosal hypertrophy, and granulation tissue formation, all of which are at least potentially reversible. If the trauma continues even beyond this point, repeated hemorrhage and inflammation can progress to permanent fibrosis and a fully *mature nodule*. *Personality factors* are also very important in the development of these lesions.◁

By far the most common and often the only *symptom* of vocal nodules is hoarseness, which may be almost unnoticeable while speaking and yet be quite remarkable when singing. Early vocal fatigue is another fairly common complaint. *Diagnosis* is almost always possible by indirect laryngoscopy. Very small lesions may not be obvious, but usually there is a telltale strand of mucus that appears between the vocal folds when nodules are present, just as they begin to separate after phonation. *Management* is primarily through *speech therapy* and voice retraining. Allergy, smoking, and other irritants may also be significant and should be identified and corrected, if possible. A trial of speech therapy should be allowed in virtually every case, even when the nodules are of long standing or when the patient's willingness or ability to cooperate is in question. Not only will this approach sometimes permit unexpected improvement without surgical intervention, but it will also be of value as a head start on the voice retraining necessary during the postoperative period. Moreover, on occasion what appeared to be bilateral vocal nodules (but was actually granulation tissue or thickening of the vocal fold in response to trauma from the nodule on the opposite fold) will regress on one side, leaving only one true nodule to be removed surgically.

In those cases that have already progressed to bilateral, mature, fibrous nodules, improvement through noninvasive means is minimal at best, inasmuch as removing the source of trauma and voice rest will not reverse scar tissue. Under these circumstances, only endoscopic *surgical removal* will offer any chance for cure. If surgical removal is carried out skillfully *and* if good vocal hygiene and voice usage are instituted postoperatively, return to normal voice can be expected in the great majority of cases. However, voice results cannot be guaranteed in any individual case, since the outcome is dependent on healing factors not entirely within the control of the surgeon.◁ Despite the best management, recurrence of nodules is frequent, especially in children. For this reason, if the diagnosis can be established indirectly, it is probably best not to intervene surgically in children with vocal nodules until they have reached an age at which they are able and willing to take part in effective voice retraining.

Contact Ulcers

The posterior third of the vocal fold is made up of the vocal process and part of the body of the arytenoid cartilage, covered only by a tightly applied mucoperichondrium. It also represents the area of the fold that undergoes greatest excursion during opening and closing of the glottis, as well as the point at which any contaminated material that may be cleared form the lungs by movement of the mucociliary blanket leaves the larynx to be swallowed. All of these factors play a part in the development of

"Clinical and research studies point to certain common characteristics among adult males who develop contact ulcer. 1) Hypertonic laryngeal musculature. . . . 2) Habitual use of an excessively low voice pitch level. 3) Explosive speech stress patterns. 4) Sharp, abrupt glottal attack. 5) Restricted pitch variability. 6) Phonation using excessively high infraglottal pressure with bursts of intensity."—AE Aronson[12]

The prednisone suppresses inflammation and, it is hoped, limits granulation tissue. The penicillin is intended to prevent opportunistic infection in a potentially contaminated area, particularly during steroid therapy. The zinc sulfate is given empirically, because inadequate levels of trace elements have been implicated in poor wound healing.—HMT

See Chapter 5.

Unless the true cords and ventricles can be visualized indirectly, direct laryngoscopy should be undertaken. Hidden lesions that prevent good approximation of the vocal folds may be responsible for development of dysphonia plica ventricularis as a compensatory mechanism and, therefore, must be ruled out.—HMT

contact ulcers. They may develop in response to certain kinds of vocal abuse, chronic coughing and throat clearing, direct trauma◁ and as a result of reflux esophagitis.[14,15] In the case of reflux esophagitis it is not clear whether the contact ulcers are the direct result of acid erosion of the interarytenoid space or due to grinding together of the arytenoid cartilages in response to referred discomfort from the vagus via the recurrent laryngeal nerves, which are irritated by gastric reflux at the lower end of the esophagus. Regardless of cause, contact ulcers are often refractory to treatment, and they may even go on to granuloma formation.

Symptoms include discomfort on swallowing and in speaking, slight hoarseness, foreign body sensation and incessant throat clearing. *Diagnosis* is usually possible by indirect laryngoscopy, although small ulcers may not be readily visible from above and may require direct laryngoscopy for confirmation. Cine barium swallow can be helpful in detecting previously unsuspected gastroesophageal reflux. In many cases, a small, sliding hiatal hernia will be identified. *Management* of most contact ulcers should be both *medical* and by *voice therapy*. If reflux is a factor, I begin a regimen designed to limit it. This includes elevation of the head of the bed 4 to 6 inches on wood blocks, bland diet, and use of antacids between meals and at bedtime. In addition, most cases require direct medical attack on the ulcer itself. Prednisone, 10 mg four times daily for 10 days, followed by tapering doses for 3 days, penicillin V, 250 mg four times daily for 30 days, and zinc sulfate, 220 mg three times daily after meals for 30 days or more has been an effective therapeutic plan in my hands.◁ Appropriate voice rest, vocal hygiene, and speech therapy are essential, in addition to medical therapy. Although these approaches usually result in healing, contact ulcers tend to recur at intervals, commonly in response to reestablishment of stressful vocal patterns. The entire regimen can be repeated at intervals, if necessary. In cases that do not respond to medical and speech therapeutic management, *laser surgery* is now regarded as the best surgical approach. The intention is carefully to remove only the diseased tissue of the ulcer, down to but not including the perichondrium, whenever possible. After removal, the entire medical and speech therapeutic regimen already mentioned should be reinstituted.

Dysphonia Plica Ventricularis

It is somewhat difficult to classify this disorder, since in many cases there are no pathologic changes in laryngeal structures. However, since there may be significant hypertrophy of the false vocal cords in prolonged and severe cases, I have elected to include it among the degenerative conditions.◁ *Dysphonia plica ventricularis* is the harsh, hoarse voice that results from phonating with the false cords. It is most commonly seen in people who are tense, aggressive, and under prolonged emotional pressure. Because it is a means of phonation that most people can employ at will, it may be habitual, due to malingering, or part of a conversion reaction. *Diagnosis* is made by observing either a normal larynx in which the patient brings the false vocal cords together during phonatory effort *before* the true folds can meet, or a larynx exhibiting significant hypertrophy of one or both of the false cords. In this latter situation, the true vocal folds are usually obscured by the hypertrophied ventricular bands, even during quiet breathing.◁ *Management* is almost always by *speech therapy* and low level *psychotherapy*. In the occasional case that is either refractory to extended speech therapy or in which false cord hypertrophy is so significant that it mechanically prevents the true cords from coming together, *laser surgical* trimming of the false cords is appropriate.

Due to Aging and Systemic Disorders

Cricoarytenoid Arthritis

Because the cricoarytenoid articulation is a true, synovial joint, it is subject to all of the diseases that can affect the larger joints of the body. Such conditions as rheumatoid arthritis, Reiter's syndrome, gout, ankylosing spondylitis, Crohn's disease, and disseminated lupus erythematosus have been associated with arthritic changes in the cricoarytenoid joint.[16–18] Laryngeal changes may be among the first signs of progression of disease or may be overlooked among the other problems of the patient with a severe exacerbation of chronic systemic disease. Most clinically recognized cases are associated with flare-ups of rheumatoid arthritis.[16]

Symptoms include vague neck fullness and discomfort, voice change, pain on speaking forcefully or on swallowing (often radiating to the ear), tenderness to palpatation of the laryngeal cartilages, and, in extreme cases, dyspnea and stridor. Laryngeal mirror examination will provide the *diagnosis* in most cases. Redness and swelling of the posterior aspect of the larynx, particularly when associated with sluggishness or limitation of motion of the arytenoids, strongly suggests cricoarytenoid arthritis. During remissions, all of the symptoms may disappear, but, in time, fixation of one or both arytenoids will result in permanent changes. Diagnosis may be confirmed by biopsy or by the inability passively to displace the vocal fold during laryngoscopy under paralytic anesthesia.

Treatment includes medical management of the underlying systemic condition. Reversal of laryngeal complaints will usually follow after control of the general disease. Once fixation has resulted, however, management must be surgical, if airway obstruction or permanent voice change ensues. In some cases, endoscopic injection of steroids into the cricoarytenoid joint can be helpful,[17] and our personal experience bears this out.◁ Bilateral fixation can be managed by tracheotomy or arytenoidectomy.

Methylprednisolone acetate can be drawn up into a control syringe, which in turn is attached to a very long, 19 gauge spinal needle. The joint can be exposed best through a slide laryngoscope and the material injected into the region of the cricoarytenoid articulation. Relief has lasted for as much as a year in some of my cases before symptoms recurred.—HMT

Flaccid Vocal Folds

There are many possible causes for the appearance of flaccidity of the vocal folds, most of which are due to neurologic problems.◁ However, it is common to observe such characteristic changes in the elderly in the absence of any demonstrable nervous system disorder. The combination of muscle atrophy, slight slow-down in coordination, and osteoarthritic changes in the laryngeal articulations can result in the typical weak, quavering voice of the elderly person. These changes are often exacerbated by lessened efficiency of the lungs and diaphragm, from which the driving force of phonatory efforts is derived. Deterioration in hearing can also contribute significantly to voice change in the elderly because of decreasing ability to monitor voice production. Finally, psychologic changes, including a perceived loss of importance of the elderly person's opinion to others may be a major factor.

The major *symptom* of vocal fold flaccidity in the elderly is a weak, higher pitched, quavering voice. Easy fatigability is another common complaint. *Diagnosis* is confirmed by observing a flaccid, but otherwise normal-appearing, larynx on indirect examination. All other possible causes for such laryngeal dysfunction must be ruled out. Audiometric assessment is also necessary. *Treatment* includes appropriate augmentation of hearing and speech therapy.◁

See Chapter 11.

"Just as elderly individuals are able to remain fit, physically active, and mentally alert into the seventh and eighth decades of life, if not longer, the voice may equally retain youth and vigor. . . . Many actors and singers retain their fine speaking voices well into old age. . . . The quavering, high-pitched piping voice often attributed to the old need never occur, or at least not until the eighth or ninth decades . . . [if] as much care is taken over preserving [vocal youth] as is over other features an aging person normally worries about—dress, hair styles, and weight gain."
—MCL Greene[19]

References

1. Atkinson L: Pharyngeal diverticula. Arch Middlesex Hosp, 2:254–254, 1952.

2. Holinger LD: Pharyngoceles, laryngoceles, and saccular cysts. In English GE (Ed). Otolaryngology, Philadelphia, Harper & Row, 1984.

3. Ward PH, et al: Laryngeal and pharyngeal pouches. Laryngoscope, 73:564–582, 1963.

4. Norris CW: Pharyngoceles of the hypopharynx. Laryngoscope, 89:1788–1807, 1979.

5. Delahunty JE, Cherry J: The laryngeal saccule. J Laryngol Otol, 83:803–815, 1969.

6. DeSanto LW, Devine KD, Weiland LH: Cysts of the larynx—classification. Laryngoscope, 80:145–176, 1970.

7. Harrison DFN: Saccular mucocele and laryngeal cancer. Arch Otol, 103:232–234, 1977.

8. Meda P: Symptomatic laryngoceles in cancer of the larynx. Arch Otol, 56:512–518, 1952.

9. MacFie WCDD: Asymptomatic laryngoceles in wind-instrument bandsmen. Arch Otol, 83:270–275, 1966.

10. Tucker HM: Surgery for Phonatory Disorders. New York, Churchill Livingstone, 1981, pp 54–56.

11. Hilger JA: Otolaryngologic aspects of hypometabolism. Trans Am Laryngol Assoc, 77:40, 1956.

12. Aronson AE: Clinical Voice Disorders, 2nd ed. Thieme, New York, 1985, Chapter 6.

13. Shechter GL, Coleman RF: Care of the professional voice. Otol Clin North Am, 17:1, 1984.

14. Delahunty JD: Acid laryngitis. J Laryngol Otol, 86:335, 1972.

15. Goldberg M, Noyek AM, Pritzker KPH: Laryngeal granuloma secondary to gastroesophageal reflux. J Otolaryngol, 7:196, 1978.

16. Montgomery WW: Cricoarytenoid arthritis. Laryngoscope, 73:801, 1963.

17. Bienenstock H, Lanyi VF: Cricoarytoid arthritis in a patient with ankylosing spondylitis. Arch Otolaryngol, 103:738, 1977.

18. Kelly JH, Goodman ML, Montgomery WW, Mulvaney TJ: Upper airway obstruction associated with regional enteritis. Ann Otol Rhinol Laryngol, 88:95, 1979.

19. Greene MCL: The voice and voice disorders. In English GM (ED): Otolaryngology, vol 3. Philadelphia, Harper & Row, 1984.

Chapter 10

Infectious and Inflammatory Disorders

The tissues of the larynx can respond to trauma in only a limited number of ways, regardless of whether the cause is infectious, allergic, toxic, thermal, or physical. Edema, inflammation, and exudation are the three main responses to acute injury, with hypertrophy or metaplasia of the mucous membrane and fibrosis of the deeper tissues of the larynx added in more chronic situations. Therefore, laryngeal symptoms of any inflammatory disorder will be essentially the same, differing only in degree, rapidity of onset, and the presence or absence of systemic findings peculiar to the specific cause. The four *major symptoms* of infectious and inflammatory disorders of the larynx are:

1. Dysphonia, most commonly hoarseness
2. Dyspnea, which may progress through stridor all the way to obstruction
3. Dysphagia
4. Pain, which may vary from a dull ache to severe, lancinating discomfort on swallowing

One very important determinant of severity and type of symptoms is the age and size of the patient. Airway compromise is much more likely in small children than in adults, even when the disease process is the same. ◁ Thus, such problems as acute epiglottitis and croup, which are major causes of significant airway obstruction in children, often go undiagnosed in adults, in whom such striking findings are usually lacking (see later).

Diagnosis is made by taking a careful history, performing an indirect laryngeal mirror examination as part of a complete physical examination, and obtaining indicated radiographic and laboratory studies. Direct laryngoscopy for cultures and biopsy may be necessary in selected cases. A speech and language pathologist should take part in the evaluation and is often critical to the management of these patients.

The *history* is particularly useful. Such factors as rapidity of onset, presence or absence of systemic symptoms, condition of family members and co-workers, exposure to noxious substances, and even psychosocial status can be important in establishing the correct diagnosis. Review of systems may reveal evidence of esophageal reflux, endocrine disorders, arthritic symptoms, previous thoracic or neck surgery, or sinus disease, any or all of which can be associated with inflammatory laryngeal problems.

The cells lining the tracheobronchial tree are of the same size and are capable of the same amount of swelling in both adults and children. However, the percent of the cross-sectional airway that will remain after the same amount of swelling is a function of the absolute size of the airway. Thus, whereas a 50 percent reduction in diameter of the trachea may be tolerated without severe compromise in a full-grown man, an infant or small child would be in dire straits under the same circumstances.—HMT

Physical examination should not be limited to the head and neck, since many of these disorders are manifestations of or are associated with systemic illnesses. Mirror laryngoscopy is essential and will often be sufficient to confirm the diagnosis. A good view must be obtained in every case, even if this requires flexible fiberoptic or direct operative laryngoscopy, since malignancies can be obscured by the inflammatory changes they sometimes induce in adjacent tissues.

Radiographic studies can be helpful, both to assess the status of the airway and to help rule out other, noninflammatory illnesses. Because dysphagia is often associated with these conditions and reflux esophagitis is frequently a cause of chronic inflammatory laryngitis (see later), cine barium swallow is a useful study. Sinus films should be considered in all patients with chronic or recurrent laryngitis.

Laboratory tests are selected, based on the working diagnosis. Throat culture may be helpful, but must sometimes be correlated with blood cultures or material obtained directly from the larynx at endoscopic examination. Endocrine evaluation, particularly regarding possible thyroid dysfunction, can be useful. Skin testing should be considered in all patients not known to be purified protein derivative-positive and who are at risk for tuberculosis. Allergic testing is essential in otherwise unexplained cases of chronic or recurrent laryngitis.[1]

Endoscopic evaluation is not always necessary, especially in obviously acute laryngitis, provided the larynx can be seen well by indirect means. However, if a biopsy or direct laryngeal culture is needed, and particularly when the airway is at risk, endoscopy must be carried out. Esophagoscopy and bronchoscopy should be performed in addition to direct laryngoscopy because of the additional valuable information that may be obtained about these adjacent structures, which are often involved in the same inflammatory disease process.

Laryngitis in Children

Children are subject to various infectious and inflammatory agents, which are usually of lesser importance in the adult, either because of he development of immunity with age or because the larger size of the adult airway masks the effects of the laryngeal swelling that results. Consequently, the management of laryngitis in the pediatric age group is largely centered around the prevention or relief of obstructive airway symptoms.

Nonobstructive

Mild, nonobstructive laryngitis in children is frequently associated with nonspecific upper respiratory tract infections (URI). These are most often the result of rhinovirus, parainfluenza, and respiratory syncytial viruses, producing the typical "cold." Nonobstructive laryngitis can also be associated with specific viral infections, such as measles, mumps, chickenpox, whooping cough, and influenza.

Regardless of the cause, the *symptoms* are usually those of a mild *croup syndrome:* hoarseness, barking cough, and low-grade fever (less than 100°F). *Diagnosis* is established on the basis of history and, in the case of the specific viral causes, systemic physical findings. Indirect laryngoscopy is rarely feasible in this age group, but if the larynx *is* examined, hyperemia, edema, and increased secretions will be observed. Purulent secretions are not a feature of this condition unless secondary bacterial infection occurs. *Treatment* includes hydration, antipyretic and anti-inflammatory drugs, such as

Most of these infections occur in the wintertime when ambient humidity is in the 50 percent range. If this cold air is heated to household temperatures, the already low humidity may be reduced by as much as half. A minimum of 35 percent humidity is desirable for healthy individuals and much higher moisture content is necessary for inflamed tracheobronchial trees. Therefore, a vaporizer should be used in the bedroom of such patients and kept running day and night, so that the room is actually slightly damp. Since the water used in vaporizers is clean but not sterile, it is imperative that the entire apparatus be emptied and cleaned using a mild disinfectant solution every 48 to 72 hours to prevent the production of a bacteria-laden aerosol.—HMT

The mucoperichondrium of the laryngeal surface of the epiglottis is tightly applied to the cartilage and really has no submucosal space to permit soft tissue edema. As a result, the epiglottis is displaced toward the glottis by the swelling of the loosely applied mucosa on its lingual surface.—HMT

See Chapter 4.

Cultures of the larynx are positive for H. influenzae *in only 25 to 50 percent of cases. Blood cultures, on the other hand, are positive in almost 90 percent.[2] It is questionable, however, whether cultures of any type are necessary, except for epidemiologic studies, since the vast majority of these children respond promptly and completely to ampicillin.—HMT*

aspirin or acetaminophen, and, probably most important, adequate humidification.◁ Topical decongestants in the form of nose drops or nasal sprays may give symptomatic relief and diminish laryngeal irritation by decreasing nasal secretions. Antihistamines are contraindicated, in my opinion, because of their drying effect. If purulent sputum or very high temperatures are encountered, secondary bacterial infection should be suspected. After obtaining appropriate cultures (*Hemophilus influenza, Streptococcus* sp., and *pneumococci* are most commonly involved), antibiotics can be prescribed.

Obstructive

The obstructive *croup syndrome* is characterized by stridor, supraclavicular and intercostal retractions, characteristic barking cough, increased respiratory and pulse rates, and often drooling and agitation. With minor variations, this symptom complex is the same regardless of the specific cause of the laryngeal obstruction that produces it.

Acute Epiglottitis

Acute epiglottitis is a specific infectious condition, most often caused by *H. influenzae*. It can occur at any age up to and including adulthood, but is usually recognized only in small children because the swelling produced in the epiglottis does not frequently cause obstructive symptoms in adults. The edema is limited to the lingual surface of the epiglottis and the adjacent false vocal folds, characteristically sparing the true vocal folds and the subglottic region.◁ The result is a *croup syndrome* with predominantly *inspiratory stridor*. "Croupy" cough is not usually a factor, since this is generally due to subglottic rather than supraglottic edema. Until exhaustion intervenes, the child will resist lying down in an attempt to keep the swollen epiglottis from falling back to obstruct the airway further. Thus, the child's willingness to assume a supine position is an *ominous* sign, unless the airway obstruction has been relieved. Onset of symptoms is quite rapid and may progress from an essentially healthy-appearing child to high temperature and severe respiratory distress in as little as 4 to 5 hours. An ashen appearance and drooling are often prominent.

Diagnosis is made on clinical grounds. Lateral soft tissue radiographs can be helpful,◁ but are needed only in cases in which the clinical findings are equivocal. They should not be obtained unless personnel capable of providing an emergency airway accompany the child to the radiology department or, better yet, the studies are carried out in the operating room. *No attempt should be made to examine the larynx until all necessary preparations have been made to stabilize the airway.* Therefore, safest *management* requires taking the child to an operating room or other facility in which immediate intubation, bronchoscopy, and tracheotomy can be carried out, with equipment and all necessary personnel to use it (otolaryngologist, anesthesiologist, etc.) being immediately available. Only under such circumstances should an attempt be made to start an intravenous line, after which a tongue blade may be used to observe the typical cherry red epiglottis, which is readily visible in most patients. Neither the intravenous nor the examination should be attempted until all necessary preparations for airway stabilization are made, since either of these stimuli may be sufficient to precipitate sudden and complete obstruction. Once intubation has been carried out, any additional studies needed may be safely obtained.◁ Electrolyte determination is usually important, since most of these small children have become dehydrated by the time stridor develops. Blood cultures are also usually obtained, since culture of the epiglottis is frequently misleading.

If the airway can be secured by intubation, tracheotomy is not necessary.[3-5] If traditional intubation cannot be accomplished, bronchoscopy may still permit secondary intubation or, if necessary, will stabilize the airway to permit an orderly rather than emergency tracheotomy. ◁

Antimicrobial therapy may then be undertaken via the intravenous route. Since virtually all cases of acute epiglottitis in children are due to *H. influenzae,* and the few other organisms that may be implicated are usually sensitive to penicillin-like antibiotics, the drug of choice has been ampicillin (100 to 250 mg/kg/day). Some have recommended adding chloramphenicol (100 mg/kg/day).[7] Steroids can also be administered to hasten resolution of the edema, thus permitting earlier extubation. Indeed, some investigators have reported successful management without routine intubation when high doses of steroids and antibiotics were employed.[3]

Supraglottic Allergic Edema

Angioedema or allergic supraglottic edema can occur rapidly after exposure to such insults as bee stings, antitoxins (horse serum), or other allergens. The clinical picture is very similar to acute epiglottitis, except for rapidity of onset and the lack of a febrile illness. If anything, this condition is at once more immediate an emergency and, providing proper treatment is instituted, less dangerous than is acute epiglottitis. The epiglottis is swollen, but is pale and watery appearing. The edema will respond almost immediately to a single subcutaneous dose of between 0.2 and 0.4 mg epinephrine or a single supramaximal dose of dexamethasone given intravenously. If necessary, a bronchoscope or endotracheal tube can be inserted for a few minutes while the medication takes effect.

Acute Laryngotracheobronchitis

This common condition of childhood is not as well understood as it might be, largely because at least two, and possibly three different conditions that produce a typical "croup syndrome" are often lumped together. All three of these conditions result in subglottic edema and thus stridor, cough, and air hunger are found in all of them. Table 10–1 compares infectious croup, bacterial tracheitis and spasmodic croup as causes of the "croup syndrome."[8]

Bacterial tracheitis has been described as a new entity, characterized by a viral prodrome, followed by high temperature and airway obstruction.[9] Pus was found below the cricoid at endoscopy in the six cases reported. However, this probably does not represent a new disease, inasmuch as there have been several previous reports of patients with thick, inspissated tracheal secretions in whom bacterial infection was incriminated.[10,11] These children require airway control and bronchoscopy, in order to aspirate the thick, often encrusted secretions. Broad-spectrum antibiotics, humidification, and hydration complete the therapeutic regimen.

Spasmodic croup has also been termed false croup and subglottic allergic edema.[12] This condition is most likely of allergic origin.[1,13] The onset is sudden, frequently at night, and there is no associated febrile illness. Episodes may recur over several consecutive nights. If the child is examined endoscopically during an attack (which rarely occurs because of the transient nature of the illness), pale, boggy subglottic edema is observed. Subcutaneous epinephrine usually relieves the symptoms within a few minutes, as will racemic epinephrine administered by nebulizer. Although the

"Prior to July 1975, all patients . . . underwent tracheostomy. Since July 1975, nasotracheal intubation has been used in all patients (61 patients . . .). The cannulation time (2 days vs 7 days) and duration of hospital stay (5 days vs 9 days) have been decreased with nasotracheal intubation. There have been no serious complications . . .).—JD Baxter.[6]

Table 10-1   Croup Syndrome: Comparison of Major Entities*

	Infectious Croup	Bacterial Tracheitis	Spasmodic Croup
Age at onset	<3 yr (mean about 21 mo)	1 month to 6 years	Childhood
Etiology	Viral	Viral/bacterial (?)	Atopy (?)
Onset	URI	URI	Sudden cough, with or without URI
Course	Wax, wane, generally mild	Rapid progression, toxicity, airway obstruction	Rapid resolution
Endoscopic findings	Edema, inflammation, crusting	Edema, inflammation, pus below cricoid	Pallor, edema
Management	See text	Artificial airway, antibiotics	Self-limited, emesis(?)

*Modified with permission from Gartner and Stool.[8]

"If the symptoms of so-called nocturnal croup have not decreased in 12 hours, the child probably has infectious laryngotracheobronchitis and treatment with corticosteroids and antibiotics should be started immediately."—Vrabec and Davison[12]

"This causes mouth breathing, and extremely dry indoor air impinges directly on the larynx without being moistened by passage through the nose. . . . Extremely dry indoor air in winter probably is one of the major predisposing factors because it dehydrates mucous membranes, stops ciliary activity, and thus permits organisms to penetrate the mucosa and produce inflammation. A majority of . . . cases occur during the months of October through March."—Vrabec and Davison[12]

latter method is probably less likely to produce unwanted systemic side effects, it is technically more difficult to administer to a struggling, unhappy child. In known cases, prospective administration of elixir of diphenhydramine has been helpful in aborting attacks.◁

Viral or infectious croup (acute laryngotracheobronchitis) is characterized by progressive inspiratory stridor, typical cough, and temperature varying between 100° and 105°F. A cold like prodrome often occurs for a few days preceding onset of airway symptoms.◁ The most common *causative agent* appears to be parainfluenza viruses 1 and 3,[14,15] but many bacterial organisms have also been implicated.[16] It may well be that all of these organisms play a part in laryngotracheobronchitis in a synergistic fashion.

Diagnosis is made primarily on clinical grounds. It is especially important to distinguish croup from acute epiglottitis because of the often extreme urgency of airway intervention in the latter. Patients with croup do not usually demonstrate the drooling or muffled voice associated with epiglottitis. Radiographic findings in croup show ballooning of the hypopharynx and narrowing of the infraglottic airway (steeple sign), as opposed to the swollen epiglottis seen in acute epiglottitis.

Management is initiated in the same way as for acute epiglottitis. As little disturbance as possible is permitted until the child has been taken to the operating room or other facility where all personnel and equipment necessary to airway stabilization have been gathered. An intravenous line is then started and the larynx examined. The absence of the cherry red swollen epiglottis and the presence of subglottic edema and crusting are diagnostic. Since most children with this condition are not in such severe respiratory distress as to demand immediate *airway intervention*, treatment usually revolves around *fluid replacement, humidification* of the airway, and use of *antibiotics* and *steroids*. Most of these children are dehydrated by the time they reach the emergency room and require fluid and electrolyte replacement. Crusting of bacteria-laden secretions below the vocal cords is a common finding and can be ameliorated by high humidity administered via face mask or mist tent. Oxygen can be administered, as well, since hypoxemia remains the major blood gas abnormality until progressive obstruction causes an increase in carbon dioxide retention.[17] Racemic enpinephrine (2.25 percent via nebulizer and mask or intermittent positive pressure breathing) has been employed with good success.[18] Although it may be used in the emergency room, it is probably better to reserve it for

"Several factors point to the need for airway support: patient fatigue and cyanosis, worsening obstruction . . . , decreasing response to racemic epinephrine, and toxicity with evidence of superinfection. As time is necessary to arrange for controlled intubation or tracheostomy, the physician must anticipate [emphasis mine— HMT] the clinical course and make arrangements so that proper personnel and equipment are available."—Gartner and Stool[8]

patients with severe enough findings to warrant admission, since unexpected rebound has been known to occur. Treatments should not be more frequent than every 30 to 45 minutes.

The use of *steroids* in this disorder is the subject of some controversy.[19–21] In our hands, a single, supramaximal dose, with perhaps one follow-up dose 4 hours later, has provided as good results as longer term therapy. *Antibiotics* (usually penicillin V or ampicillin) are useful to reduce the secondary infection frequently associated with this condition and are mandatory if steroids are used.

If this regimen is insufficient to control the subglottic edema, serious consideration should be given to *intubation.* In those cases in which airway support becomes necessary,◁ we now use nasotracheal intubation whenever possible. *Tracheotomy,* although still supported by some investigators in the literature as the procedure of choice,[8] is probably no safer than properly managed nasotracheal intubation.[4,22]

Diptheria of the Larynx

Although this former scourge of childhood is now quite uncommon because of the widespread use of diptheria-pertussis-tetanus immunizations, it remains a consideration in the differential diagnosis of upper airway obstruction. It is *caused* by *Corynebacterium diptheriae* infection. A membrane in the nasopharynx is typical, but laryngeal involvement may occur as an isolated phenomenon. Dyspnea and stridor usually do not develop for 2 or 3 days after onset of a febrile illness and hoarseness, but once airway compromise begins, it may progress to severe obstruction very rapidly. *Diagnosis* is based on observation of the laryngeal membrane, but requires smear and culture for confirmation. However, when a membrane is present or smears are suggestive of *C. diptheriae,* immediate treatment is indicated without waiting for final cultures. Paralysis of one or more of the cranial nerves◁ occurs in about 10 percent of cases, but almost invariably resolves completely in successfully treated cases.

Dysphagia secondary to palatopharyngeal paralysis is most common of these.—HMT

Treatment includes *airway stabilization, antitoxin,* and *antibiotic* therapy. If diagnosis is established early enough in the course of the disease, airway intervention may be limited to humidification, administration of oxygen, and careful observation while other measures take effect. However, if there is any doubt, *tracheotomy* remains the method of choice for control of the airway in diptheria.[23] Antitoxin should be administered in doses appropriate for age and weight (20,000 to 100,000 U) by either the intravenous or intramuscular route, after first determining any history of sensitivity to horse serum. Although penicillin or erythromycin are highly effective in eradicating the bacterial infection, they do not deal with the toxin already released into the system. If palatopharyngeal weakness is present, nasogastric tube feedings will be necessary.

Juvenile Laryngeal Papillomatosis

Strong et al[24] noted that only 52 percent of new cases were first detected before the age of 15 years.

Although this disease entity is by no means limited to childhood,[24]◁ it does usually begin at an early age and its management is most difficult in a small larynx. Therefore, I will consider it here among the obstructive laryngitides.

The *cause* of laryngeal papillomatosis is as yet unproved, but most evidence suggests a *viral* cause.[25,26] A possible correlation with maternal condylomata acuminata has also been noted in retrospective studies.[27,28] Because papillomatosis is often seen within a few weeks of birth and has a high incidence in offspring of women with condyloma acuminata, a contact phenomenon, such as swallowing infected meconium or vaginal secretions at a time when the fetal immune mechanism may be as yet incapable of responding to such an antigen, is an attractive explanation for the viral cause of this disease. Later onset of symptoms could be due to quiescence of the virus contracted at birth, with later "breakout" because of hormonal or local changes. Clearly, however, this theory cannot explain many cases, such as those of late adult onset or in children whose mothers do not have a history of venereal warts. Moreover, one would expect an equally high incidence of oral and nasal mucosal infections if the aspiration contact theory were correct, and such extralaryngeal involvement is much less common. At the very least, therefore, the aspiration contact theory implies the concomitant existence of some local laryngeal phenomenon on the part of the infant, as well as recognition that there must be more than one means of obtaining the infection. However, it is clear that other factors, such as hormonal changes, inadequate levels of trace elements (magnesium[29]), and disadvantaged socioeconomic status play a part in the etiology of this condition. Regardless of the cause, approximately 2000 new cases a year are seen in the United States alone.[30]

There are probably *two forms* of the disease, *juvenile* and *adult,* which cannot be distinguished from each other on histologic grounds.[30] The juvenile form is usually multiple, recurs frequently, and tends to undergo spontaneous involution. The adult variety is usually singular, can often be eradicated with one attempt at removal, and has tendency for malignant transformation. *Diagnosis* is made by history and direct laryngoscopy in a newborn infant or small child with progressive hoarseness or stridor. Biopsy confirmation is necessary, since other lesions may mimic papillomas.

The three aims of *management* are maintenance of an airway, maintenance of voice, and eradication of the disease. Most infants and small children with juvenile papillomatosis do not require tracheotomy for airway maintenance, especially since the advent of the carbon dioxide laser, which has permitted removal of obstructing disease without edema or severe bleeding. This is fortunate, because those children that *do* require tracheotomy are often condemned to wear one for several years. Moreover, in more virulent cases, there is a tendency for growth of papilloma at the site of trauma, such as tracheotomy, which may in turn lead to obstruction of the trachea at lower levels.◁ Initially, therefore, the aim of therapy is to establish a tissue diagnosis and to determine if airway intervention is required. If airway is not at risk or can be satisfactorily maintained by periodic endoscopic removal, the next issue of importance is preservation of as normal a voice as possible. Finally, although it is seldom possible, the surgeon can attempt to eradicate all disease.

The carbon dioxide *laser* has revolutionized the management of juvenile laryngeal papillomatosis, although it has not proved to be the universal panacea that its early use suggested. Rather, it permits precise removal of lesions with little or no edema or tissue destruction beyond what is necessary for disease control, with bleeding much reduced from that which generally follows cup forceps removal. Voice preservation is more likely after laser surgery, since very precise removal of mucosal lesions is possible without damaging any of the underlying muscle. Finally, since cup forceps removal may lead to seeding of previously uninvolved adjacent tissue due to unavoidable trauma, the laser may be more successful in achieving complete removal with fewer recurrences. In practice, however, most of the surgeons with whom I have spoken agree that complete eradication is still more often the exception than the rule. Many of the cases that appear to be "cures" are probably spontaneous remissions.◁ In actuality, the laser only permits better ongoing management of recurrences without long-term

In occasional cases, rapid growth beyond a tracheostomy site along the traumatized tracheal wall can become life-threatening. I have successfully managed two cases by transecting the trachea below the level of papillomatous growth and creating a double-barreled tracheostoma that did not require a tube.[31] Both of these children were eventually reconstructed after the papilloma had disappeared. The use of the laser should preclude the need for such "heroic" intervention in most cases.—HMT

"[A]ssessment of therapeutic effect in a nonstandardized fashion may result in considerable distortion. . . . Although spontaneous remissions do occur, there is no evidence that any mode of therapy yields complete cure; thus, the standard assessment of therapeutic effect is the length of time between endoscopic excisions. However, while some therapists perform excisions at the first sign of recurrent growth, others wait until phonatory or even respiratory embarrassmet becomes clinically obvious. This variability itself may account for some of the effects attributed to the various modalities investigated."—RC Bone[32]

laryngeal damage and less frequent need for tracheotomy than did any previously available method.

Other means of treatment have included cryosurgery, ultrasound treatments, use of various caustic agents, and radiotherapy. In my opinion, none of these modalities is still feasible when the laser can be used instead. Radiotherapy has been incriminated in malignant degeneration of papillomas and, therefore, should no longer be considered.[33] Adjunctive therapy using autogenous vaccines has not resulted in reliable improvement.[34] Human interferon, on the other hand, has shown some early promise in the management of refractory cases.[35] However, it remains experimental at this writing. There appears to be a good response during therapy, but recurrence is common when treatment has stopped.

Laryngitis in Adults

Many of the conditions of the larynx discussed in the previous section also occur in the adult, but there are several others that are seen mainly in individuals beyond childhood. Moreover, the primary focus of concern in these older patients is not the airway, as is true in childhood, but the voice and the other systemic problems of which the laryngeal complaint is often only one symptom. Laryngitis may occur as a local finding in systemic illnesses, due to infection, hormonal derangements, autoimmune and allergic conditions, and degenerative disorders, as well as an illness limited to the larynx, itself.

Acute Laryngitis

See Chapter 7.

This common complaint may be due to viral or bacterial infections, allergy, or inhalation of irritants.◁

Viral

As is true in children, the most common organisms responsible are the rhinoviruses. Laryngitis is usually part of a "cold" syndrome. Other contributing factors include lack of adequate humidification, smoking, and voice abuse. Fever may occur when there is secondary bacterial infection. *Diagnosis* is made by history and laryngeal examination, which shows diffuse erythema and patchy, dry exudate. Swelling is usually not a major factor, but, if present, may result in a prominent cough. *Treatment* is largely symptomatic in this generally self-limited disease. Humidification, steam inhalations, voice rest, increased fluid intake, and the use of aspirin or other anti-inflammatory drugs is sufficient in most cases. Antibiotics are indicated only if there is a high temperature and culture evidence of bacterial involvement.

Bacterial

Bacterial laryngitis is most commonly secondary to purulent rhinosinusitis. *Diagnosis* is made by identifying the underlying infection and by mirror examination, which shows purulent erythema.

Acute epiglottitis can occur in adults and is often due to *H. influenzae,* as it is in children.[36] Because the swelling produced is usually insufficient to cause significant airway obstruction in the adult's larger larynx, symptoms are usually limited to a muffled voice, dysphagia, and vague discomfort in the throat. Fever is usually prominent in adult bacterial laryngitis, regardless of the cause. *Treatment* is the same as for viral laryngitis, with the addition of appropriate antibiotic therapy. Penicillin V or ampicillin are good empiric choices, but culture and sensitivities should be obtained before beginning antibiotic therapy, whenever possible.

Laryngeal abscess can occur spontaneously, but is usually the result of malignancy,[37] radiation, or trauma. Airway compromise is rapid and severe, so that prompt tracheotomy, institution of intravenous antibiotics appropriate to the offending organism, and surgical drainage must be undertaken as soon as the diagnosis is suspected. Mortality as high as 30 percent has been reported even recently when tracheotomy was delayed.[38]

Allergic

Sudden onset of significant laryngeal edema can result from exposure to any allergen. Usually the edema is mild, with only slight hoarseness and a "scratchy" sensation, but such challenges as bee stings, certain food allergies and *angioedema* (Quincke's disease) can produce rapid airway obstruction that may even, in some cases, require intubation or tracheotomy. *Diagnosis* is made by history and laryngeal mirror examination, which demonstrates pale, boggy edema of the soft tissues, mainly limited to the supraglottic structures. Immediate *treatment* includes subcutaneous administration of epinephrine, 0.2 to 0.5 ml. Intravenous steroids can also be helpful in some cases. If there is not a prompt improvement in the airway, short-term intubation will usually allow the patient to "get over the hump." Once the acute episode is over, allergic evaluation should be carried out and appropriate long-term management begun, since subsequent attacks of allergic edema of the larynx may be more severe than the first one.

Chronic Laryngitis

Infectious

Various organisms can be responsible for chronic, infectious laryngitis. Most of these produce granulomatous lesions of one kind or another.

Tuberculosis of the larynx, although much less common now than in the past, must still be considered (along with syphilis) the "great imitator." With rare exception, it is always the result of preexisting pulmonary involvement.[39]◁ Peak incidence is in the third and fourth decades of life, with children and the elderly uncommonly involved. Any debilitating systemic illness, preexisting chronic pulmonary disease (i.e., anthracosilicosis), and malnutrition are important predisposing factors.

Symptoms include hoarseness, odynophagia (sometimes referred to the ear), and, less prominently, cough, weight loss, night sweats, and hemoptysis. *Diagnosis* depends on the suspicion raised by laryngeal examination and history, which is heightened in the presence of an abnormal chest radiograph or known previous tuberculosis. Although the appearance of the larynx is not specific, selective involvement of the posterior third of the larynx should raise the examiner's suspicions.◁ Diagnosis is confirmed by smear and culture of acid-fast organisms obtained from sputum, but, since other similar-appearing diseases (such as syphilis and carcinoma) may coexist with tuberculosis, biopsy of the larynx should be carried out in every case. *Treatment* is by systemic use of appropriate antituberculous drugs.

Syphilis of the larynx, although now a relative rarity, still must be considered in the differential diagnosis of chronic inflammatory and, for that matter, mass lesions of the larynx. *Primary syphilis* can occasionally

Most cases of so-called primary laryngeal tuberculosis are eventually proved to be associated with indolent and undetected pulmonary disease at autopsy. There have been a few scattered reports of bovine tuberculosis, apparently contracted by drinking unprocessed milk from infected cattle, that was limited to the larynx and the stomach and with no pulmonary lesions.—HMT

The predilection for posterior involvement can be explained by the probable pathophysiology whereby pulmonary tuberculosis infects the larynx. The mucosal blanket, bearing active organisms from the lungs, is propelled upward by the endobronchial cilia. As the larynx is approached, the mucus is concentrated toward the posterior commissure, where, once it has cleared the glottis, it spills over into the postcricoid area and is swallowed.—HMT

I have seen one case of a young woman who presented with vague laryngeal discomfort of about 1 week's duration. Examination revealed a shallow, grayish ulceration of the free border of the epiglottis. Smears from this lesion were dark-field positive and biopsy demonstrated typical granuloma. On questioning, she admitted to having performed fellatio on a new sex partner about 10 days previously. He was also found to have a positive fluorescent treponemal antibody absorption test. Theoretically, primary leutic ulcers are supposed to be painless. However, when they occur in the upper aerodigestive tract, secondary infection is common and often results in some discomfort.—HMT

be responsible for transient lesions of the epiglottis. ◁ The more commonly encountered form of luetic laryngeal involvement is *secondary syphilis*. This stage is usually associated with generalized lymphadenopathy and multiple lesions in the mouth as well. Examination shows diffuse hyperemia and mucous patches. The lesions typically clear within 1 or 2 weeks, even without treatment. *Tertiary* gummas can also be seen, usually resulting in or concomitant with chondritis and eventual cicatrization and stenosis. *Diagnosis* is made by serologic means, although spirochetes can often be seen on dark-field examination of material from primary lesions. Since nonluetic spirochetes are often resident in the mouth and possibly the larynx as well, serologic confirmation is necessary. *Treatment* consists of an adequate course of penicillin.

Scleroma is a chronic granulomatous infection of the upper aerodigestive tract (classically the nose) caused by *Klebsiella rhinoscleromatis*. It can, on occasion, involve the larynx,[40] but seldom in the absence of other lesions. It is endemic in the region of the Mediterranean and South America, but is rare in individuals who have not traveled outside the United States. Slowly progressive, painless submucosal swellings are typical. *Diagnosis* is made by biopsy, with confirmation using specific complement fixation or flourescent antibody testing. *Treatment* is by such antibiotics as chloramphenicol, tetracycline, and, more recently, the cephalosporin group. Prolonged antibiotic treatment is usually advised.

Other granulomatous infections that may occasionally exhibit laryngeal involvement include leprosy,[41] granuloma inguinale, yaws, lymphogranuloma venereum, and leishmaniasis.[42]

Mycotic infections of the larynx are relatively uncommon, but must be considered in the differential diagnosis of any case of indolent, treatment-refractory laryngitis, especially in patients with other debilitating diseases, diabetes, or who are on long-term steroid treatment, all of which favor fungal overgrowth.

Actinomycosis (now recognized as a bacterial rather than a fungal disease) results in chronic, draining infections of the submandibular area. The portal of entry is usually the teeth in patients with poor dental hygiene. The drainage classically contains "sulfur granules," which are small aggregations of the bacterial colonies. The causative agent is usually *Actinomyces israelii*, although *A. bovis* is sometimes involved. These are grampositive, branching, filamentous bacteria that do not produce spores. The larynx is seldom involved alone, except in postirradiation or surgical situations.[43,44] *Diagnosis* is made by biopsy and recovery of the organisms from drainage or tissue. *Treatment* requires 3 months or more of therapeutic doses of penicillin (or tetracycline when penicillin cannot be used). Devitalized tissue or cartilage sequestra (which are common in postsurgical laryngeal involvement) should be debrided.

Blastomycosis occurs in two forms: *North American* and *South American*. The former is caused by *Blastomyces dermatitidis* and the latter by *B. brasiliensis*. The North American variety is fairly common in the southeastern United States and Mississippi Valley areas, but the South American type (also called paracoccidioidomycosis) is rare in this country. Both types produce miliary nodules with caseation, often mimicking pseudoepitheliomatous hyperplasia in gross appearance. The lesions are indistinguishable from those of tuberculosis. Either of them can occur in the larynx,[45] but the lungs are almost always involved as well. *Diagnosis* is made by recovering the organisms from tissue and by culture. *Treatment* is with amphotericin B[46] or with ketoconazole.

Candidiasis of the larynx can occur, but is almost always in association with typical oral or vaginal infections (thrush, moniliasis). It is rarely

Like most fungi, Candida *prefers a basic pH. Since most of the saprophytes usually present in the mouth or vagina tend to create a slightly acid environment,* Candida *cannot get a foothold unless something disrupts homeostasis. As a result, thrush can often be treated with simple acetic acid mouthwash or douche.—HMT*

seen in the absence of debilitating disease, immunosuppression, steroid usage, or broad-spectrum antibiotic treatment. The causative organism, *Candida albicans,* is an opportunistic agent, which is widely available in the environment.◁ *Diagnosis* is suspected by observing widespread erythema and swelling, with typical cheesy-white exudate. The epithelium bleeds easily when the membrane is removed. Potassium hydroxide preparation of the exudate usually reveals yeast forms, which can be identified by culture. *Treatment* is with nystatin as a topical agent and with amphotericin B when systemic medication is needed.

Coccidioidomycosis (valley fever) is a fungal disease that is endemic in the San Joaquin Valley of California and in other parts of the southwestern United States. It is caused by *Coccidioides immitis,* a thick-walled fungus with endospores. The route of infection is by inhalation of the spores and probably does not take place from individual to individual. The incubation period is 1 to 4 weeks, after which there are fever, night sweats, arthralgias, pleuritis, cough, and sore throat. *Diagnosis* is usually made by skin test, with complement fixation tests providing confirmation. Biopsy reveals granulomas very similar to those of tuberculosis. Typical endospore-filled organisms must be seen to distinguish them histologically. The larynx may be involved selectively.[47] *Treatment* with amphotericin B is usually successful, but must be used with great care in small children, because of the risk of renal toxicity.

Histoplasmosis primarily affects the lungs, but the larynx and tongue are also frequent sites of involvement. Concomitant oral ulcerations are common. The causative organism is *Histoplasma capsulatum.* The lesions resemble tuberculosis, both microscopically and clinically, although histoplasmosis tends to involve the epiglottis and false cords, whereas tuberculosis seems to have a predilection for the posterior third of the larynx. *Diagnosis* is usually made by complement fixation test and by culture of the organism. Amphotericin B (given intravenously, 30 to 50 mg over a 4- to 6-hour period daily to a total dose of 950 to 5000 mg) is the *treatment* of choice, although ketoconazole has been introduced recently as an alternative.

Noninfectious

There is a group of chronic laryngitides that are thought to be autoimmune disorders, represent local manifestations of systemic disease, or are of unknown cause.

Amyloidosis may be primary or secondary. The primary type (not associated with systemic disease) has a predilection for the tongue and the larynx.[48] Deposits of amyloid (an amorphous, pink-staining material) are found as subepithelial nodules, usually quite circumscribed, and are *diagnosed* upon biopsy. Long-standing, hyalinized vocal nodules or polyps may give a similar histologic appearance, but special stains for amyloid can be used to differentiate them. The condition is usually without symptoms unless the deposits interfere with phonation by position, in which case, simple endoscopic removal will suffice for *treatment.*

Pemphigus and pemphigoid are of unknown etiology. Both diseases produce impressive bullae of the skin and mucous membranes, usually seen about the lips, oral cavity, and vagina. Pemphigus produces intraepithelial bullae, whereas those of pemphigoid are subepithelial. Circulating antibodies can be demonstrated by immunoflourescent techniques to confirm the *diagnosis.* Both pemphigus and benign mucous membrane pemphigoid can affect the larynx. (Bullous pemphigoid, the second variety of the disease, seldom involves mucous membranes.) In the acute phases, recently ruptured bullae may appear as superficial, whitish ulcers of the epiglottis and false cords. In later stages, after many relapses, laryngeal stenosis can result. *Treatment* of both diseases is primarily with steroids, although pemphigus has also been treated with immunosuppressants like cyclophosphamide or methotrexate.[49]

Relapsing polychondritis is a condition of unknown cause that is thought to be an autoimmune disorder. It is characterized by recurring episodes of inflammation and eventual destruction of cartilaginous structures, especially the ears, nose, and larynx. Costal cartilages are also sometimes involved. There are fever, erythema, swelling, and arthritic symptoms, although the findings may be limited to only one structure at a time. As the name implies, the illness typically exhibits exacerbations and spontaneous remissions. *Diagnosis* is made by recording the typical history and by eventual biopsy of an involved cartilaginous structure. Histologic findings include replacement of the basophilic cartilage matrix by eosinophilic material and infiltration of acute and chronic inflammatory cells. In later stages, fibrosis and chondronecrosis become more prominent. Hoarseness, painful swelling of the larynx and trachea, and dysphagia are the symptoms of laryngeal involvement (which occurs in just over half of all cases[50]) in this disease. Airway problems as a result of laryngeal involvement are the most common cause of death. *Treatment* is with steroids and dapsone.[51,52] Tracheostomy is sometimes necessary in late stages of the disease. Attempts at reconstruction of nasal or auricular collapse are generally of limited value, since the disease is usually progressive.

Sarcoidosis results in laryngeal involvement in only a small percentage of cases,[53] but its manifestations can be of great importance, since severe edema is often the result. Many other types of laryngeal involvement have been reported, including ulcerations, granuloma formation, and scarring. *Diagnosis* is made by biopsy of a typical noncaseating granuloma and by ruling out tuberculosis. *Treatment* includes periodic use of steroids and, occasionally, laser surgery for management of the laryngeal lesions.

Systemic lupus erythematosus can produce many types of laryngeal findings during active phases of the disease. Epiglottitis,[54] acute and chronic laryngitis, granuloma formation, and vocal cord paralysis have all been associated with it. *Diagnosis* and *treatment* are those of the disease. Local management of the laryngeal problems may be attempted using the laser, which not only permits extirpation of various lesions, but can be used to alleviate the pain that is sometimes associated with ulcerations.

Wegner's granulomatosis and lethal midline granuloma were once thought to be the same disease. It is now well established, however, that they are distinct entities, but their laryngeal manifestations are essentially indistinguishable. It is rare for there to be laryngeal symptoms in the absence of previous or concomitant nasal or sinus involvement in these illnesses. In addition to nasal obstruction, chronic sinusitis, nonhealing ulcerations of the septum, often with perforation, there are usually systemic symptoms, such as fever, malaise, and weight loss. Laryngeal lesions include necrotic ulceration and pseudoepitheliomatous hyperplasia. It is seldom possible to observe the typical vasculitis of lethal midline granuloma in laryngeal biopsies, because of the relative paucity of soft tissue. Repeated biopsies are needed, as a rule, before a definitive *diagnosis* can be reached. Both of these conditions may eventually prove fatal, but *treatment* can now be undertaken with some hope of control or cure. Steroids and immunosuppressive agents have shown some good results in the management of Wegener's granulomatosis,[55] and radiotherapy has been helpful for lethal midline granuloma.

References

1. Pang LQ: Allergy of the larynx, trachea, and tracheobronchial tree. Otol Clin North Am, 7:719–733, 1974.
2. Baxter JD, Pashley NRT: Acute epiglottitis: 25 years' experience in management, the Montreal children's hospital. J Otolaryngol, 6:473, 1977.
3. Strome M, Jaffe B: Epiglottitis: Individual management with steroids. Laryngoscope, 84:921, 1974.
4. Schuller DE, Birk HG: The safety of intubation in croup and epiglottitis: An eight year follow-up. *Laryngoscope,* 85:33, 1975.
5. Cantrell RW, Bell RA, Morioka WT: Acute epiglottitis: intubation vs tracheotomy. Laryngoscope, 88:994, 1978.
6. Baxter JD: Acute epiglottitis. In English GE (Ed): Otolaryngology, vol 3. Philadelphia, Harper & Row, 1984.
7. Faden HS: Treatment of *Hemophilus influenzae* type B epiglottitis. *Pediatrics,* 63:402, 1979.
8. Gartner JC Jr, Stool SE: Acute laryngotracheobronchitis. In English GE (Ed): *Otolaryngology,* vol 3. Philadelphia, Harper & Row, 1981.
9. Jones R, Santos JI, Overall JC Jr: Bacterial tracheitis. JAMA 242:721, 1979.
10. Orton HB, Smith EL, Bell HO, et al: Acute laryngotracheobronchitis: Analysis of sixty-two cases with a report of autopsies in eight cases. Arch Otol, 33:926, 1941.
11. Brighton GR: Laryngotracheobronchitis. Ann Otol Rhinol Laryngol, 49:1070, 1940.
12. Vrabec DP, Davison FW: Inflammatory diseases of the larynx. In English GE (Ed): *Otolaryngology,* vol. 3 Philadelphia, Harper & Row, 1980.
13. Wolf IJ: Allergic factors in the etiology of spasmodic croup and laryngotracheitis. Ann Allergy, 24:79, 1966.
14. Buchan RA, Marten KW, Kennedy DH: Aetiology and epidemiology of viral croup in Glasgow, 1966-1972. J Hyg (Lond), 73:143, 1974.
15. Glezen WP, Denny FW: Epidemiology of lower respiratory diseases in children. N Engl J Med, 288:498, 1973.
16. Loda FA, Clyde WA Jr, Glezen WP, Senior RJ, Shaeffer CI, Denny FW Jr: Studies on the role of viruses, bacteria and *M pneumoniae* as causes of lower respiratory tract infections in children. J Pediatr, 72:161, 1968.
17. Newth CJL, Levison H, Bryan AC: The respiratory status of children with croup. J Pediatr, 81:1068, 1972.
18. Westley CR, Cotton EK, Brooks JG: Nebu-

lized racemic epinephrine by IPPB for the treatment of croup. Am J Dis Child, 132:484, 1978.
19. Eden AN, Kaufman A, Yu R: Corticosteroids and croup: Controlled double-blind study. JAMA, 200:403, 1967.
20. Leipzig B, Oski FA, Cummings CW, et al: A prospective randomized study to determine the efficacy of steroids in treatment of croup. J Pediatr, 94:194, 1979.
21. Tunnessen WW, Jr, Feinstein AR: The steroid-croup controversy: An analytic review of methodologic problems. J Pediatr, 96:751, 1980.
22. Shann FA, Phelan PD, Stocks JG, et al: Prolonged nasotracheal intubation or tracheostomy in acute laryngotracheobronchitis and epiglottitis? Aust Paediatr J, 11:212, 1975.
23. Lang WS: Diptheria at the present time. Laryngoscope, 75:1092, 1965.
24. Strong MS, et al: Recurrent respiratory papillomatosis: Management with the CO2 laser. Ann Otol Rhinol Laryngol, 85:508, 1976.
25. Uhlman EV: On the etiology of laryngeal papilloma. Acta Otolaryngol (Stockh), 5:317, 1923.
26. Resler DR, Snow JB: Cell-free filtrate transplantation of human laryngeal papillomata to dogs. Laryngoscope, 77:397, 1967.
27. Cook TA, Brunschwig JP, Butel JS, et al: Laryngeal papilloma: Etiologic and therapeutic considerations. Ann Otol Rhinol Laryngol, 82:649, 1973.
28. Quick CA, et al: Relationship between condylomata and laryngeal papillomata. Ann Otol Rhinol Laryngol, 89:467, 1980.
29. Shilovtseva AS: Complex treatment of patients affected with papillomatosis of the larynx and trachea. Arch Otol, 89:552, 1969.
30. Batsakis JG: *Tumors of the Head and Neck: Clinical and Pathologic Considerations.* Williams & Wilkins, Baltimore, 1974, pp 82–85.
31. Tucker HM: Diversionary (double-barrelled) tracheotomy in the management of juvenile laryngeal papillomatosis. Ann Otol Rhinol Laryngol, 89:504, 1980.
32. Bone RC: Laryngeal papillomatosis. In English GM (Ed): *Otolaryngology,* vol 3, Philadelphia, Harper & Row, 1978, p 6.
33. Walsh TE, Beamer PR: Epidermoid carcinoma of the larynx occurring in two children with papilloma of the larynx. Laryngoscope, 60:1110, 1950.
34. Gross EW, Hubbard R: Management of juvenile laryngeal papilloma: Further observations. Laryngoscope, 84:1090, 1974.

35. Hagland S, et al: Interferon therapy in juvenile laryngeal papillomatosis. Arch Otol, 107:327, 1981.

36. Hawkins DB, Miller AH, Sachs GB, Benz RT: Acute epiglottitis in adults. Laryngoscope, 83:1211, 1973.

37. Canalis RF, Jenkins HA, Osguthorpe JD: Acute laryngeal abscesses. Ann Otol Rhinol Laryngol, 88:275, 1979.

38. Heeneman H, Ward KM: Epiglottic abscess: Its occurrence and management. J Otolaryngol, 6:31, 1977.

39. Lell WA: Laryngeal tuberculosis: Diagnosis, incidence and present day treatment. Arch Otolaryngol, 60:350–366, 1954.

40. Miller RH, Shulman JB, Canalis RF: *Klebsiella rhinoscleromatis:* A clinical and pathogenic enigma. Otolaryngol Head Neck Surg, 83:212, 1979.

41. Sandberg P, Shum TK: Lepromatous leprosy of the larynx. Otolaryngol Head Neck Surg, 91:216, 1983.

42. McNeil R: Nonsurgical conditions of the larynx. In Bailey BJ, Biller HF (Eds): *Surgery of the Larynx.* Philadelphia, WB Saunders, 1985.

43. Brandenburg JH, Finch WW, Kirkham WR: Actinomycosis of the larynx and pharynx. Otolaryngol Head Neck Surg, 86:739, 1978.

44. Koegel L Jr, Tucker HM: Postoperative actinomycotic infection of the larynx. Otolaryngol Head Neck Surg, 91:213, 1983.

45. Stachowsky L: Primary paracoccidioidomycosis of the larynx. Arch Otolaryngol, 78:205, 1963.

46. Restrepo A, et al: Paracoccidioidomycosis (South American blastomycosis). Am J Trop Med Hyg, 19:68, 1970.

47. Ward PH, Berci G, Morledge D, Schwartz H: Coccioidomycosis of the larynx in infants and adults. Ann Otol Rhinol Laryngol, 86:655, 1977.

48. Beasley P: Localized amyloidosis of the larynx. J Laryngol Otol, 85:83, 1971.

49. Block LJ, et al: Pemphigus of the air and food passages. Ann Otol Rhinol Laryngol, 86:584, 1977.

50. Esdaile J, et al: Vascular involvement in relapsing polychondritis. Can Med Assoc J, 116:1019, 1977.

51. Barranco UP, et al: Treatment of relapsing polychondritis with dapsone. Arch Dermatol, 112:1286, 1978.

52. Damiani JM, Levine HL: Relapsing polychondritis—report of ten cases. Trans Am Laryngol Soc, 5: 1979.

53. Mayock RL, et al: Manifestations of sarcoidosis: Analysis of 145 patients with a review of 9 series selected from the literature. Am J Med, 35:67, 1963.

54. Toomy JM, Snyder GG 3rd, Maenze RM Rothfield NF: Acute epiglottitis due to systemic lupus erythematosus. Laryngoscope, 84:522, 1974.

55. Pashley RT, Levitt MN: Some aspects of therapy in the nonhealing granulomas of Wegener and Stewart. J Otolaryngol, 8:53, 1979.

Chapter 11

Neurologic Disorders

See Chapter 2.

In order to function properly as a valve at the crossroads between the airway and food passages,◁ the larynx must achieve near-perfect synchrony of its intricate sensory and motor capabilities. In similar fashion, the ability to phonate depends on a delicate and continually adjusted balance between the afferent and efferent limbs of the larynx's intrinsic and extrinsic neurologic connections. It is a small wonder, then, that these complicated functions operate as reliably as they do, even in the presence of increasing incidence of trauma and the need for sometimes destructive surgery in the region. The otolaryngologist must have a thorough understanding of the conditions that can interfere with orderly function of the larynx if prompt diagnosis and appropriate management are to be instituted.

Sensory Disorders

See Chapter 1.

Sensation from the supraglottic larynx, including both surfaces of the epiglottis, aryepiglottic folds, false vocal cords, and the roof of the ventricle, is transmitted centrally via the internal branch of the superior laryngeal nerve.◁ The surface of the true vocal folds, the subglottis, and the trachea are served by sensory fibers of the recurrent laryngeal nerve (Fig. 11–1), including both proprioceptive fibers from muscle spindles and joint capsules and surface sensation from the mucosa. Most of these fibers synapse in the nodose ganglion of the vagus nerve and have central connections to the nucleus of the tractus solitarius and to the cerebellum. As a result, tactile sensation, vocal fold position, and tension can be monitored continuously.

Loss of sensation can occur as a separate problem, but is almost always associated with some degree of motor deficit as well. Incompletely recovered stroke, Guillain-Barré syndrome, diabetes, and "idiopathic" superior laryngeal nerve paralysis are some of the conditions that can result in isolated sensory losses. *Unilateral sensory loss* of the supraglottic larynx may produce few, if any, problems, especially in a young, otherwise uncompromised patient. Subtle *symptoms,* such as frequent *throat-clearing,* unexpected paroxysmal *coughing,* easy *voice fatigue,* and vague *foreign body sensations* may be encountered in the absence of any motor

Figure 11–1. Sensory distribution of superior and recurrent laryngeal nerves within the larynx.

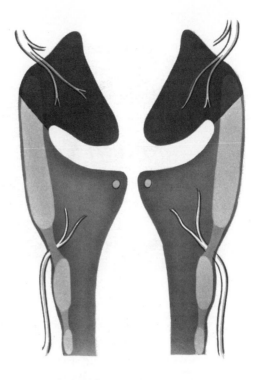

Loss of supraglottic sensation permits accumulation of normal secretions that would otherwise be cleared by reflex swallowing, throat-clearing, or cough. Sudden spill-over into the subglottic area, whose sensory innervation is mediated via the intact recurrent laryngeal nerve, causes sudden, paroxysmal coughing. Incomplete or recovering sensory loss can also produce paresthesias, which may be interpreted as the presence of secretions needing to be cleared or even vague discomfort.—HMT

Several previous investigators[3,4] have maintained that it is the anterior commissure that deviates toward the side of the paralysis. Abelson and Tucker[2] clearly demonstrated that it was the thyroid cartilage that remains fixed and the cricoid cartilage that deviates, carrying the posterior commissure structures with it.—HMT

losses.◁ Fortunately, *bilateral sensory loss* is uncommon. It can result in severe *aspiration* and subsequent pneumonia.

Superior laryngeal nerve paralysis usually presents with both supraglottic sensory loss and visible rotation of the larynx with phonatory effort, because this nerve includes an external motor branch to the cricothyroideus muscle in addition to its sensory component (See later). It almost always occurs as an isolated palsy, not associated with other findings or progression to more general neurologic disorders,[1] and is thought to be due to a viral neuropathy. In addition to the *symptoms* noted for unilateral sensory loss, there is usually a slight, but noticeable *voice change,* which the patient may interpret as hoarseness. In fact, the most common finding is *diplophonia,* especially in higher pitched voices or when trying to sing. *Examination* reveals what appears to be a normal larynx at rest. On phonatory effort, however, the posterior commissure will be seen to rotate *toward* the side of the palsy[1,2] (Fig. 11–2).◁ Thus, P-P-P is a useful mnemonic to remember that the *p*osterior commissure *p*oints to the side of the *p*aralysis. This causes apparent shortening, flaccidity, and slight limitation of motion of the focal fold on the affected side and accounts for the diplophonia and easy fatigability noted by the patient. Approximately 50 to 60 percent of cases resolve spontaneously within 1 year of onset, without intervention. Most of the rest compensate to a greater or lesser extent. This is fortunate, since there is really no effective treatment. May[5] has suggested reinnervation of the cricothyroideus muscle by nerve-muscle pedicle technique, but this seems inappropriate except in very unusual cases. Speech therapy may allow the patient to compensate more effectively.

Motor Disorders

Motor disorders of the larynx can be *spasmodic* or *paralytic. Spasmodic dysphonia* and *dysphonia plica ventricularis* are discussed in Chapters 5 and 9. *Paralytic disorders* can be further classified as *central* or *peripheral,* depending on the site of the lesion.

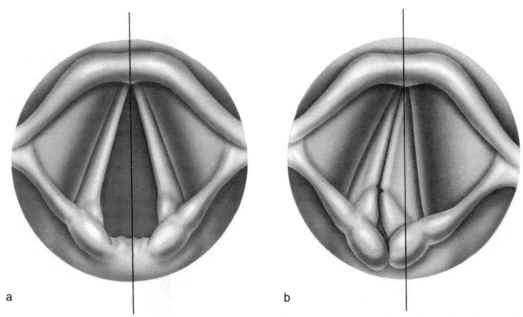

a   b

Figure 11–2. **a,** Normal-appearing larynx at rest in unilateral superior laryngeal
nerve paralysis. **b,** Posterior commissure deviates toward the side of paralysis.

Central Neurologic Lesions

These account for a relatively small percentage of all laryngeal
paralyses[6] (Table 11-1 and 11-2). They may be of congenital origin, or
may be secondary to trauma, infection, neoplasm, or vascular accident.
Depending on the relationship of the lesion to the nucleus ambiguus, they
may be further classified as *supranuclear, nuclear,* or *infranuclear.*

Table 11–1   Etiology of Unilateral Vocal Cord Paralysis*

	Parnell and Brandenburgh (1970)		Maisel and Ogura (1974)		Titche (1976)		Tucker	
	No.	%	No.	%	No.	%	No.	%
Thyroidectomy	17	21	10	8	5	4	10	5
Other trauma	2	2	27	21	18	13	77	37
Neurologic	3	4	10	8	21	16	5	2
Malignancy	32	40	23	18	51	38	46	22
Miscellaneous	27	33	57	45	39	29	72	34
Total	81	100	127	100	134	100	210	100

*Reprinted with permission from Tucker.[6]

Table 11–2   Etiology of Bilateral Vocal Cord Paralysis*

	Maisel and Ogura (1974)		Holinger et al		Tucker	
	No.	%	No.	%	No.	%
Thyroidectomy	22	41	138	58	82	46
Other trauma	17	32	7	3	54	30
Neurologic	4	7	52	22	10	6
Malignancy	4	7	16	6	14	7
Miscellaneous	7	13	27	11	20	11
Total	54	100	240	100	180	100

*Reprinted with permission from Tucker.[6]

Supranuclear Lesions

Massive insult to the cortex can produce an upper motor neuron lesion that results in bilateral spastic paralysis of the larynx.[7,8] Patients so affected exhibit disordered mentality, major neurologic deficits, slow, dysarthic speech, and monotonous voice. Occasionally, both because of the spastic paralysis and the other neurologic problems, tracheotomy may be necessary.

Nuclear Lesions

"Discrete areas of the nucleus ambiguus may be affected, causing a paralysis of only one or two muscles. In practice, however, most lesions involve contiguous brainstem structures such as nuclei of cranial nerves IX, XI and XII, producing additional findings that implicate the area of the nucleus ambiguus."—Holinger and Wolter[7]

Insult to the area around the nucleus ambiguus results in combined superior and recurrent laryngeal nerve paralysis. This is a bulbar or lower motor neuron type palsy and is frequently associated with involvement of other nuclei in the medulla.◁ Until recently, these and the infranuclear lesions, to be discussed, were referred to as "syndromes of associated laryngeal paralyses" and often by specific eponyms (Villaret's, Vernet's, etc.). As is true of most eponyms, they are better replaced by descriptive nomenclature.

Infranuclear Lesions

See Chapter 4.

Infranuclear lesions may be located at or near the jugular foramen and are usually associated with other lower cranial nerve palsies. They comprise the rest of the so-called syndromes of associated laryngeal paralyses, or *jugular foramen syndrome*. Both the superior laryngeal nerve (SLN) and the recurrent laryngeal nerve (RLN) are usually involved. Consideration of the other neurologic and physical findings can often pinpoint the lesion. Computed tomography (CT) scanning, with and without digital subtraction angiography, can delineate the location and extent of the mass.◁

Two generalized neurologic disorders of unknown cause are frequently associated with laryngeal paralysis or dysfunction.

1. *Amyotrophic lateral sclerosis* (Lou Gehrig's disease) occurs mostly in adults in the fifth or sixth decades. Progressive loss of anterior horn cells in the bulbar region results in muscle wasting in the tongue, pharynx, and larynx. Unexplained *spastic paralysis* of the larynx, especially when coupled with *weakness* and *fasciculations* of the tongue and severe *dysphagia*, strongly suggests the diagnosis. In the early stages, speech and swallowing therapy can be very helpful. Many of these patients eventually require a tracheotomy.

"There is some urgency to treating the disease effectively from the beginning. If one considers this diagnosis, one should either make it or refer the patient quickly to someone who can determine whether it is or is not myasthenia gravis. Patients can change rapidly with this illness when untreated. It is named myasthenia "gravis" with good reason. The usual cause of death is respiratory failure or inspiration difficulties, which are preventable if the patient is under treatment. I consider the making of this diagnosis (and initiating treatment) a neurological emergency.—HR Tyler[9]

2. *Myasthenia gravis* can occur at any age, although it is most common in the young adult. Thymic enlargement with prominent germinal centers are present in a high percentage of patients.[9] Typically, the laryngeal *symptoms* of this disease are related to easy *fatigability* and *weakness* of the voice. The larynx appears normal on routine examination, but will show poor approximation of the vocal folds with prolonged phonatory effort. These findings are usually associated with weakness of the muscles of the upper face and around the eyes. Neostigmine or edrophonium bromide can be used as a diagnostic test, but since only approximately 30 seconds of improvement may result even in patients who do respond, these tests are not often useful in evaluating isolated laryngeal involvement. Prompt referral to a neurologist who has been alerted to the otolaryngologist's findings is strongly recommended.◁

Peripheral Neurologic Lesions

Any or all possible combinations of paralysis of the SLN or RLN, or both, can be encountered in clinical practice. Determination of the nerve or nerves involved is important not only to diagnose the cause of paralysis accurately (when possible), but also in determining best management.

Diagnosis

Peripheral vocal fold paralysis can present with a single symptom (such as voice change, airway restriction) or with a bewildering combination of symptoms relating not only to the larynx itself, but also to swallowing capability, pulmonary function, and even electrolyte balance (see later). For this reason, it is imperative that the physician obtain as detailed and accurate a history as possible, since such factors as time and circumstances of onset, intermittency, progression, or severity, and association with other symptoms, previous illnesses, or exposure to drugs or toxic materials may be essential to the ability to make a correct diagnosis.

Examination

Subtle abnormalities of movement are often missed even by experienced examiners, but if alerted to the potential diagnosis beforehand, it is less likely that such paralyses or weaknesses will be overlooked.—HMT

Before the larynx is examined, a "voice diagnosis" should be undertaken.◁ Patients tend to classify all voice changes as "hoarseness," largely because they do not have the vocabulary to describe what has happened with a more appropriate term. The examiner, however, can learn to distinguish between roughness, diplophonia, breaking, hoarseness, harshness, etc., with sufficient practice. As a general rule, and particularly if any surgical intervention is contemplated, baseline voice recordings and consultation with a speech pathologist is strongly recommended.

In most cases of laryngeal paralysis the diagnosis can be made by noting the position of the vocal folds at rest and during phonatory effort.

Superior laryngeal nerve paralysis (Fig. 11–2) demonstrates normal vocal fold position during quiet respiration, but noticeable deviation of the posterior commissure to the paralyzed side occurs during phonatory effort (see before). The superior laryngeal nerve not only provides sensation from the supraglottic region via its internal branch, but also is the motor nerve to the cricothyroideus muscle through its external branch. This muscle can serve as a tensor of the glottic musculature and, when unopposed because of paralysis of the other side, rotates the larynx.[2] As a result, the vocal fold on the paralyzed side becomes slightly flaccid, may be depressed below the level of the normal side, and may even permit prolapse of the affected arytenoid forward into the laryngeal introitus. *Bilateral superior laryngeal nerve paralysis* can occur, but is fortunately rare. Because the lesion is symmetrical, there may be no significant laryngoscopic findings, although in some cases aspiration can be observed.

Recurrent laryngeal nerve paralysis results in nonfunction of the intrinsic muscles on the affected side or sides. If the superior laryngeal nerve is intact, the vocal fold will assume the *paramedian position* (Fig. 11–3) Nevertheless, patients with recurrent laryngeal nerve palsies often exhibit what appears to be active adduction to the midline during phonatory effort, which may account for the failure of some observers to recognize such a paralysis and the relatively good voice that is preserved in most bilateral cases. This apparent adduction is due to the unopposed action of the cricothyroideus muscles, which, although they are normally tensors of the vocal fold, can act as adductors when not opposed by other intrinsic laryngeal

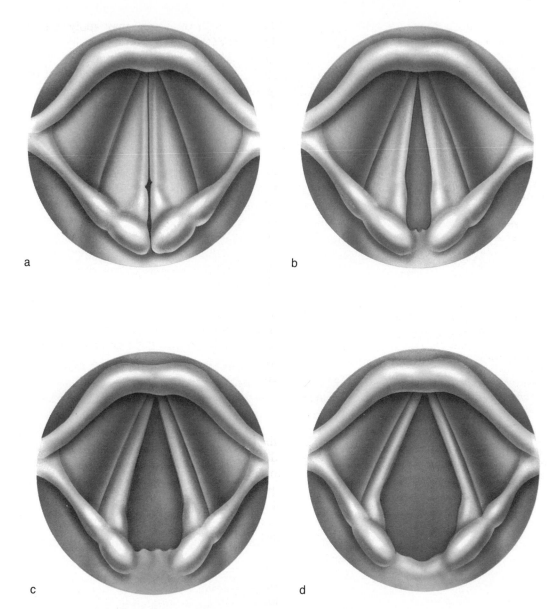

a

b

c

d

Figure 11–3. Vocal fold positions. **a,** Midline (phonation). **b,** Paramedian. **c,** Intermediate (position of rest). **d,** Full abduction.

All patients who anticipate neck surgery in which either recurrent laryngeal nerve may be at risk should undergo a preoperative laryngeal mirror examination.[10,11] *Such a practice not only can help prevent unjustified medicolegal complications, but may alert the surgeon that the vocal fold on the side opposite the contemplated neck surgery is nonfunctional so that the patient can be prepared for possible tracheotomy if the remaining recurrent nerve is compromised.—HMT*

"In 1881, Sir Felix Semon stated that abductor fibers of the recurrent laryngeal nerve are more susceptible to injury than the adductor. This theory may be an

muscle activity. As a result, although *breathiness, rapid air escape,* and *diplophonia* (because of the difference in tension between the two vocal folds) are hallmarks of *unilateral vocal fold paralysis,* such lesions sometimes result in very little apparent voice change and may even go unnoticed for years. ◁

In cases of *high vagal* or *complete unilateral paralysis* in which both the recurrent and the superior laryngeal nerves are not functioning, absence of the adduction usually provided by the unopposed cricothyroideus muscle allows the vocal fold to assume the *intermediate position.* As a result, such patients often have a *very breathy* voice and are more likely to *aspirate* than are those with isolated recurrent laryngeal nerve paralysis, both because of greater incompetency of the glottis and the loss of sensation associated with the superior laryngeal nerve paralysis. ◁

Although most nonmoving vocal folds are, in fact, due to recurrent laryngeal nerve paralysis, some may be secondary to *fixation* of the *cri-*

coarytenoid joint, or both conditions may apply. On observing an immobile vocal fold, most examiners speak of "paralysis," even though the actual cause can be determined only by palpation of the arytenoid under general, paralytic anesthesia. Since the management of a fixed vocal fold may differ significantly from that which is appropriate for a paralyzed one, this differentiation must be kept in mind in every case (see later).

Etiology

Vocal cord paralysis may result from injury or other disease process impinging on the vagus or recurrent laryngeal nerves anywhere from the brainstem to the point of entry into the larynx. Because of its long cervical and (particularly on the left side) intrathoracic course, as well as proximity to vascular structures and other viscera, the recurrent laryngeal nerve is subject to many types of trauma. Tables 11–1 and 11–2 compare the causes of unilateral and bilateral paralyses as recorded in several series.[6]

As can be seen from Table 11–1, *unilateral vocal fold paralysis* is usually idiopathic, but when the cause *can* be determined, it is most likely to be the result of trauma. Thyroid surgery is becoming steadily less common as a cause for unilateral palsy. On the other hand, Table 11–2 shows that thyroid surgery remains the single most common identifiable cause of *bilateral paralysis* and that nonsurgical neck trauma is the next most common and becoming steadily more so.◁

Evaluation

When the cause of vocal cord palsy is evident from the history or physical findings, the physician can proceed directly to appropriate management. However, many cases of unilateral paralysis and even some bilateral ones present with no apparent cause. Such idiopathic lesions should be evaluated in an orderly fashion in order to illucidate the cause, if possible. To this end, a series of screening evaluations can be carried out that should at least raise suspicion of a detectable cause, if one exists (Table 11–3).

After careful examination has established the presence of a nonmoving vocal cord and has ruled out obvious evidence of either a tumor or other neurologic findings, the three radiologic studies will address the possibility of mass lesions of the chest, esophagus, and mediastinum, jugular foramen, and parapharyngeal space, in essence examining the entire course of the recurrent laryngeal nerve. Radioactive iodine uptake and scan is intended to identify malignancies or other mass lesions of the thyroid gland, and the glucose tolerance test and serology should rule out diabetic mononeuropathy or late syphilis as possible causes of vocal cord paralysis. Although these screening tests are by no means foolproof, they should suggest an underlying cause when one is sufficiently far advanced to be identified.

Table 11–3   Evaluation of Idiopathic Vocal Cord Paralysis

1. Otolaryngologic examination (including fiberoptic endoscopy, if needed)
2. Chest radiograph
3. Cine barium swallow
4. CT scan (or tomograms) of the skull base and parapharyngeal spaces.
5. Radioactive tracer uptake and scan of the thyroid
6. Glucose tolerance test
7. Serology

Management

Once the diagnosis of vocal cord paralysis has been made and its cause identified, if possible, the laryngologist can proceed to appropriate management.

Unilateral paralysis rarely results in significant airway obstruction or aspiration, unless there are other deficits as well (see before). The major symptom is diminution in voice strength and quality. The patient's voice typically is hoarse, breathy, exhibits rapid air escape,◁ and may be diplophonic. In idiopathic cases and in those of known cause in which there remains any possibility of spontaneous recovery, surgical intervention should be withheld for at least 6 months to 1 year to allow for recovery or compensation. Approximately 60 percent of idiopathic cases will recover within 1 year of onset[6] and many of those that do not recover will compensate to satisfactory voice levels within the same period.

The only valid *indications* for surgical intervention early after onset of *unilateral paralysis* are:

1. Intractable aspiration
2. Ventilatory insufficiency because of inability to maintain expiratory back-pressure (such as in severe emphysema)
3. Psychologic inability to wait for recovery or compensation
4. Professional or financial factors that demand prompt restoration of voice

Even under these circumstances, nothing irreversible should be carried out that might interfere with spontaneous recovery if it should be destined to take place.

All approaches to rehabilitation of unrecovered and uncompensated unilateral paralysis seek to displace the paralyzed vocal fold from the paramedian position to or near the midline so that the functioning vocal fold can meet it effectively. Besides speech therapy to maximize compensation, the three approaches to vocal fold medialization are:

1. Teflon (Gelfoam) injection
2. Surgical medialization of the vocal fold
3. Vocal fold reinnervation

1. *Teflon injection* is generally regarded as the procedure of choice for most cases of uncompensated unilateral vocal fold paralysis.[13–15] When used properly, this approach is safe, inexpensive, results in almost immediate improvement, and usually provides a very satisfactory voice. It should be carried out under topical anesthesia, unless there is some strong reason to the contrary. If temporary results are desirable or if a "test" to see what kind of voice results might be achieved with Teflon injection is appropriate, Gelfoam paste may be substituted, otherwise using the same technique and equipment.[15]

The *technique* of *Teflon injection* is as follows.[16] Topical anesthesia◁ is preferred because monitoring of the voice and observation of improving glottic competence are the only ways to judge when sufficient paste has been injected.◁ With the patient in the supine position, a straight laryngoscope is introduced. The larynx is exposed and the tip of the laryngoscope is advanced to a point just above the surface of the vocal folds (Fig. 11–4). The tip of the laryngoscope is rotated toward the paralyzed side to displace the false cord and expose as much of the surface of the true cord as possible. Using a Bruning syringe and a side delivery needle (Fig. 11–5a) the needle tip is inserted into the surface of the paralyzed vocal fold as far posteriorly and as far laterally as possible. In essence, the tip of the

Rapid air escape during speech may be responsible not only for the patient's impression that he or she is short of breath, but can produce hypocalcemic tetany *if the patient is aready in a borderline metabolic state.—HMT*

See Chapter 6 for technique of topical anesthesia.

Teflon can be removed from the vocal fold only with difficulty and generally poor voice results. Therefore, if any error is made in judging the amount of Teflon to be injected, it should be on the side of too little rather than too much. Additional Teflon can be added a few weeks after initial placement, if needed.—HMT

Figure 11–4. Laryngeal
exposure for Teflon injection.
a, Tip of laryngoscope is
positioned just above vocal
fold. **b,** Laryngoscope is rotated
to expose entire upper surface
of vocal fold and to displace
false cord.

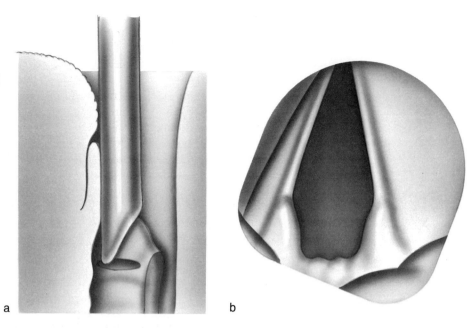

a   b

needle should be placed between the vocal process of the arytenoid and the
posterior aspect of the thyroid ala (Fig. 11–5b). In this manner, the injected Teflon will be contained in its lateral dimension between the two
cartilaginous structures and will displace the movable arytenoid medially,
as desired. Once proper placement of the needle has been achieved, the
necessary depth is estimated by advancing the needle until the lateral projection (which is 1 cm from the delivery port) is just above the surface of

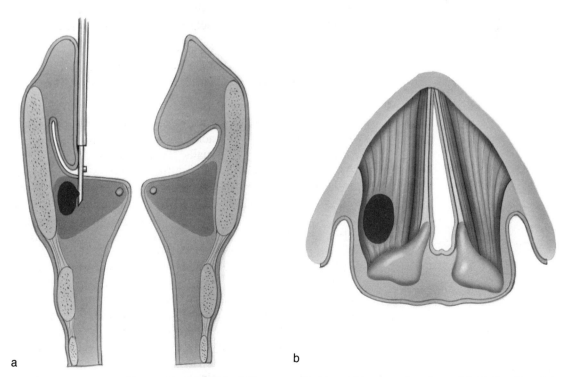

a   b

Figure 11–5. **a,** Side delivery needle inserted into paralyzed vocal fold. Small metal
guard is opposite the direction of delivery of Teflon and permits estimating depth
of injection. **b,** Teflon properly placed as far laterally and posteriorly as possible.

Figure 11–6. Misplacement of
Teflon. **a,** Anterior to tip of
vocal process. **b,** Too close to
surface of vocal fold. This leads
to distortion of free margin of
fold and favors granuloma
formation.

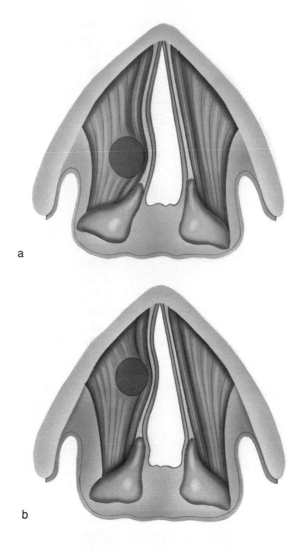

a

b

the vocal fold. Teflon (or Gelfoam) paste is delivered one click at a time
while medialization of the vocal fold is observed. The patient may be asked
to phonate while the needle and laryngoscope are in place, but care must
be taken that the instruments are not restricting the movement of the remaining vocal fold. When good apposition of the vocal folds is observed,
the instruments are withdrawn. Approximately four clicks of Teflon are
usually adequate. In very carefully selected cases, one or two clicks can
be placed more anteriorly in the membranous vocal fold to "plump up" a
flaccid or wasted cord, but this must be positioned as far laterally as possible (Fig. 11–6). At times, some of the Teflon will extrude from the needle
hole and should be suctioned away. This usually implies that too much
Teflon has been placed and that there is excess tension, forcing the paste
out.

Voice improvement may be dramatic, even while the patient is still
on the operating room table, although immediate voice results are often
quite variable and do not necessarily have any implications for eventual
outcome. The voice will vary from day to day or even from hour to hour
for several days after Teflon injection before the final result is achieved.

2. *Surgical medialization* may be preferable in patients with un-
usually large gaps between the vocal folds (as, for example, in cases of
combined superior and recurrent nerve palsies), since Teflon injection is
not as reliable in achieving satisfactory results when the deficit at the pos-

terior commissure exceeds 3 to 4 mm. If the arytenoid is fixed rather than simply paralyzed, Teflon injection may not be able to displace it adequately. In this latter situation, surgical medialization may be the only alternative. The *disadvantages* of this approach are that it requires an open surgical procedure under general anesthesia and it must usually be preceded by a tracheotomy, not only to provide a safe airway, but also so that the cartilage graft will not be displaced at the end of the operation by removal of an endoctracheal tube. On the other hand, almost any size gap can be reliably corrected and, if optimal voice results are not achieved, a subsequent small Teflon injection can be used as a "tuning" procedure.

The *technique* of *surgical medialization* that I have found most useful is as follows.[16]

With the patient in a supine position, a tracheotomy is carried out in the usual manner. A horizontal neck-crease incision is made at the level of the mid-thyroid cartilage on the side of paralysis (Fig. 11–7.) The strap muscles are retracted laterally to expose the thyroid ala at its upper border. An incision is made through the perichondrium along the upper edge of the thyroid cartilage and part way down the posterior margin (Fig. 11–8). The perichondrium is mobilized inferiorly to the level of the thyroid notch on both external and internal surfaces of the cartilage. The upper portion of the thyroid ala thus exposed is removed and trimmed to a triangular shape (Fig. 11–9). The inner perichondrium is carefully elevated to a point well below the estimated level of the paralyzed vocal fold to prepare a pocket for the cartilage graft and to free up the muscles around the arytenoid from their lateral attachments (Fig. 11–10). The prepared cartilage graft is placed in the pocket at the level of the paralyzed vocal fold with the apex of the triangle oriented anteriorly (Fig. 11–11). The cartilage may be anchored with absorbable sutures, but usually simple closure of the perichondrial leaflets to each other will suffice. Since the larynx is not actually entered, no antibiotics are needed and a simple Penrose drain is usually sufficient. The tracheotomy can be removed in just a few days, in most cases.

3. *Reinnervation* of the unilaterally paralyzed vocal fold[17,18] is a procedure that should be reserved for "valuable" voices that are absolutely critical to the patient's livelihood and emotional well-being.◁ Of all the procedures available to deal with unilateral vocal fold paralysis, only reinnervation offers the possibility of restoration of the ability to adjust tension in the vocal fold and, with it, better pitch control. The *drawbacks* of reinnervation include: the need for general anesthetic, open surgery, and a delay of from 4 months to as much as 1 year before the ability to move the vocal fold is restored, even if the operation is ultimately completely successful. The longterm success rate for this technique of voice restoration is about 85 percent.[18]

The *technique* for *unilateral* vocal fold *reinnervation* is as follows.[16] Since the vocal fold must be passively mobile in order for reinnervation to succeed, laryngoscopy is first performed without intubation and with the patient under general, paralytic anesthesia to permit palpation of the arytenoid cartilage (see later under Bilateral Paralysis). If the vocal fold is passively mobile (which is almost always true in unilateral paralysis,[6]) the patient is prepared and draped for sterile surgery of the neck. Tracheotomy is not required. With the patient in a supine position, a neck-crease incision is made at approximately the level of the lower border of the thyroid cartilage on the paralyzed side. The sternocleidomastoid muscle is mobilized posteriorly to expose the jugular vein and its overlying fascial sheath. The ansa hypoglossi nerve is identified by direct vision, or by dissecting posteriorly along the upper border of the omohyoid muscle, progressing from medial to lateral. A nerve-muscle pedicle, measuring 2 to 3 mm on

All voices are "valuable," of course, but there are some patients (such as professional singer, actor, clergyman, orator, teacher) whose livelihood requires not only a satisfactory voice, but one that can be relied on to project or otherwise be used under stressful conditions. Such patients may find it worthwhile to accept the greater cost, hospitalization, and the approximately 6-month delay in rehabilitation that are inherent in reinnervation of the unilaterally paralyzed vocal fold in order to realize the potentially superior voice result this procedure can provide.—HMT

Figure 11–7. Incision for
surgical medialization of vocal
fold.

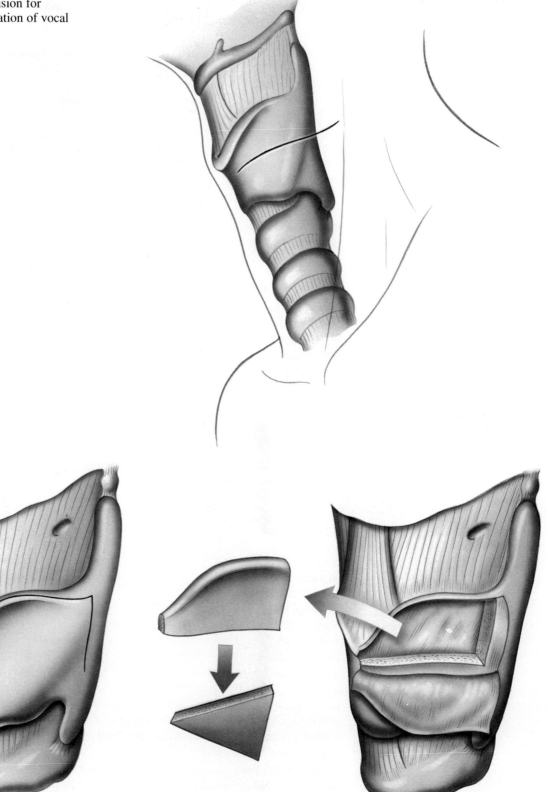

Figure 11–8. Perichondrial incision.

Figure 11–9. Upper portion of thyroid ala is removed
subperichondrially and trimmed to appropriate shape.

Figure 11–10. Dissection of
inner perichondrium to form a
pocket.

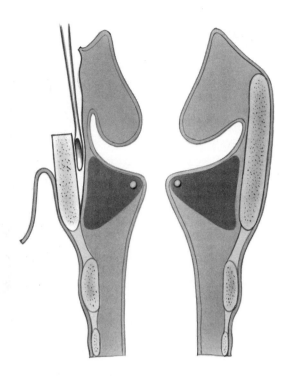

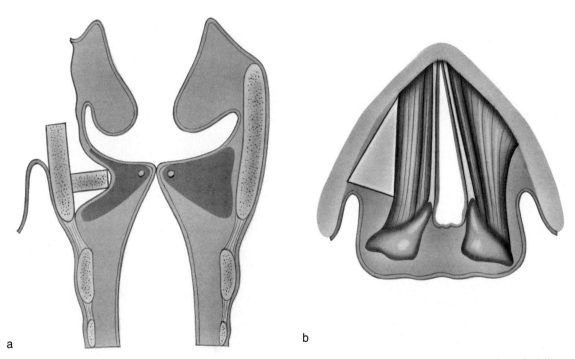

a

b

Figure 11–11. Placement of cartilage wedge into pocket. **a,** Coronal view. **b,** View
from above. Note that shape of wedge tends to force the wider end posteriorly.

Figure 11–12. Development of
nerve-muscle pedicle from
anterior belly of omohyoid
muscle.

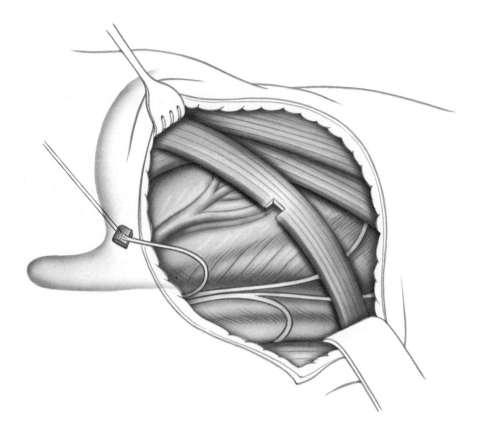

a side is developed from the branch of the ansa hypoglossi to the anterior
belly of the omohyoid muscle (although any other strap muscle will serve
as well) (Fig. 11–12). The lateral aspect of the thyroid ala is identified and
the overlying strap muscles are displaced anteriorly. An anteriorly based
flap of perichondrium is developed from the lower 50 percent of the thyroid cartilage and a window of the cartilage is removed in order to preserve
an inferior and posterior strut for support (Fig. 11–13). This maneuver will
expose the inner perichondrium overlying the insertions of the lateral thyroarytenoideus muscle, a major vocal fold adductor and tensor. The inner
perichondrium is incised and the nerve-muscle pedicle is sutured to the
muscle with one or two 5–0 nylon sutures (Fig. 11–14). The perichondrium is returned and the wound closed with a small Penrose drain. Antibiotics are unecessary.

Bilateral vocal fold paralysis usually affects voice quality only to a
small degree because the paralyzed vocal folds assume a position very close
to that necessary for phonation when the superior laryngeal nerves are intact. The real *problem* is *airway compromise*, which, in occasional cases,
can be so slight that the patient may even be unaware of it. It is much
more common, however, that the patient is quite *dyspneic* and *stridorous*,
especially on exertion, and may even be in severe airway distress.

Management of this problem falls into one of three broad approaches:
tracheotomy, vocal fold lateralization, or vocal fold reinnervation.

1.   *Tracheotomy* will be part of the management of most patients with
bilateral vocal fold paralysis, if only as a temporary measure. For many
patients, it may be the best means of long-term management because it
restores control of the airway to the patient with relatively little additional
reduction in voice quality or strength. It has the further advantages that it
is quick, inexpensive, reversible, and can be carried out under local anesthesia, if desired.◁ Tracheotomy can solve the problem of inadequate air-

*For most patients with bilateral
vocal fold paralysis, a tracheotomy
may be corked much of the time,
thus avoiding the need to occlude
the tube digitally while speaking.
Most people are seldom called on
to speak a great deal except when
they are sitting or standing quietly
(such as at mealtimes, in social
circumstances). On the other hand,
during active exertion, while
sleeping, or because of further
airway compromise during a cold
or allergy attack, the tube can
simply be left open to provide
improved breathing capability.—
HMT*

Figure 11–13. Cartilage window removed from thryoid ala.

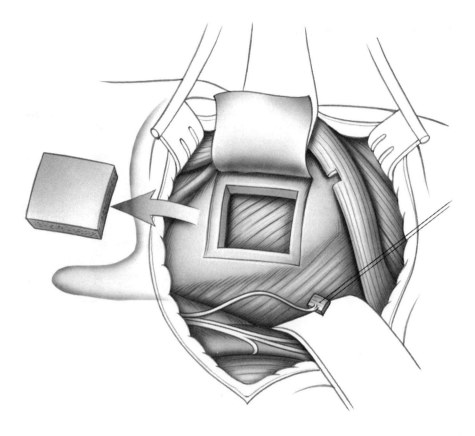

way by providing a prompt bypass. On the other hand, patients do not generally prefer to have the cosmetic and long-term care problems that are inherent in wearing a tracheal cannula, even in light of the much-improved, lighter weight tubes that are available.

Figure 11–14. Nerve muscle pedicle sutured to lateral thyroarytenoideus muscle fibers.

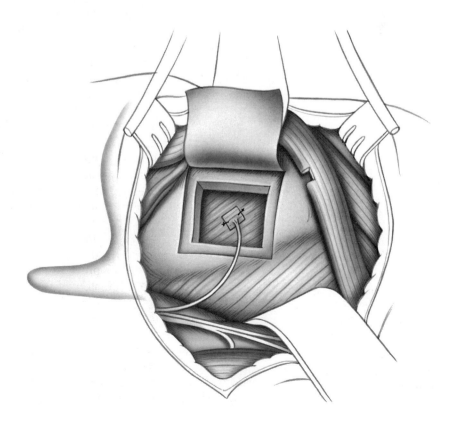

2. *Vocal fold lateralization* is the next approach. If the glottis can be widened by removing or displacing one of the vocal folds, adequate airway can be restored to patients with bilateral vocal fold paralysis. However, all of the procedures designed to achieve this end will do so at some expense to the residual voice. There are many techniques for reestablishing adequate airway and ridding the patient of the need for tracheotomy.[19-22] These can be classified as arytenoidopexy (lateralization), arytenoidectomy, and cordectomy.

Arytenoidopexy represents vocal cord lateralization in its purest sense. None of the vocal fold or arytenoid is actually removed; the structures are simply displaced and fixed in the abducted position. In theory, at least, this is intended to preserve as normal a vibratory vocal fold as possible in hopes of maintaining a good voice. The procedure has the *advantage* of avoiding open surgery or tracheotomy and can even be carried out under local anesthesia (although general anesthesia will probably be preferred by most surgeons). The major *drawback,* at least in my hands, is that adequate improvement does not ensue in many cases. One *technique* for this procedure is as follows.

The endolarynx is topically anesthetized and the skin of the neck overlying the thyroid ala on one side is infiltrated with local anesthesia. With a flexible, fiberoptic laryngoscope in place (under general anesthesia a direct laryngoscope is used from the outset), a small skin incision is made down to the surface of the cartilage. A 16 guage needle is passed through the thyroid ala, just above and just below the vocal fold at a point approximating the position of the tip of the vocal process (Fig. 11–15). A 2–0 monofilament nylon suture is passed through the lower of the two needles. The fiberoptic instrument is partially withdrawn and a hand-held direct laryngoscope is introduced. The end of the suture is grasped endoscopically and manipulated into the opening of the upper needle until it can be grasped outside the neck. The needles are withdrawn and the suture tied firmly down at the level of the thyroid cartilage. The small incision may be closed or

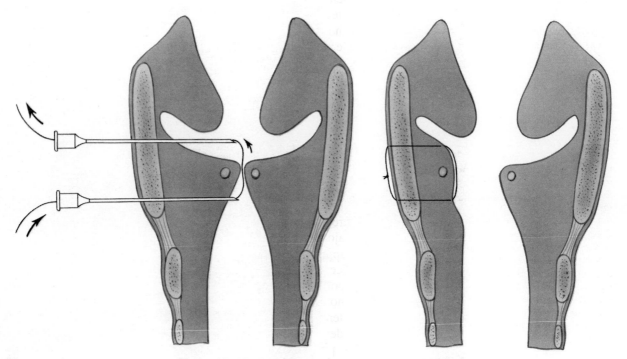

Figure 11–15. Suture technique to lateralize paralyzed vocal fold.

left open, as desired. The tightened suture lateralizes the vocal fold permanently.

The term *"arytenoidectomy"* covers a somewhat broader spectrum of procedures designed to gain a better airway by removing some or all of the arytenoid cartilage. Classic arytenoidectomy can be accomplished endoscopically by microsurgical technique (Thornell[20]) or with laser surgery (Jako,[22] and others), by thyrotomy approach (Scheer[16] and others), or by lateral neck approach (Woodman [21]). All of these can be coupled with suture lateralization of the remaining vocal fold, either as described in the previous section for the endoscopic techniques or under direction vision for the open surgical approaches. When suture lateralization is not employed, eventual spontaneous lateralization is expected to occur as a result of scarring in the bed of the excised arytenoid. Although all of these techniques have their proponents and can be successful in practiced hands, they all suffer from less than universal reliability. All of them should include a tracheotomy at the time of surgery, if one is not already in place. My personal preference is for the *Woodman technique,* which I perform as follows.

Even though the procedure is carried out under general anesthesia via tracheotomy, a large-bore endotracheal tube is passed into the glottis to force the vocal cords as far lateral as possible. This maneuver is very helpful in stabilizing the arytenoid during later dissection. The neck is prepared and draped for sterile surgery. A lateral neck-crease incision is made at the level of the midpoint of the thyroid ala. The sternocleidomastoid muscle and the great vessels are mobilized and retracted laterally. The retropharyngeal space is entered behind the thyroid cartilage and bluntly dissected to allow rotation of the larynx. The posterior edge of the thyroid ala is grasped with a double hook and the larynx rotated as far anteriorly as possible to expose the inferior constrictor muscle and, eventually, the cricoid lamina. The fibers of the inferior constrictor muscle are separated near the lesser cornu of the thyroid cartilage to expose the reflection of the pyriform sinus (Fig. 11–16). The pyriform is dissected upward to expose the posterior aspect of the cricoid lamina and the posterior cricoarytenoid muscle. Palpation identifies the junction of the superior aspect of the cricoid lamina with the arytenoid cartilage at the cricoarytenoid joint. The muscle is transected and the joint is identified. The entire arytenoid is carefully denuded of all muscle attachments on both its medial and lateral surfaces (Fig. 11–17). A single hook can be used to manipulate and stabilize the arytenoid cartilage during this maneuver. Finally, the joint space is entered and transected. Once the cartilage is completely mobilized, a doubled 2–0 silk suture is passed through the vocal process or into the membranous vocal fold just anterior to it. The remainder of the arytenoid is removed (Fig. 11–18), leaving the suture in place. The suture is then led around the lesser cornu of the thyroid cartilage or is driven through the posterior aspect of the thyroid ala at the level of the vocal fold (Fig. 11–19). The suture is tied firmly to lateralize the vocal fold. The wound is closed in the usual fashion with a drain. Antibiotics are not used unless the larynx has been entered during the procedure. ◁

The major *disadvantage* of all lateralization procedures, including the Woodman approach, is that airway is invariably gained at the expense of residual voice. In effect, the adequacy of the airway achieved will be inversely proportional to the quality of voice retained. For this reason, tracheotomy should be considered a preferable solution to long-term management of bilateral vocal fold paralysis, especially in children and young adults. I will consider performing vocal fold lateralization only after tracheotomy has been in place for at least 6 months to 1 year and then only if I am satisfied that the patient really cannot tolerate ongoing tracheotomy. *It is*

Although the Woodman procedure is among the technically most difficult operations I know, it is well worth mastering, inasmuch as it is by far the most reliable technique for vocal cord lateralization. It has the advantage over those techniques that require anterior thyrotomy (i.e. Scheer[16]) that the anterior commissure is not blunted, which can further diminish both airway and voice results. Moreover, if the membranous vocal fold remnant is fixed at the level of the opposite vocal fold (not depressed by fixing it to the lesser cornu as Woodman[21] described) the voice results are really quite satisfactory in most cases.—HMT

Figure 11–16. Separation of
fibers of inferior constrictor
muscle to expose posterior
cricoarytenoid muscle.

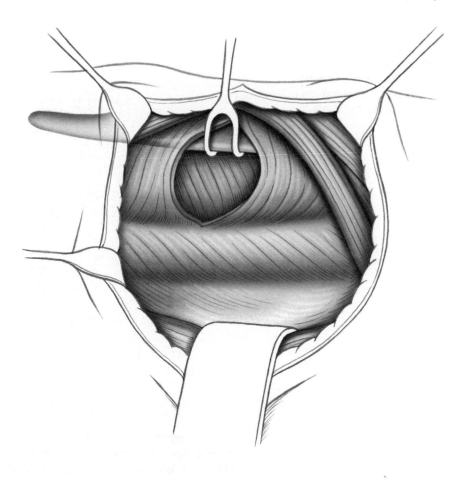

Figure 11–17. Exposure of
cricoarytenoid joint. All muscle
attachments should be removed
before the joint is transected.

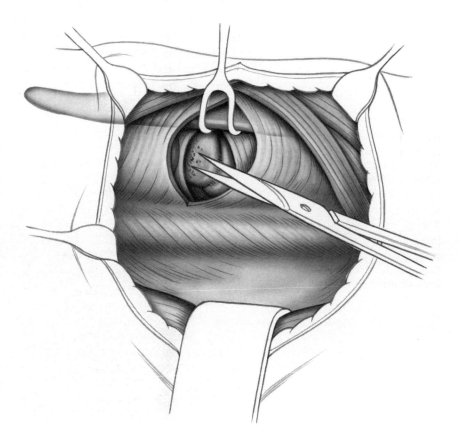

Figure 11–18. Vocal process is transected after entire arytenoid cartilage has been mobilized. Suture will be placed through the remaining vocal process to allow lateralization of vocal fold.

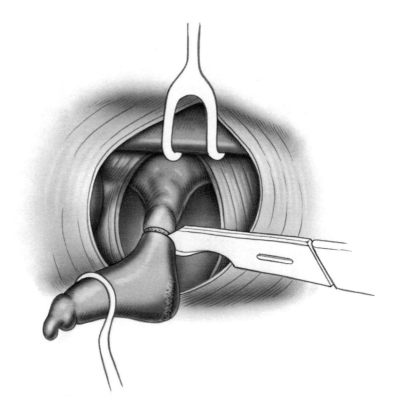

critically important that the patient accurately comprehend the impact that *loss of voice* will have in his or her life before arytenoidectomy or other irreversible lateralization procedure is considered.

3. *Reinnervation:* If one or both paralyzed vocal folds are passively mobile and if the cause of the paralysis has not also made the nerves needed unavailable, active restoration of abduction of at least one vocal fold can be achieved by nerve-muscle pedicle reinnervation.[23–26] This approach, when successful, is theoretically superior to other means of restoration of glottic airway because there is no further loss of voice. At present, long-term success with this procedure has been about 80 percent.[12] The *disadvantages*

Figure 11–19. Suture fixation of lateralized arytenoid remnant. The vocal fold can be depressed below the level of the glottis by suturing it to the lesser cornu of the thyroid cartilage (inset). This maneuver can provide better airway results, but also compromises the voice more than fold lateralization at the level of the glottis.

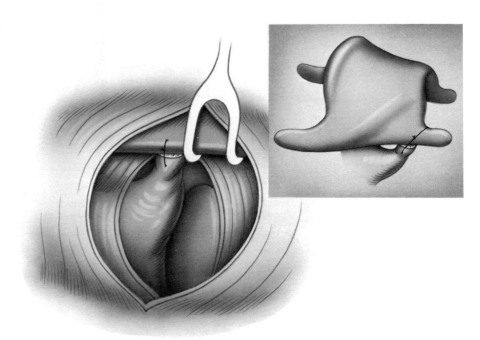

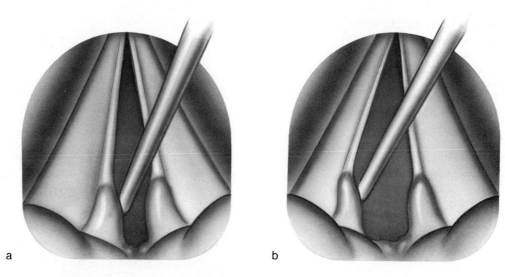

a   b

Figure 11–20. Palpation of arytenoid cartilage to determine passive mobility. **a,** Placement of suction tip against vocal process. **b,** Note widening of posterior commissure in normally mobile cricoarytenoid joint.

Another possible disadvantage is the apparent difficulty many well-trained and competent otolaryngologists have encountered in obtaining consistently successful results with this approach.[27] Some of these can be explained, perhaps, as misunderstanding some of the potential pitfalls of the procedure (as discussed in the main text); but clearly, any procedure that does not provide reliable results in the hands of the majority of competent practitioners is of questionable value to our surgical armamentarium.—HMT

of reinnervation include a delay of from 4 to 6 months after the surgery is carried out before active abduction may begin and the fact that it cannot be used if both cricoarytenoid joints have become fixed. This latter problem is present to at least some degree in 30 percent of all patients with bilateral vocal fold paralysis within 6 months of onset.[6]◁

The *technique* for reinnervation of the posterior cricoarytenoid muscles in bilateral vocal fold paralysis is as follows.[16]

The patient's *suitability* for reinnervation must first be determined by performing *direct laryngoscopy* under general, paralytic anesthesia, since fixation of the arytenoids is a contraindication to the procedure. Anesthesia should be by apneic technique without an endotracheal tube, if the patient does not already have a tracheotomy in place. A straight laryngoscope is introduced, taking care to position it so that the arytenoids are in view but there is no displacement or restriction of arytenoid mobility by the scope. A spatula or suction tip (with suction blocked off) is used to determine if the arytenoid cartilages can be displaced laterally (Fig. 11–20). Care must be taken to avoid misplacement of the suction tip and to note that the posterior glottic chink is actually widened by this maneuver. (Fig. 11–21). If at least one of the vocal folds is passively mobile and if no other uncorrected airway obstruction is encountered, the procedure may be carried out. The neck is prepared and draped for sterile surgery. A midline tracheotomy is placed if one is not already present. An incision is made in a horizontal skin crease at the lower border of the thyroid ala, extending from just posterior to the anterior border of the sternocleidomastoid muscle to the midline of the neck. The sternocleidomastoid muscle is retracted and the fascia overlying the jugular vein is inspected. Often, the ansa hypoglossi nerve can be seen shining through it on the surface of the vein. An alternative method to identify the nerve is to mobilize the anterior belly of the omohyoid muscle from anterior to posterior. The branch of the ansa to this muscle will usually be encountered entering the superior aspect of the muscle's deep surface.

When an appropriate nerve has been identified (any of the strap muscles will do, although the omohyoid is usually used), a nerve-muscle pedicle measuring approximately 2 to 3 mm on a side is developed. The pos-

Figure 11–21. Pitfalls in palpation of paralyzed vocal fold. **a,** Only membranous vocal fold is displaced. Fixed arytenoid does not move. **b,** Too deep placement of palpating suction tip impacts on cricoid lamina below vocal fold, giving false impression of fixation.

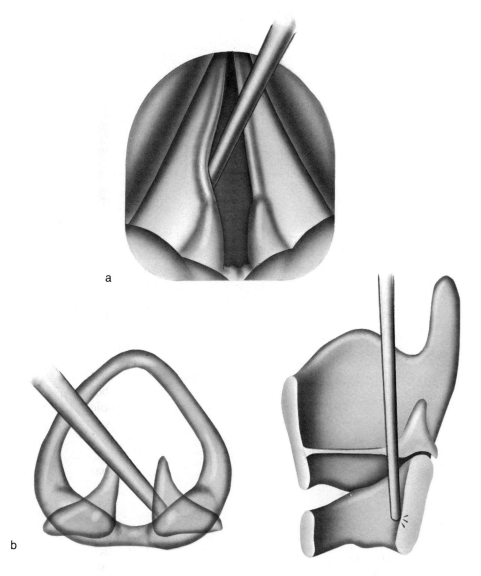

a

b

terior aspect of the thyroid ala is grasped with a double hook and the retrolaryngeal space is mobilized to permit rotation of the larynx. The fibers of the inferior constrictor muscle are separated at a point close to the base of the inferior cornu of the thyroid cartilage, thus exposing the reflection of the pyriform sinus. (Fig. 11–22) If this mucosa is reflected carefully, the posterior cricoarytenoid muscle will be exposed. This muscle can be recognized either by the fact that its fibers are oriented at right angles to those of the overlying inferior constrictor muscle, or by noting that the next deeper structure is the posterior cricoid lamina. The nerve-muscle pedicle is sutured to the denuded surface of the posterior cricoarytenoid muscle with one or two 5–0 nylon sutures (Fig. 11–23). The incision is closed after placement of a Penrose drain. Antibiotics are unnecessary.

Postoperative assessment is important in evaluating success in this procedure. Approximately one-third of patients whose surgery is ultimately successful will exhibit improved exercise tolerance and visible, spontaneous abduction of the reinnervated vocal fold on inspiratory effort within 2 to 6 months of surgery. Another third will report good exercise tolerance, but vocal cord motion will not be apparent unless the patient is stressed by being made to run in place for several minutes with the tracheotomy tube corked. After such exertion, the reinnervated vocal fold will either be

Figure 11–22. Nerve-muscle
pedicle prepared, inferior
constrictor fibers separated, and
pyriform sinus mucosal
reflection exposed. This
structure must be carefully
elevated to permit access to
posterior cricoarytenoid muscle.

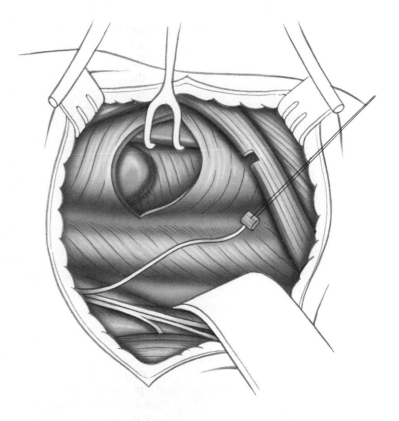

noted to move spontaneously or there will be tonic lateralization that persists as long as the patient's oxygen demand remains above resting levels.
This phenomenon occurs because some patients with bilateral vocal fold
paralysis have sufficient airway while at rest and do not stimulate activity
in the reinnervated vocal fold unless they are stressed. Finally, approximately one-third of patients who are successfully reinnervated will dem-

Figure 11–23. Nerve-muscle
pedicle is transposed and
sutured to the posterior
cricoarytenoid muscle.

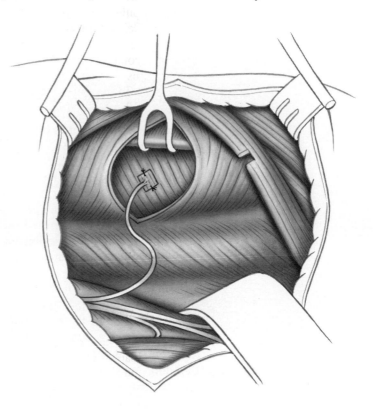

onstrate obviously improved exercise tolerance, but movement of the vocal fold will not be apparent even under stress. Since the aim of the procedure is to reestablish airway capability adequate to the patient's daily needs without worsening the voice, this last group of patients are considered successful, even though the results cannot be documented by observation of movement.

Management of the Patient with an Incompetent Glottis

Isolated unilateral or even bilateral paralysis of the vocal folds are not usually sufficient to result in significant aspiration. Almost without fail, some other airway or swallowing compromise must be present before the patient will be unable to manage his own secretions and swallow effectively. Such concomitant deficits as sensory loss or dyscoordination of the entire swallowing mechanism must occur in conjunction with vocal fold paralysis before these problems become significant. Best management requires accurate assessment of the lesion responsible, not only so that the full extent of airway and swallowing compromise can be appreciated, but also so that a good estimate of potential recovery or compensation can be made.

Assessment requires (1) accurate visualization of the larynx (indirect or direct); (2) cine barium swallow; (3) esophageal manometry; (4) chest radiographs; and (5) pulmonary function studies. These studies permit evaluation of the *need* for intervention (evidence of aspiration, pneumonia, decreasing pulmonary function) as well as the *cause* of dysfunction, so that appropriate intervention can be selected.

1.   If the patient is able to handle his own secretions without significant pulmonary compromise, simple passage of a nasogastric tube may suffice initially, with either esophagostomy[28] or gastrostomy as potential long-term solutions.

2.   Placement of a tracheotomy to gain access for pulmonary toilette and/or the ability to limit aspiration during feedings by blowing up the balloon may be considered, if inability to handle saliva and other secretions results in pulmonary soilage or pneumonia.

3.   Gelfoam or even Teflon injection may be enough to improve glottic competence and provide better ability to clear the airway by restoring an effective cough. Gelfoam is chosen either when the possibility of some spontaneous recovery exists (i.e., stroke) or to determine whether a more permanent Teflon injection is likely to be effective.

4.   When aspiration remains intractable and is likely to last for some time, laryngeal diversion should be considered.[29] Although drastic, such a maneuver absolutely prevents pulmonary soilage by directing aspirated material either back into the esophagus or to the outside. If the patient should later recover sufficiently, the trachea can be anastomosed again. Procedures recommended for suturing of the vocal folds to prevent aspiration are generally unsuccessful.

References

1.   Ward PH, Berci G, Calcaterra TC: Superior laryngeal nerve paralysis: An often overlooked entity. Trans Am Acad Opthalmol Otolaryngol, 84:78, 1977

2.   Abelson TI, Tucker, HM: Laryngeal findings in superior laryngeal nerve paralysis: A controversy. Otolaryngol Head Neck Surg, 89:463–470, 1981

3.   Thornell WC: Vocal cord paralysis. In Paparella MM, Shumrick DA (Eds): Otolaryngology, vol 3: Head and Neck. Philadelphia, WB Saunders, 1973, pp 650–651

4.   Faaborg-Anderson K, Munk-Jensen A: Unilateral paralysis of the superior laryngeal nerve. Acta Otolaryngol (Stockh), 57:155, 1964

5. May M: Rehabilitation of the crippled larynx. Laryngoscope, 90:1–18, 1980

6. Tucker HM: Vocal cord paralysis—1979: Etiology and management. Laryngoscope, 90:585, 1980

7. Holinger LD, Wolter RK: Neurologic disorders of the larynx. In English GM (Ed): Otolaryngology, vol III. Hagerstown, MD, Harper & Row, 1979

8. Hart CW: Functional and neurological problems of the larynx. Otol Clin North Am, 3:609, 1970

9. Tyler HR: Neurology of the larynx. Otolaryngol Clin North Am, 17:75–79, 1984

10. Hertzer NR, Feldman BJ, Beven EG, Tucker HM: A prospective study of the incidence of injury to the cranial nerves during carotid endarterectomy. Surgery 151:781–784, 1980

11. Astor FC, Santilli P, Tucker HM: Incidence of cranial nerve dysfunction following carotid endarterectomy. Head Neck Surgery 6:660–663, 1983

12. Levine HL, Tucker HM: Surgical management of the paralyzed larynx. In Bailey BJ, Biller HF, (Eds): Surgery of the Larynx. Philadelphia, WB Saunders Co, 1985, pp 117–134

13. Lewy R: Glottic rehabilitation with Teflon injection: The return of the voice, cough, laughter. Acta Otolaryngol (Stockh), 58:214, 1964

14. Tucker HM: Management of the patient with an incompetent larynx. Am J Otol, 1:47, 1979

15. Schramm VL, May MM, Lavorato AS: Gelfoam paste injection for vocal cord paralysis: Temporary rehabilitation of glottic incompetence. Laryngoscope, 88:1268, 1978

16. Tucker HM: Surgery for Phonatory Disorders. New York, Churchill Livingstone, 1981

17. Tucker, HM: Reinnervation of the unilaterally paralyzed larynx. Ann Otol, 86:789, 1977

18. Rusnov M, Tucker HM: Laryngeal reinnervation for unilateral vocal cord paralysis: Long-term results. Ann Otol, 90:1981

19. King BT: A new and function restoring operation for bilateral abductor cord paralysis: Preliminary report. JAMA, 112:814, 1939

20. Thornell W: Transoral intralaryngeal approach for arytenoidectomy in bilateral vocal cord paralysis with inadequate airway. Ann Otol, 66:364, 1957

21. Woodman G: A modification of the extralaryngeal approach to arytenoidectomy for bilateral vocal cord paralysis. Arch Otolaryngol, 43:63, 1946

22. Jako G: Microsurgery of the larynx with the carbon dioxide laser. In English GM (Ed): Otolaryngology, vol 3. Philadelphia, Harper & Row, 1978

23. Tucker HM: Human laryngeal reinnervation: Long-term experience with the nerve-muscle pedicle technique. Laryngoscope, 88:598–604, 1978

24. Appelbaum EL, Allen GW, Sisson GA: Human laryngeal reinnervation: The Northwestern experience. Laryngoscope, 89:1784–1787, 1979

25. Tucker HM: Complications after surgical management of the paralyzed larynx. Laryngoscope, 93:295–298, 1983

26. Tucker HM: Congenital bilateral recurrent nerve paralysis and ptosis: A new syndrome. Laryngoscope, 93:1405–1407, 1983

27. Crumley R: New perspectives in laryngeal reinnervation. In Bailey BJ, Biller HF (Eds): Surgery of the Larynx. Philadelphia, WB Saunders, 1985

28. Tucker HM, Broniatowski M: Tube esophagostomy. Laryngoscope, 1985

29. Tucker HM: Double-barrelled (diversionary) tracheostomy in the management of juvenile laryngeal papillomatosis. Ann Otol Rhinol Laryngol, 89:504–507, 1980

Chapter 12

Benign Neoplasms

"Certain tumors have a predilection for anatomic sites within the larynx. A number of tumors are typically found in the supraglottis -paragangliomas, neurofibromas, neurilemmomas, adult hemangiomas, oncocytic tumors, and lipomas. Granular cell tumors are nearly always glottic. Pediatric hemangiomas, chondromas, and pleomorphic adenomas tend to grow subglottically." –Jones et al[1]

See also Chapter 10.

Glottic webbing and subglottic stenosis are distressing, but ever more frequent findings in these patients and may be responsible for symptoms similar to those produced by the papillomas themselves. However, such scarring is most often the result of aggressive efforts at treatment and not of the disease process.—HMT

With the exception of papillomas, benign neoplasms of the larynx are rather uncommon, especially if a strict pathologic definition is followed and such non-neoplastic growths as polyps and nodules are excluded.[1] Table 12–1 outlines the *incidence* of these lesions in a series from the Eye and Ear Hospital of Pittsburgh and Presbyterian-University Hospital (1955–1982). Many previous studies have included various non-neoplastic conditions, rendering their statistical findings less useful when considering these lesions.[2,3]

As a rule, the *symptoms* produced by benign neoplasms are a function of size and location relative to voice production and airway. Thus, *voice change* and/or *stridor* are the most common complaints. Occasionally, a feeling of a *mass in the throat* or a visible *external swelling* will be encountered.◁ Clearly, the location of the lesion will determine any presenting complaints to a large degree.

Papillomas

It can be argued that these friable, wartlike growths should be considered among the infectious lesions of the larynx◁ because of strong evidence suggesting a viral etiology.[4,5] Whether they are associated with maternal condyloma acuminata or not, there is very convincing evidence to suggest that the cause is the DNA human papilloma virus.[6]

The juvenile onset type and the adult type behave differently despite their indistinguishable histologic appearance. The *juvenile type* is more common in females (2:1), multiple, recurs frequently, and sometimes "metastasizes" to recently traumatized areas of the larynx and trachea. When unchecked in their growth below the vocal folds, these benign neoplasms can be life-threatening.[7] The *adult-onset type,* on the other hand, is more common in males, usually solitary, and can often be eradicated by appropriate surgery. There is, however, a certain incidence of *malignant degeneration* among those that exhibit marked keratinization.[8] Regardless of age at onset papillomas are seen most often on the vocal folds, although any part of the upper aerodigestive tract can be affected. They produce *hoarseness* as the most common presenting complaint, but *airway obstruction* is often a problem, especially in children.◁

Although many other methods for control of papillomatosis have been

Table 12–1   Benign Neoplasms of the Larynx*

Papilloma	227 (87%)
Oncocytic tumor	15 (6%
Granular cell tumor	7 (3%)
Hemangioma	5 (2%)
Lymphangioma	3
Paraganglioma	2
Neurilemoma	2
Neurofibroma	2
Lipoma	1
Chondroma	1
Pleomorphic adenoma	1
Nodular fasciitis	1
Fibrous histiocytoma	1
Fibromatosis	1
Rhabdomyoma	1
Total	270

*Reprinted with permission from Jones et al.[1]

"The development of the CO2 laser has revolutionized the management of this difficult lesion. . . . [It] prevents most bleeding and therefore papilloma can be removed under direct vision with better preservation of normal laryngeal structures. . . . [B]ecause the laser is capable of removing large volumes of papilloma without producing significant edema in the residual tissues, tracheotomy can now be avoided in many more cases than was previously possible, thus avoiding . . . papilloma formation at the tracheotomy site and all of the other well-recognized complications."—Tucker[9]

advocated,[4] *surgical excision* remains the mainstay of *management*. Microlaryngoscopy with "cold knife" forceps removal is adequate, but many otolaryngologists now feel that laser surgery is preferable.[9,10]◁ Early hopes that this modality would promptly eradicate the disease have, however, not been borne out. Although the laser has greatly improved our ability to avoid tracheotomy and to limit damage to residual laryngeal structures, it is the exception rather than the rule when the disease does not recur and require long-term and repeated management.

The aims of *treatment* in papillomatosis are the following.

1.   Airway maintenance. Tracheotomy is to be avoided at all costs, since growth of papilloma at the stoma site, difficulties in extubation, and later stenoses are frequent problems. The laser has permitted airway maintenance without tracheotomy in many such patients. It is generally advisable to remove only as much neoplasm as is necessary for this purpose, especially in massively involved larynges, since it is often impossible to determine what is normal tissue in such cases. Overly vigorous attempts at complete removal increase the likelihood of damage to normal structures. If tracheotomy *is* required in very severe cases, the laser may be used in retrograde fashion eventually to clear the subglottic and tracheal disease.

2.   Preservation of voice. Once the airway can be maintained, the treating physician may then turn attention to preserving as normal a voice as possible. Although a "normal" voice is rarely achieved even with maximal effort, these children usually develop reasonably normal speech patterns. It is important to preserve some intact mucosa on one side of the larynx (even if it is covered with papilloma) when removing lesions from the other. This is especially true at the anterior commissure where webbing tends to develop as a result of fusion of denuded adjacent surfaces. Since it is rarely possible to eradicate extensive disease completely, multiple laser treatments will be needed in any event and removal of residual disease can be delayed until the first area treated has healed.

3.   Eradication of Disease. Although it is occasionally possible to remove all apparent papilloma, *recurrence is the rule*. Those cases of juvenile onset that "disappear" after several laser treatments probably represent natural involution of disease rather than cure. Attempts at use of autogenous vaccines, steroids, ultrasound, cryosurgery, and other nonsurgical means of treatment have generally been unsuccessful, although inter-

feron has shown some initial promise.[11,12] Unfortunately, at this time (1986) it is still not readily available except as an experimental drug.

For most children with this disease, a *"good" management result* will be: (1) a stable airway without need for tracheotomy; (2) an abnormal but serviceable voice; and (3) the need for repeated laser treatments only once or twice a year until puberty, at which time many patients' disease undergoes spontaneous involution. In other cases, simple growth of the larynx will minimize the need for surgical intervention while vigorous regrowth of papilloma slows down, thus arriving at an acceptable situation. Adult-onset papilloma, on the other hand, can often be eradicated with one or two laser treatments. If it persists or recurs after a significant disease-free interval, the otolaryngologist should be suspicious of malignant change.

Oncocytic Tumors

Oncocytomas are found most frequently in the salivary glands. Like the more common Warthin's tumor (papillary cystadenoma lymphomatosa), they have the ability to take up radioactive gallium or technetium, thus permitting noninvasive diagnosis by imaging.—HMT

These uncommon tumors always appear in the supraglottic area, which supports the view that they probably arise from mucous glands. They are also referred to as papillary cystadenoma,◁ and several other designations, all of which recognize the common feature of the oncocyte.[13] They are slightly more common in females and tend to appear after the age of 50 years.[1] They are often confused with oncocytic metaplasia of supraglottic mucoserous glands, which occurs frequently in elderly patients.[14]

Oncocytic tumors appear as smooth, mucosal-covered, often cystic lesions involving the supraglottic larynx. *Treatment* should be by adequate but nonmutilating *surgical excision*. Most of them can be handled satisfactorily by endoscopic means, but the occasional larger lesion may require open pharyngotomy or even partial laryngectomy. Less than adequate excision leads to recurrence,[1] possibly because of multicentricity.[15]

Granular Cell Tumors

This lesion is much more common in the oral cavity, only about 10 percent of all cases (less than 200 total) having been found in the larynx. There is controversy as to its cell of origin, but it is now generally agreed that it is derived from the Schwann cell.[16] These lesions tend to present in young people, usually between the ages of 10 and 40,[1] twice as commonly in males as in females. They are most often found in the posterior glottis, with symptoms and even appearance similar to contact granuloma, although these tumors are not bilateral. A sessile or pedunculated, white to yellow mucosal-covered mass is the usual gross appearance. *Biopsy* specimens must be distinguished from squamous cell carcinoma, with which they may easily be confused. *Treatment* is by adequate endoscopic removal, in which the laser can be very helpful. Recurrence is unusual.

Hemangiomas

"There has been some controversy whether hemangiomas represent true neoplasms or congenital anomalies. Their behavior, which at times may be fairly aggressive, is consistent with a neoplastic process."—Jones et al[1]

See also Chapter 7.

Although congenital subglottic hemangiomas◁ are well-recognized in the literature, they comprise only about 10 percent of all such lesions in the larynx.[17] They may be cavernous or capillary in histologic type, the latter being more common. Those of juvenile onset have a distinctly higher preponderance in females and there are associated cutaneous hemangiomas in 50 percent of cases.◁ In newborn infants, the lesion most often causes *obstructive symptoms,* such as inspiratory and expiratory stridor, hoarseness, and poor feeding, which appear within a few weeks of birth. Xeroradiography or soft tissue plain films often will show subglottic narrowing. *Diagnosis* is usually confirmed by the appearance of the lesion at laryngoscopy and biopsy should be avoided because of threat of serious bleeding.

Treatment should be conservative whenever possible, but the airway must be maintained and this will sometimes necessitate tracheotomy. More commonly, systemic steroids and local humidification are enough to avoid the need for surgical intervention; this is fortunate, since tracheotomy often cannot be removed from small children for several years. The carbon dioxide laser can sometimes be used to excise some of an obstructing lesion and thus avoid tracheotomy as well.[18] Other means of management have been suggested, (sclerosing agents, cryosurgery, radiotherapy) but all of them are either ineffective, capable of producing complications even worse than the disease itself, or unecessary. In most cases, spontaneous involution takes place between 18 months and 3 years of age.

Lymphangiomas

These are rare in the larynx and almost always represent only part of a much larger lesion involving many head and neck structures.[19] They are usually detected in the newborn and present with *symptoms* similar to those of hemangioma—stridor, poor feeding, dysphagia. Unlike hemangiomas, lymphangiomas to not tend to involute and *treatment* must, therefore, center around judicious surgical removal. Since it is rarely possible to remove them totally because of involvement of vital structures, only *airway stabilization, swallowing* capability, and *cosmesis* should be considered when deciding on appropriate surgical intervention. Tracheotomy is frequently necessary, at least during childhood, but judicious use of the carbon dioxide laser may minimize the need for airway bypass and can also be helpful in reducing tumor size in the oral cavity and hypopharynx.

Paragangliomas

These rare lesions (in the larynx) are also referred to as chemodectomas and glomus tumors. They are found most frequently in association with parapagliar tissue near the carotid and jugular bodies, but can occur almost anywhere in the body. There have been 27 cases of paraganglioma limited to the larynx reported in the English language literature.[20] Three-quarters of the patients are male and the supraglottic area is almost always the area of involvement.◁ There appears to be some potential for malignant change or for a malignant variant of this neoplasm.[21] Typical *symptoms* include *hoarseness,* inspiratory *stridor,* and, occasionally, *hemoptysis.* These lesions are not usually hormonally functional.

Diagnosis is made by observing the lesion and, if its potentially vascular nature is appreciated, by digital substraction angiographic (DSA) studies. Biopsy can result in severe bleeding and is best accomplished at the time of *definitive resection.* In some cases, laser excision may be possible,[22] but most patients will require open pharyngotomy or partial laryngectomy.

This is due to the anatomic relationship of paired paraganglia to the superior laryngeal nerves, thus accounting for the propensity for these lesions to be associated with the aryepiglottic folds and false vocal cords. There are also less constant paraganglia related to the recurrent laryngeal nerves near the first tracheal ring, but only two cases of paraganglioma have been reported from this location.[1]—HMT

Neurilemmomas and Neurofibromas

These tumors of nerve sheath origin involve the larynx with some frequency,[23] but almost always either as part of systemic neurofibromatosis (von Recklinghausen's disease) or by extension of a larger lesion from outside the larynx. Isolated laryngeal neurofibroma is uncommon. Neurilemommas, on the other hand, although less common than neurofibromas, tend to be solitary.

Both are slow-growing lesions that produce *symptoms* because of location. In the larynx they can result in slow progression of *stridor, voice change, dysphagia,* and, in the case of isolated neurilemomas, *pain. Diagnosis* is made by observing a *mass* that is usually visible within the larynx and, if it extends from the neck, may be *palpable,* as well. *Computed tomography (CT)-scanning* with DSA or contrast usually demonstrates the mass, which often exhibits a slight vascular blush.

Treatment is by adequate *surgical excision,* most often requiring sacrifice of the nerve from which the tumor arose. Since they to not usually produce preoperative paralysis or loss of feeling in the involved nerve (slow growth allows the nerve to compensate), it is imperative that the patient be warned about the necessary neurologic deficits that may ensue after removal. Lateral pharyngotomy, partial laryngectomy, and, occasionally, endoscopic laser surgery are the usual approaches to excision. In von Recklinghausen's disease, the surgeon should avoid mutilating or debilitating procedures in light of almost certain recurrence and the systemic nature of the illness. In such cases, *aim of treatment* should be limited to *maintenance of airway* and *deglutition* and, where possible without destructive surgery, of *voice.* Simple tracheotomy and esophagostomy or gastrostomy may be in the patient's best interest in severe systemic cases.

Lipomas

Although lipomas can occur anywhere in the body where there is fat, they are uncommon in the larynx.[24] Most of them occur in relationship to the epiglottis and false cords, where there is normally the most fat in the larynx. They are slow-growing and produce gradual onset of *obstructive symptoms,* which may be *intermittant* because of a "ball-valve" effect from pedunculated lesions. *Diagnosis* is made by observing a *yellowish, submucosal mass.* CT scanning or xeroradiography can confirm the extent of the lesion. *Treatment* by endoscopic removal is usually adequate.

Chondromas

These benign tumors of cartilage are slow-growing and occur predominantly in males (4:1) of middle age. They arise most often from the posterior cricoid lamina (70 percent), but can involve any of the laryngeal cartilaginous structures and can even arise from the vocal fold itself.[25] Routine radiographs and CT scans demonstrate the lesion and its extent.◁

Some texts in radiology allege that punctate calcification virtually guarantees malignancy when seen in films of suspected chondromatous lesions. Our experience in three such cases, however, has been that none of them was histologically malignant, although one recurred as a malignant chondrosarcoma some 6 years after initial resection.—HMT

Treatment is by temporary tracheotomy and adequate surgical excision, avoiding total laryngectomy wherever possible.[26] Since the most common involvement is of the cricoid cartilage (the major supporting structure of the larynx and the only complete ring in the upper airway), it can be difficult to maintain a patent airway after complete excision of a chondroma. In such cases, one may even consider subtotal removal, with the understanding that repeated procedures and eventual total laryngectomy are likely to be necessary. Tracheotomy alone may be a suitable means of preservation of airway while maintaining a functional voice as long as possible.

Although *malignant transformation* of chondroma can occur, it is often difficult to distinguish benign lesions from chondrosarcomas on histologic grounds. Since conservative management of lesions that eventually prove to be malignant gives essentially the same survival as initial radical excision, only those lesions that are histologically high-grade malignancies should be subjected to total laryngectomy.[27]

Pleomorphic Adenomas

These so-called benign mixed tumors are most frequent in the salivary glands, particularly the parotid. In the larynx, where they are uncommon, they tend to occur subglottically and produce obstructive symptoms as one would expect from a lesion in this area. Because of the location and propensitiy for local recurrence, this lesion may require fairly extensive surgery (even including total laryngectomy) for complete removal.[28]

Fibrous Histiocytoma

See Chapter 3.

Also called fibroxanthoma, the term ''fibrous histiocytoma'' really denotes a group of fibroproliferative disorders, some of which are neoplastic and others probably reactive.◁ *Nodular fasciitis,* which has been reported only once in the larynx,[1] is a benign proliferative disorder that can easily be mistaken for a sarcoma. Growth is rapid and often prodigious, but endoscopic excision is usually adequate. *Fibromatosis* comprises a group of benign proliferative tumors that can sometimes behave in an aggressive manner. They tend to occur in infants and small children and may be part of systemic disease, in which case the condition is frequently fatal.[29] *Fibrous histiocytoma* has been recorded 12 times in the Armed Forces Institute of Pathology Tumor Registry. These have been largely pedunculated, yellow-orange masses, most of which have appeared in males between 30 and 60 years of age. Local wide excision has been adequate, although some do recur.

Rhabdomyoma

This is a benign neoplasm arising from striated muscle. Nine have been recorded in the larynx.[30] Only the adult type occurs in this location, where they tend to be solitary and lobulated. The most frequent site is the vocal fold itself. Local surgical excision is appropriate, although it can be quite difficult because of lobular extension into adjacent sites.[1]

References

1. Jones SR, Myers EN, Barnes L: Benign neoplasms of the larynx. Otolaryngol Clin North Am, 17:151–178, 1984
2. New GB, Erich JB: Benign tumors of the larynx: A study of 722 cases. Arch Otolaryngol, 28:841–910, 1938
3. Holinger P, Johnston K: Benign tumors of the larynx. Ann Otol Rhinol Laryngol, 60:496–509, 1951
4. Alberti PW, Dykun R: Adult laryngeal papillomata. J Otolaryngol, 10:463–470, 1981
5. Resler DR, Snow JB: Cell-free filtrate transplantation of human laryngeal papillomata to dogs. Laryngoscope, 77:397, 1967
6. Quick CA, Watts SL, Krzysek RA, Faras AJ: Relationship between condylomata and laryngeal papillomata. Ann Otol Rhinol Laryngol, 89:467, 1980
7. Tucker HM: Diversionary (double-barrelled) tracheotomy in the management of juvenile laryngeal papillomatosis. Ann Otol Rhinol Laryngol, 89:504–507, 1980
8. Kleinsasser O, Cruz EO: Juvenile and adult papillomas of the larynx. HNO, 21:97–106, 1973
9. Tucker HM: Surgery for Phonatory Disorders. New York, Churchill Livingstone, 1981, pp 42–43
10. Strong MS, Vaughan CW, Cooperband SR, Healy GB, Clemente MA: Recurrent respiratory papillomatosis—management with the CO2 laser. Ann Otol Rhinol Laryngol, 85:508–516, 1976
11. Hagland S, et al: Interferon therapy in juvenile laryngeal papillomatosis. Arch Otol, 107:327, 1981
12. McCabe BF, Clark KF: Interferon and laryngeal papillomatosis: The Iowa experience. Ann Otol Rhinol Laryngol, 92:2–7, 1983
13. Olveira CA, Roth JA, Adams GL: Oncocytic

lesions of the larynx. Laryngoscope, 87:1718–1725, 1977

14. Holms-Jensen S, Jacobsen M, Tommesen N, Ferreira O: Oncocytic cysts of the larynx. Arch Otolaryngol, 83:366–371, 1977

15. Gallagher JC, Puzon BQ: Oncocytic lesions of the larynx. Ann Otol Rhinol Laryngol, 78:307–318, 1969

16. Agarwal RK, Blitzer A, Perzin KH: Granular cell tumors of the larynx. Otolaryngol Head Neck Surg, 87:807–814, 1979

17. Thomas RL: Non-epithelial tumors of the larynx. J Laryngol Otol, 93:1131–1141, 1979

18. Healy GB, Fearon B, French R, McGill T: Treatment of subglottic hemangioma with the carbon dioxide laser. Laryngoscope, 90:809–813, 1980

19. El-Serafy S: Rare benign tumors of the larynx. J Laryngol Otol, 85:837–851, 1971

20. Hordyk GJ, Reuter DJ, Bosman FT, Mauw BJ: Chemodectoma (paraganglioma) of the larynx. Clin Otolaryngol, 6:249–254, 1981

21. Schaefer SD, Blend BL, Denton JG: Laryngeal paragangliomas: Evaluation and treatment. Am J Otolaryngol, 1:451–455, 1980.

22. Wetmore RF, Tronzo RD, Lane RJ, Lowry LD: Nonfunctional paraganglioma of the lar-

ynx: Clinical and pathological considerations. Cancer, 48:2717–2723, 1981

23. Supance JS, Quenelle DJ, Crissman J: Endolaryngeal neurofibromas. Otolaryngol Head Neck Surg, 88:74–78, 1980

24. Manson I, Wilske J, Kindblom LG: Lipoma of the hypopharynx. A case report and a review of the literature. J Laryngol Otol, 92:1037–1043, 1978

25. Hyams VJ, Rabuzzi DD: Cartilaginous tumors of the larynx. Laryngoscope, 80:755–767, 1970

26. Damiani KK, Tucker HM: Chondroma of the larynx. Arch Otolaryngol, 107:399–402, 1981

27. Lavertu P, Tucker HM: Chondrosarcoma of the larynx: Case report and management philosophy. Ann Otol Rhinol Laryngol, 93:452–456, 1984

28. Som PM, Nagel BD, Feuerstein SS, Strauss L: Benign pleomorophic adenoma of the larynx. Ann Otol Rhinol Laryngol, 88:112–114, 1979

29. Rosenberg HS, Vogler C, Close LG, Warshaw HE: Laryngeal fibromatosis in the neonate. Arch Otolaryngol, 107:513–517, 1981

30. Modlin B: Rhabdomyoma of the larynx. Laryngoscope, 92:580–582, 1982

Chapter 13

Malignant Tumors

Although sarcomas, adenocarcinomas, and metastatic neoplasms occur in the larynx, more than 90 percent of all laryngeal malignancies are squamous cell carcinoma. The surgeon who seeks to care for patients so afflicted must have a thorough understanding of the pertinent anatomy, pathology, epidemiology, radiobiology, and surgical concepts that permit the improved cure rates and rehabilitation that are now possible.

Historical Background and Development

From the time of its mention by the early Greek physicians (Aretaeus, ca AD 100, Galen ca AD 200) until the middle of the 19th century, little understanding and no progress were gained in the diagnosis and management of laryngeal carcinoma.[1,2] To begin with, until the development of *mirror laryngoscopy* by Garcia in 1854, it was essentially impossible to observe the larynx. Moreover, the *histopathology* of laryngeal disease was poorly understood until Virchow published his landmark treatise on the subject in 1858. Largely as a result of these critical developments, interest in laryngeal cancer burgeoned. By 1879, Krishaber had recognized the differences in the behavior of the slower growing and late metastasizing "intrinsic" (glottic) carcinoma, as opposed to the more rapid growth and aggressive course of "extrinsic" (supraglottic and hypopharyngeal) tumors.

Efforts to manage laryngeal carcinoma with *surgery* can be dated to the attempt at *laryngofissure* carried out in 1851 by Gurdon Buck in the United States, although he did not realize initially that the lesion was malignant, and the patient had a prompt recurrence. Jacob DaSilva Solis-Cohen was the first to record a long-term cure of documented laryngeal carcinoma by this approach in 1867. Although the initial results of laryngofissure were poor both in terms of cure rates and surgical mortality, improvements in anesthesia, postoperative care, and patient selection eventually led to satisfactory survivals by the first two decades of the 20th century.

Vertical partial laryngectomy was first performed by Billroth in 1878, but was popularized by his assistant Gluck. In 1903, Semon redefined the procedure and its indications. Since that time, it has been refined by many investigators until it has become one of the mainstays in the management of glottic carcinoma.

The tragic story of Crown Prince Frederick of Germany and the management of his laryngeal carcinoma by Morell Mackenzie, the leading laryngologist of his time, is well told by Stevenson.[3] Morell Mackenzie insisted upon biopsy confirmation of the suspected cancer and would not concur with the decision to perform surgery without it. Virchow examined several specimens and was unable to confirm the diagnosis. Although much controversy still exists about this case, it is probably true that the outcome would have been even worse had the dangerous and poorly supported surgery available at the time (1887–1888) been carried out. The Crown Prince, later briefly Kaiser Frederick III, eventually succumbed to what was probably both syphilis and carcinoma of the larynx. Because Frederick was a liberal and his successor Kaiser Wilhelm II led Germany into World War I, Morell Mackenzie has at times been accused of indirectly precipitating that war by his failure to advise surgery. The outcome would almost certainly have been the same had an operation been attempted and might well have set surgical development back for many years.—HMT

See Chapter 5.

Although *pharyngotomy* for resection of supraglottic cancer was developed by Von Langenbeck and others in the latter part of the 19th century, the procedure was not of much clinical value until Trotter described a lateral pharyngotomy approach to *partial laryngopharyngectomy* in 1913. After World War II, Alonso revitalized and extended both the technique and indications for *supraglottic laryngectomy*. More recently, Ogura et al, Som, and many others have further extended and refined this approach until there are relatively few cases of supraglottic cancer that cannot be considered for *conservation* or *voice-sparing procedures* with cure rates that approximate those for total laryngectomy.

Total laryngectomy was first performed in the human by Billroth in 1873. The procedure was done in stages and a large laryngotracheal defect was created. A special valved tracheotomy and speaking tube was devised by Gussenbauer, Billroth's assistant, and the patient survived for 7 months before dying of recurrent tumor. Bottini carried out the first fully successful total laryngectomy in 1875 for a sarcoma. The patient survived for 10 years. Solis-Cohen was the first to divert the tracheal remnant to the skin as a permanent and separate tracheostoma in 1892, and Sorenson devised a one-stage pharyngeal closure. With these two innovations, both before 1900, the operation had reached its current state of development, for all intents and purposes.

Radiation therapy as a means of treatment of laryngeal carcinoma had become effective by 1922, when Coutard recommended fractionated treatment as an alternative to total laryngectomy in an effort to preserve the voice. In the 1950s, cobalt-60 improved radiotherapy as an alternative to surgery and led to the attitude that carcinoma of the larynx could be treated with *radiation for cure* and *surgery* be reserved *for salvage* of failures with as good results as surgery alone or combined radiotherapy-surgery, but with preservation of many more larynges.[4] On the other hand, *planned combined radiation and* definitive *surgery* for management of advanced carcinomas of the larynx has also gained widespread support.[5] The issue of whether radiation is more effective given preoperatively, postoperatively, or as the sole means of treatment still remains unresolved.

Rehabilitation of voice after total laryngectomy has revolved around pharyngeal speech and artificial larynges until recent years. Conley suggested a mucosally lined *tracheoesophageal shunt* as a means of voice restoration in 1959.[6] Further development of this concept, both as a direct shunt[7,8] and via intervening *valved prostheses*,[9,10] never received widespread support because of unsatisfactory long-term results and other late complications. Construction of a *neoglottis* was recommended by Arslan and Serafini[11] and Staffieri and Serafini.[12] This approach was well received but has been largely supplanted because of the ease of performance and good results that have been achieved with the "duck-bill" prosthesis technique popularized by Singer and Blom.[13]

Transplantation of the larynx has been an attractive concept ever since successful replacement of other organs has become a reality. Laryngeal *reimplantation* has been performed successfully in dogs,[14,15] and it has also been possible to restore glottic function to these organs.[16] The single reported attempt at transplantation (actually a nonvascularized cadaver graft) in a human resulted in miliary spread of cancer, probably secondary to immunosuppressive drugs.[17] In light of our ability to preserve voice in most cases of laryngeal cancer and to restore it in many others, it seems unlikely that the larynx will be routinely transplanted in the forseeable future, unless some safe means can be found to render either the transplant or the host immunologically neutral.[18]

Epidemiology

Carcinoma of the larynx is the fifth or sixth most prevalent malignancy (2.3 percent of all cancers in males and 0.4 percent in females) in the adult, with an approximate *incidence* of 5.6 new cases per 100,000 population per year in the United States.[19] Estimates are that there were approximately 11,800 new cases of laryngeal cancer in the United States in 1985. The actual incidence varies greatly from one country to another, with the highest reported from India (more than 50 new cases per 100,000 population each year).

The disease is *five times more common in males* than in females, but this ratio has dropped from 10:1 only 10 years ago with the increase in number of females who smoke.[19,20] Peak *age incidence* is *between 40 and 70 years,* with the majority of cases occurring in the sixth and seventh decades. Only a small percentage of laryngeal cancers occur before the age of 20 years.[21] *Mortality* from laryngeal cancer has remained stable (despite hoped-for improvements in survival because of better diagnosis and treatment) at about 2.4 per 100,000 person-years from 1950 through 1977.[19]

Etiologic factors that have been incriminated in carcinogenesis in the larynx include cigarette smoking, alcohol abuse, radiation exposure, asbestos, and genetic factors.

1.   Cigarette smoking. Exposure to tobacco smoke is the epidemiologic factor most strongly implicated in the development of cancer of the larynx.[22–24] Carcinoma has been induced experimentally in susceptible laboratory animals exposed to cigarette smoke and dose-related studies have demonstrated that degree of exposure is also important.[25] In a large group of heavy smokers, 70 percent developed keratotic changes of the larynx and 20 percent of those at risk eventually developed cancer, whereas only 0.3 percent of the control group did so.[26] There is also evidence that the mucosal changes induced by smoking are reversible if the patient will stop using tobacco before actual malignancy has occurred.[27]◁

2.   Alcohol. Heavy alcohol intake seems to potentiate the development of laryngeal cancer, especially when it is abused in conjunction with heavy smoking (25 percent higher death rate for those who also drank heavily).[29,30] Since it is unusual to encounter an alcoholic who is not also a heavy smoker, studies to show the effects on the development of laryngeal cancer of alcohol intake alone are difficult to do.

3.   Radiation. Radiation to the head and neck in young individuals has been implicated in later development of carcinoma of the larynx.[31,32] A second primary cancer was noted to develop twice as often in patients who had received radiotherapy as part of the management of a previous primary lesion when compared with those who had only surgery.[33] These statistical findings may have importance in considering alternate modalities for management of laryngeal carcinoma, especially in younger individuals.

4.   Asbestos. Exposure to asbestos seems to result in an increase in incidence of carcinoma of the larynx over the normal population.[34] The risk may be limited to those who are also smokers, however.[35]

5.   Genetic factors. It is clear that some factor other than exposure to known carcinogens must be involved in the development of cancer of the larynx, since only about 20 to 30 percent of those exposed eventually develop a malignancy. Whether these factors include some impairment of the immune mechanism (systemically or locally) or simply familial predisposition is not well understood. A positive family history for malignancy has been found in approximately half of patients with laryngeal carcinoma,[22] but only a small percentage of these were of the larynx.

Pathologic Considerations

Premalignant Lesions

The normal squamous epithelium of the larynx can undergo a continuum of changes when subjected to trauma or other noxious stimuli. Some of these changes are nonspecific and are not necessarily related to eventual development of carcinoma, whereas others are clearly precursors to ultimate malignant change. These include: leukoplakia, hyperplasia, keratosis without atypia, keratosis with atypia, carcinoma in situ, and microinvasive carcinoma.

1.   Leukoplakia. Properly used, this term is not a pathologic diagnosis. Rather, it is a *descriptive clinical term* denoting any white plaque (a direct translation from the Greek). Leukoplakia of the larynx can signify any of the other pathologic conditions that follow, but it may also represent relatively innocuous circumstances, such as adherent secretions or fungus infection, as well.

2.   Hyperplasia. This thickening of the mucosa with otherwise normal cellular proliferation is a common response to chronic irritation. It is an absolute increase in the number of cells with no real change in character or maturation.

3.   Keratosis without atypia. The mucosa normally found on the surface of the vocal folds is nonkeratinizing stratified squamous epithelium, and on the rest of the larynx, it is pseudostratified, ciliated, columnar epithelium with goblet cells (respiratory epithelium). In response to trauma or chronic irritation, *metaplasia* to keratinizing epithelium can take place.◁ If the process is orderly and proceeds from the basal layers out to the surface without abnormality, the *keratosis* is *without atypia*. Clinically, this change has the appearance of *leukoplakia*, which, if it involves large areas of the larynx and is exuberant, is referred to as *pachydermia laryngis*. This condition is reversible in most cases,[28] especially if the irritant can be avoided, and is *not premalignant*.

4.   Keratosis with atypia. When metaplasia to keratinizing epithelium is associated with *dysplastic changes*, particularly in the basilar layers, the condition is referred to as keratosis with atypia. The clinical appearance is commonly *leukoplakic*, but may also exhibit *erythroplakia* (reddish patches of raised epithelium), which is more often suggestive of severe atypia or even early malignancy. This pathologic finding is considered *premalignant*,[36,37] since reports indicate that between 15 and 55 percent of cases of keratosis with atypia will eventually result in frank invasive squamous cell carcinoma.[38,39]

5.   Carcinoma in situ. This *malignant* condition is also referred to as *intraepithelial carcinoma*. There is replacement of the entire thickness of the epithelium with dysplastic and malignant cells, but *without invasion* of the *basement membrane*. Although it is beyond premalignancy and one would expect all such cases to progress to invasive carcinoma if untreated, there are suggestions that even this condition may still be reversible if the irritant or irritants are avoided.[40]◁

6.   Microinvasive carcinoma. This lesion is identical to *carcinoma in situ*, except for the finding of discrete and *limited* areas of *invasion through* the *basement membrane*. Not all pathologists are willing to distinguish this finding from invasive carcinoma, although there is good evidence that appropriate treatment can be much the same as for carcinoma in situ.[43,44] It is not unlikely that many cases of apparent carcinoma in situ would be found

The common but incorrect term "hyperkeratosis" is frequently used for this condition. Since no keratin should be present in vocal fold mucosa under normal, healthy conditions, its very presence (keratosis) is pathologic and there is nothing "hyper" about the keratinization that ensues.—HMT

"Batsakis[41] feels that although progression from keratosis to carcinoma is by no means obligatory, the risk is small yet significant. Keratosis without atypia is benign in its behavior, with little tendency to progress further to atypia or to carcinoma. [It] has [been] noted . . . that progression from keratosis without atypia to carcinoma in situ and finally infiltrating carcinoma is rarely seen.[42] The pathway most likely to be followed is from normal epithelium to keratosis with atypia to invasive carcinoma."—CE Silver[2]

to be microinvasive if a more thorough stripping and examination of the specimen were carried out.

Invasive Squamous Cell Carcinoma

Once the basement membrane or underlying musculature is clearly invaded with malignant cells, the diagnosis of invasive or infiltrating squamous cell carcinoma can be made. The patterns of spread, likelihood of nodal metastasis, appropriate treatment, and prognosis are all related to location within the larynx.

1. Pertinent laryngeal anatomy.◁ The larynx can be divided into several regions in relation to the glottis (Fig. 13–1). The *supraglottic region* includes the laryngeal surface of the epiglottis, aryepiglottic folds, laryngeal surfaces of the arytenoid cartilages, false cords, and roof of the ventricles. The *glottic region* is made up of both vocal folds, the vocal processes of the arytenoids, and the anterior and posterior commissures. The *subglottic region* begins approximately 2 to 4 mm below the free margin of the vocal fold at the anterior commissure and increases to about 5 to 7 mm at the point below the tip of the vocal process.◁ It extends inferiorly to the lower border of the cricoid cartilage. The *marginal region* (superior hypopharynx) includes the lingual surface of the epiglottis, the valleculae, and the posterior third of the tongue up to the line of circumvallate papillae. The *pyriform fossae* (inferior hypopharynx) are made up of the lateral surfaces of the arytenoid cartilages and the aryepiglottic folds medially, the pharyngeal wall laterally, and are open to the hypopharynx posteriorly. The apices (inferiormost point) are below the level of the vocal folds. These last two regions are actually outside of the larynx proper, but are always considered when discussing laryngeal cancer because they are really subject to the same disease processes.

Laryngeal compartments have been defined by Pressman[45] and the various membranes and ligaments that determine them were described by

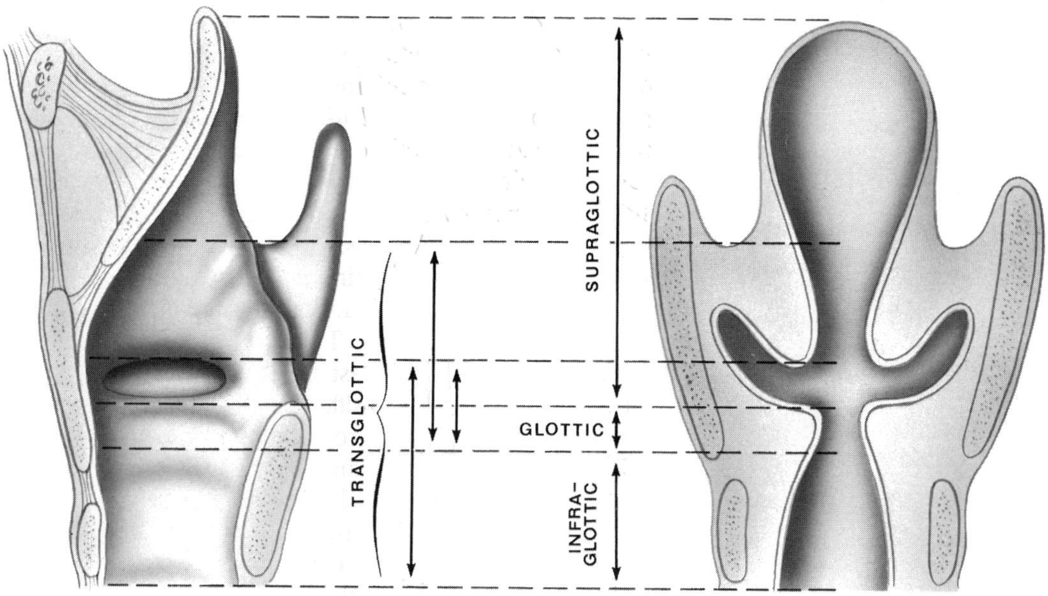

See also Chapter 1.

This dividing line between the glottis and the subglottic region is not agreed on by all investigators, most of whom do not define it clearly. The majority simply say that the subglottis begins approximately 1 cm below the free margins of the vocal folds.—HMT

Figure 13–1. Regions of the larynx. Although many of these designations are arbitrary and not consistent from one author to the other, they are used extensively in the literature and can be helpful in discussion of malignant disease.

Tucker and Smith.[46] These compartments tend to *contain* laryngeal malignancy for some time and to determine the *pattern of spread*. When extension does occur, it is usually along predictable lines of least resistance, as defined by these connective tissue structures. As a result, *glottic cancer* tends not to cross the midline (although once the anterior commissure is involved, it not only can spread to the opposite cord, but also may escape from the larynx via Broyles' ligament), the ventricle, or to spread into the subglottic region. *Supraglottic tumors* usually remain localized to the laryngeal surface of the epiglottis (although they often extend through the perforations in that cartilage into the *preepiglottic space*),◁ or to either false cord. *Subglottic carcinoma* tends to spread inferiorly either into the upper trachea when it is confined to the mucosa or to escape from the larynx via the cricothyroid membrane, if it is deep to the conus elasticus (paraglottic space). *Transglottic lesions* are those that extend across at least one of the dividing lines to *involve two or more regions*. There is frequent cartilage invasion and spread into the paraglottic space, so that transglottic carcinoma generally carries a poor prognosis. Carcinoma in any of these regions can become *deeply invasive* and produce *fixation of* the *arytenoid* or direct involvement of the thyroid or cricoid cartilages.

2. Involvement of cervical lymph nodes. Most studies agree that *regional node involvement* is the *most critical prognostic factor* in cancer of the larynx.[47–50] Uncontrolled nodal involvement is the single most common cause for failure of primary treatment, especially in supraglottic disease.

Primary site is a major determining factor in cervical node metastasis.[47] The *lowest* incidence is seen with *glottic* involvement, probably because of the relatively poor lymphatic supply to the true vocal folds and to early detection of carcinoma because of voice change. Indeed, nodal involvement in what appears to be uncomplicated glottic cancer should raise suspicion of extension of tumor outside the larynx.◁ *Transglottic* lesions have the *highest* incidence of nodal metastasis (about 55 percent), with *supraglottic* (30 to 40 percent) and *subglottic* (20 to 25 percent) *less* commonly involved in descending order. Well-differentiated lesions are less likely to metastasize than are poorly differentiated ones.

The *jugular chain* of lymph nodes is *most commonly* involved. The *posterior triangle* is an *infrequent* site for metastases from the larynx.[47] Spinal accessory nodes, although they can occasionally be involved with massive disease, drain toward the larynx, thus permitting salvage of the spinal accessory nerve branch to the trapezius muscle in most cases. *Contralateral* involvement, whether synchronous or occurring after primary treatment, is a *grave prognostic finding*. Supraglottic and transglottic lesions with positive ipsilateral nodes will eventually be found to involve the other side in almost 50 percent of cases.[47]

3. Staging. Staging of laryngeal cancer is undertaken in an effort to provide similar criteria for selection of best treatment and to permit comparison of results. As such, it is a *clinical* system that must be applied *before surgical intervention* (other than biopsy) or other modalities and that should not be changed later in light of postsurgical pathologic findings. The American Joint Committee for Cancer Staging and End Results Reporting revised its criteria in 1977.[51] These are outlined in Tables 13–1[50,51] through 13–4.[51]

Verrucous Carcinoma

This uncommon variant (1 or 2 percent) of laryngeal squamous cell carcinoma has presented a dilemma to pathologists and head and neck surgeons alike: to the former because of the very high differentiation of this

See also Chapter 1.

Glottic carcinoma can escape the larynx by direct extension along Broyles' ligament if the anterior commissure is involved. Once this has happened, spread to the Delphian node and, thereafter, metastasis to either midjugular chain of lymph nodes can occur.
—HMT

Table 13–1   T Classifications for Carcinoma of the Larynx

Supraglottis

TIS	Carcinoma in situ
T1	Tumor confined to region of origin with normal mobility
T2	Tumor involves adjacent supraglottic site(s) or glottis without fixation
T3	Tumor limited to larynx with fixation and/or extension to involve postcricoid area, medial wall of pyriform sinus, or preepiglottic space
T4	Massive tumor extending beyond the larynx to involve oropharynx, soft tissues of neck, or destruction of thyroid cartilage

Glottis

TIS	Carcinoma in situ
T1	Tumor confined to vocal cord(s) with normal mobility (includes involvement of anterior or posterior commissure)
T2	Supraglottic and/or subglottic extension of tumor with normal or impaired vocal cord mobility
T3	Tumor confined to the larynx with vocal cord fixation
T4	Massive tumor with thyroid cartilage destruction and/or extension beyond the confines of the larynx

Subglottis

TIS	Carcinoma in situ
T1	Tumor confined to the subglottic region
T2	Tumor extension to vocal cords with normal or impaired mobility
T3	Tumor confined to larynx with vocal cord fixation
T4	Massive tumor with cartilage destruction or extension beyond the confines of the larynx or both

Marginal

TIS	Carcinoma in situ
T1	Limited to aryepiglottic fold; normal mobility
T2	Limited to aryepiglottic fold *and* one of the following: ventricular bands, medial wall of pyriform sinus, epiglottis; normal mobility
T3	Aryepiglottic fold with vocal fold fixation *or* two of the following: medial or anterior walls of pyriform sinus *not* involving apex, ventricular bands
T4	Aryepiglottic fold *and* three walls of pyriform sinus or apex or extends beyond larynx

Pyriform Sinus

TIS	Carcinoma in situ
T1	One site only (i.e., medial or lateral wall)
T2	Two sites (i.e., two walls or one wall and aryepiglottic fold)
T3	Three sites involved
T4	Tumor extends beyond hypopharynx (i.e., postcricoid or base of tongue)

Table 13–2   Cervical Lymph Node Classification

N0	No clinically positive nodes
N1	Single clinically positive homolateral node less than 3 cm in diameter
N2a	Single clinically positive homolateral node, 3 to 6 cm in diameter
N2b	Multiple clinically positive homolateral nodes, none over 6 cm in diameter
N3	Massive homolateral node(s), bilateral nodes, or contralateral node(s)
N3a	Clinically positive homolateral node(s), none over 6 cm in diameter
N3b	Bilaterally clinically positive nodes (stage each side separately)
N3c	Contralateral clinically positive node(s) only

Table 13–3   Distant Metastases

M0	No (known) distant metastases
M1	Distant metastasis present

Table 13–4   Stage Grouping

Stage I	T1N0M0
Stage II	T2N0M0
Stage III	T3N0M0, T1-3N1M0
Stage IV	T4NanyM0, TanyN2-3M0, TanyNanyM1

tumor, which can make a firm diagnosis of malignancy quite difficult, and to the latter because of controversy about its proper treatment. Clinically, verrucous carcinoma appears as a warty, papillomatous lesion, which is often bulky but well circumscribed. Metastasis is rare,[52] but growth is inexorable if untreated and the tumor can result in the patient's death. Demographics are similar to other types of squamous cell carcinoma.

Pathologic *diagnosis* can be very *difficult,* especially if the biopsy material provided to the pathologist does not show an area of junction between tumor and normal tissue. Because of the bulkiness of these lesions, frozen section monitoring of repeated biopsies is often necessary in order to obtain tissue that will permit a firm diagnosis. ◁

Once the diagnosis has been made, most otolaryngologists agree that adequate *surgical excision* (usually subtotal laryngectomy) is the proper approach to management.[53] There is *controversy* about whether or not these lesions can be safely treated with *radiotherapy*. To begin with, verrucous carcinoma appears to have limited radiosensitivity,[54,55] which can be expected in well-differentiated tumors; perhaps more important, there is some evidence that lesions treated with primary radiotherapy can undergo conversion to anaplastic carcinoma.[55,56] Since properly performed surgery has a very high cure rate, most practitioners still avoid radiotherapy for this type of laryngeal cancer.

On one or two occasions, I have even found it necessary to proceed with definitive excision of what was strongly suspected to be a verrucous carcinoma, but which had defied firm histologic diagnosis despite repeated biopsies of multiple recurrences. The pathologist observed the lesion in situ at laryngoscopy and concurred in the presumptive diagnosis and proposed excision, pending his ability to section the entire lesion. Needless to say, the patients were fully aware of the unusual circumstances and agreed to the surgery.—HMT

Pseudosarcoma

This rare variant of carcinoma of the larynx is best thought of as a "collision tumor," representing the interface between malignant connective tissue and epithelial elements.[57] Although it was originally thought to have a fairly benign prognosis, Hyams[58] reported mortality of 40 percent at 2 years, despite aggressive treatment. Radiation alone is clearly inadequate for these tumors, which may require radical surgery for best management.

Adenocarcinoma

These are rare neoplasms of the larynx, which occur primarily in the subglottic and supraglottic regions because of the presence in these areas of the minor salivary gland elements from which they are derived. *Adenoid cystic carcinoma* behaves much as it does in major salivary glands: *locally aggressive,* late or nonmetastasizing, and relatively unresponsive to radiotherapy. Therefore, these lesions are best *managed by partial* or total *laryngectomy,* with neck dissection reserved for clinically evident disease.[59] Distant metastases are not necessarily a contraindication to laryngeal surgery, since these patients often survive for years with metastases if local disease can be controlled. *Nonspecific adenocarcinomas,* on the other hand, are *highly malignant* with virtually no survivors at 2 years.[60]

Chondrosarcoma

This *uncommon* malignancy of the laryngeal cartilages most often arises in the posterior lamina of the *cricoid* cartilage, but can occur in any of the other skeletal elements of the larynx or even in soft tissue structures, such as the vocal fold.[61] *Computed tomography (CT) scanning* will delineate the extent of the tumor and allegedly suggest a malignant chondroma if speckled *calcification* is present within the mass. Obtaining a successful *biopsy* of this hard, mucosal-covered lesion at laryngoscopy requires that a second, *deeper piece* be obtained through the same mucosal defect created by the first cup forceps removal. It is frequently difficult to *distinguish chondrosarcomas from* benign *chondromas* on histologic grounds alone. Moreover, chondrosarcomas are generally slow growing and do not metastasize and therefore can be managed initially by the same *conservative surgical approach* as would be appropriate for chondromas.◁ Subtotal laryngeal conservation surgery or even ''shelling out'' procedures are usually adequate. Total laryngectomy should be reserved for recurrent lesions that do not permit less radical surgery.[62]

See Chapter 12.

Diagnosis and Evaluation

When presented with a patient suspected of a laryngeal malignancy, an orderly approach to diagnosis and evaluation is essential if the best choice of available treatment options is to be made. The necessary elements of proper evaluation include: (1) history; (2) physical examination; (3) radiologic evaluation; (4) medical and laboratory evaluation; (5) oral panendoscopy and biopsy, and (6) staging.

1. History. Such factors as time of onset of symptoms, smoking and other carcinogen exposure, family history, and previous radiation treatment or surgery may be important not only in determining best treatment, but also for future demographic and epidemiologic studies that may lead to preventive measures. *Symptoms* such as *voice change* and the presence of a *neck mass* (particularly with supraglottic lesions) are common presenting complaints. However, unexplained *weight loss, dysphagia, halitosis,* and *earache* (often a presenting symptom in lesions of the pyriform sinus and base of tongue) may also be important.

2. Physical examination. Besides a thorough otolaryngologic examination, the patient should have a complete general physical evaluation, as well. Indeed, it may be advisable for this to be carried out by an appropriate internist who can appreciate and treat other physical deficits that may have an impact on the patient's future management. The head and neck surgeon should consider the use of flexible fiberoptic endoscopy if there is any question about the adequacy of indirect mirror examination.

3. Radiologic assessment. This is fully discussed in Chapter 4.

4. Other appropriate evaluation. Suitable laboratory studies to permit *assessment* of the patient's general health and state of *nutrition* should be carried out. Hooley and associates[63] showed that nutritional status not only could be evaluated, but that preoperative intervention could have a significant impact on postoperative healing.

Some effort should also be made to *assess* the patient and family from a *psychologic* standpoint, inasmuch as all concerned will undoubtedly face serious emotional stress during and after treatment.◁

5. Oral panendoscopy and biopsy. When all other matters regarding assessment of patients suspected of carcinoma of the larynx have been at-

The importance of establishing both frankness and rapport among the patient, his family, and the surgeon who will manage the case cannot be stressed too strongly. Not only is it imperative to provide all of the parties with a realistic understanding of the prognosis and treatment options available for medicolegal reasons, but my colleagues and I have repeatedly observed that patients who manage a confident attitude toward the medical necessities as well as good familial support generally do better than those who do not.—HMT

tended to, careful oral panendoscopy (laryngoscopy, esophagoscopy, bronchoscopy) should be carried out. This evaluation, which will usually be performed under general anesthesia, is intended to: (1) rule out concurrent malignancy elsewhere in the upper aerodigestive trace;◁ (2) confirm the histologic diagnosis of cancer of the larynx; and (3) permit careful mapping and delineation of the precise extent of the primary lesion.

Biopsy should be generous and should straddle a margin of tumor and apparent normal tissue, if possible, since this may be of great assistance to the pathologist in determining tumor type and invasiveness. It is also advisable to ask for a *frozen section,* not so much to make the diagnosis, but to be certain that adequate tissue has been obtained to permit diagnosis. When appropriate, carefully mapped biopsies can be taken from what appear to be clear areas in order to determine the actual extent of the lesion better. This may be critical in later deciding on the advisability of conservation versus radical surgery. If the tumor is very bulky or if *airway is compromised, subtotal laser excision* can be carried out at this time, perhaps avoiding the need for tracheotomy in some cases.

6.   Staging. Once all other evaluative procedures have been carried out, the lesion can be staged (Table 13–1 to 13–4). It is imperative, however, that *tumor maps, photographs* (where possible), and a *detailed narrative description* of the extent of the lesion *as it was* when first seen be included in the record. These are important not only to remind the surgeon of the original tumor size and extension after other treatment may have changed them, but to permit restaging by others, if necessary.◁

Treatment

Premalignant Lesions, Carcinoma-in-situ, and Microinvasive Carcinoma

Keratosis with atypia, carcinoma in situ, and very early malignancies of the glottis can be considered as a continuum of disease that will lead ultimately to invasive squamous cell carcinoma if not arrested or reversed. The *aims of treatment* of these lesions are: (1) to determine the current stage of disease; (2) to eradicate that disease; (3) to prevent recurrence; and (4) to detect persistence, recurrence, or progression to a more highly malignant stage as early as possible. The modalities available to achieve these ends include: (1) microlaryngoscopic stripping, (2) laser surgery, (3) radiotherapy, (4) removal of irritants.

1.   *Microlaryngoscopy and stripping* is the mainstay of treatment by most surgeons[28,43]. Supravital *staining* with *toluidine blue* can be helpful in identifying suspicious areas that might otherwise go unnoticed.[65] Meticulous attention to removal of all of the mucosa allows identification of areas of greater progression toward malignancy and helps to minimize recurrence. If pathologic examination demonstrates *keratosis without atypia,* only *careful follow-up* is needed. If *keratosis with atypia, carcinoma in situ,* or *microinvasive carcinoma* are found, it is advisable to *restrip* the same areas in 8 to 12 weeks, regardless of whether there is apparent recurrence or not. If the repeat stripping demonstrates normal tissue or keratosis without atypia, only careful follow-up is needed. On the other hand, stripping should be repeated at least once more after any finding of keratosis with atypia or greater progression toward malignancy. Stutsman and McGavran[66] reported long-term cure without the need for radiotherapy or invasive surgery and with no mortality in virtually all of a group of patients who had microinvasive carcinoma managed in this way.

2. *Laser surgery* is a valuable addition to our armamentarium in the management of premalignant and early malignant disease of the larynx. After meticulous stripping has been carried out, the *laser* can be used to assure *complete removal* of all mucosa through Reinke's space without damage to underlying muscle. Strong[65] has advocated use of the laser not only for premalignant lesions, but also for early, superficially invasive carcinomas, providing that excellent exposure can be obtained.

3. *Radiation* has been proposed as a primary treatment modality for *premalignant lesions,* carcinoma in situ, and early invasive carcinomas[4] on the grounds that there is great variability in the diagnosis of these lesions from one pathologist to another, which may lead to underdiagnosis in some cases, and that it is difficult to be sure that a more invasive lesion has not been missed by the biopsy of extensive disease. *Results* of this approach have been *approximately* the *same* as for similar T classifications in invasive disease. DeSanto[67] compared radiation, transoral procedures and open surgical approaches to the management of these lesions. He found comparable cure rates, but *radiation* was the *most expensive, time consuming,* and resulted in the greatest ultimate *loss of larynges* (due to salvage of failures). Since radiotherapy remains the treatment of choice for early invasive carcinomas of the larynx, it seems reasonable to reserve it for these more advanced cases and to continue to approach premalignant lesions with endoscopic methods, especially since results are generally good.

4. *Removal of carcinogens* and other conservative measures cannot be stressed too strongly. *Smoking and alcohol abuse must be stopped* if there is to be any hope of long-term control and prevention of recurrence.[40] It is important to realize that the mucosa of the entire upper aerodigestive tract has become "distressed" by the combination of exposure to carcinogens and whatever genetic or acquired depression of immune competence may be operational in an individual who has developed a premalignant lesion. Such a patient is not only subject to recurrence of a previous lesion if smoking and drinking continue, but is also at risk for development of separate new lesions elsewhere.

Invasive Squamous Cell Carcinoma

There is an understandable tendency, particularly on the part of physicians in training, to want to learn "how to" perform surgical procedures; however, the really difficult part of learning to manage patients with cancer properly is "when to" and "when not to". Because so many parameters must be considered, I have found it very helpful to decide first on the best modality for the lesion alone, as if it existed in an otherwise ideal patient. Thereafter, each of the other factors can be considered and the final treatment plan modified as needed. With this approach, important aspects of planning are not likely to be overlooked and the best available treatment can be selected.—HMT

In general, invasive carcinoma of the larynx can be *treated* in three ways: *radiation* alone, *surgery* alone, and *planned combined radiation* (and/or chemotherapy) *and surgery. Chemotheray* has not yet been shown to affect survivorship in carcinoma of the larynx.[2,102] Each modality has its advantages and disadvantages (not to mention proponents and detractors), and no one of them is ideal for all patients. The decision as to which approach offers the best chance for cure and preservation of as much normal function as possible depends on site and extent of lesion, degree of nodal involvement, general state of health, availability of types of care, and physician and patient preference, to mention just a few. The physician to whom the responsibility for planning treatment falls must be prepared to consider all of these parameters, each in its proper place, if best choices are to be made.

So many factors can impact on choice of management for carcinoma of the larynx that it is helpful to consider each of them separately, at least at first. Once this has been done (i.e., best approach selected for the lesion), the plan can be modified to take other factors (i.e., state of health) into account.◁ Treatment selection for each of the regions of the larynx will be considered separately, because anatomic location is such an important determining factor in these decisions.

Glottic Carcinoma

Proper treatment for glottic carcinoma is largely *dependent on T stage*, since extralaryngeal spread is rarely seen early and the treatment of the later stages is essentially that of transglottic disease (Table 13–5).

Most investigators agree that the treatment of choice for *T1 glottic* carcinoma is *radiotherapy*.[68–72] If the primary cure rates in large series (excluding surgical salvage) are averaged, they show that approximately 80 to 85 percent of all T1 cancers of the glottic larynx are cured by radiotherapy alone. If subsequent surgical salvage is added, overall 5-year tumor-free survival in excess of 95 percent can be achieved. ◁

The *advantages* of radiotherapy for cure, when successful, include avoidance of surgery and voice results that are generally better than those achieved with partial laryngectomy. The *disadvantages* of this approach are side effects of radiotherapy (i.e., dryness of the mouth, skin changes), higher likelihood that salvage surgery will necessitate loss of voice than if surgery had been chosen initially,[67,74] and possibility of development of second primary, either because of preservation of already distressed mucosa or as a result of long-term effects of radiotherapy (younger individuals).

Vertical partial laryngectomy is a good alternative for *T1 cancer* of the glottis,[67,75] offering primary cure rates averaging about 90 to 92 percent. Surgical salvage brings the ultimate survival to more than 95 percent.[76] Because cure rates for radiotherapy alone are less satisfactory in lesions of the *anterior commissure* and in which there is *extension to* the *arytenoid* (i.e., T1b),[67] *conservation surgery* should be considered for these lesions. As much as one entire vocal fold with its arytenoid cartilage and all of the opposite membranous cord and vocal process can be removed and reconstructed in a single procedure[77] and still result in good airway, swallowing, and a useful voice. In addition to better cure rates for more extensive T1 lesions, the *advantages* of partial laryngectomy include total treatment time of approximately 2 weeks (in uncomplicated cases) as opposed to 8 weeks with radiotherapy, higher probability of avoiding total laryngectomy, and avoidance of radiotherapy side effects. *Disadvantages* are the requirement for surgery and temporary tracheotomy and the average voice result is not as good as after radiotherapy (although individual results may vary greatly). In general, the decision between radiotherapy and surgery as primary modalities for early carcinomas of the larynx should be made *with* the patient, after weighing all of the parameters just listed, since overall survival is almost identical for either approach.

T2 glottic carcinoma (subglottic or transglottic extension) can be treated with radiotherapy for cure, but the results are considerably less satisfactory than for earlier stages.[78] Average failure rates are approximately 35 to 45 percent for primary treatment and 15 to 45 percent even with surgical salvage. Therefore, partial vertical laryngectomy should be selected for glottic carcinoma with *subglottic extension* and for *limited transglottic* lesions. Since *extensive transglottic* lesions are not suitable for partial laryngectomy, they should be managed with *radiotherapy*, with total laryngectomy held in reserve to salvage failures.

T3 glottic carcinoma (fixed cord) is clearly a surgical lesion. Radiotherapy alone offers only a 20 to 30 percent cure rate, and with surgical

"There are . . . factors that also make apparent curability of glottic carcinoma by radiotherapy falsely high. The finding of Stutsman and McGavran[66] that in about 20 percent of the patients undergoing hemilaryngectomy there was no tumor in the specimen suggests that the lesion was totally removed by the biopsy. Also, when radiotherapy end results are reported, distinction is often not made between carcinoma in situ, superficially invasive carcinoma, and invasive carcinoma."—Lawson and Biller[73]

Table 13–5 Treatment Modalities for Carcinoma of the Glottis

T1	Radiotherapy (vertical partial laryngectomy a good alternative)
T2	Surgery (usually vertical partial laryngectomy)
T3,T4	High-dose *planned* radiotherapy and surgery (usually total laryngectomy)

Before it was established that radiotherapy was as effective as neck dissection in controlling subclinical nodal disease,[81] the clinician was often faced with the dilemma of deciding which side to subject to node dissection. Even though most advanced cancers of the larynx have a predominant side, the incidence of contralateral metastasis is almost as high as ipsilateral once the lesion has escaped from the confines of the cartilage. It is now possible to irradiate both sides of the neck, if necessary, and to reserve surgical node dissection for proved disease.—HMT

salvage about 50 percent. *Total laryngectomy* with *neck dissection* if there are palpable nodes is the treatment of choice, although some studies suggest that good results can be achieved with *partial laryngectomy*.[78,79]

T4 carcinoma (cartilage destruction or extralaryngeal extension) offers a poor prognosis by any means of treatment.[80] Since cure rates for either radiation alone or surgery alone leave much to be desired, *planned combined radiation and surgery* seems the best approach, offering approximately a 60 percent 5-year survival.

Nodal metastasis is uncommon (less than 5 percent overall) in glottic carcinoma, although the incidence increases with advancing stage. In T4 lesions, for example, it may reach 15 to 20 percent. This incidence is not high enough to warrant prophylactic neck dissection,◁ but it is usually convenient to *irradiate the neck* to adequate prophylactic levels in the course of providing combined therapy for the primary lesion. Formal *neck dissection*, whether radical or conservative, can thus be reserved *for palpable disease.*

Supraglottic Carcinoma

Carcinoma of the *supraglottic larynx* generally has a worse prognosis than comparable stages of glottic cancer. This is because: (1) the supraglottic larynx has a rich lymphatic supply, permitting early metastasis, and the glottis does not; (2) supraglottic lesions are often silent in early stages; and (3) there is a less complete cartilaginous "box" enclosing the supraglottic structures than that which confines lesions of the vocal cords. For all these reasons, supraglottic cancer is generally detected later in the progression of the disease. Indeed, the most common presenting complaint for many supraglottic lesions is a metastatic mass in the neck. As a result, with the possible exception of very limited lesions of the laryngeal surface of the epiglottis or of the false cords, radiotherapy alone does not yield survival rates comparable either to surgery alone or to planned combined therapy.[82,83]

A large body of literature exists supporting each of these therapeutic approaches. Unfortunately, statistical results are confusing and contradictory, largely because of inconsistencies in types of tumors included, differences in staging from one study to another, and lack of controls. It is clear from all of these studies, however, that *prognosis* depends on (1) stage and location of primary disease; (2) choice of primary treatment; and (3) most important, presence or absence of nodal involvement.

1.   Stage and location of primary disease. It is apparent that the more advanced a lesion is when first treated, the less likely it is to be controlled. *Location* is also important, exclusive of stage. Tumors of the so-called *"marginal zone"* (suprahyoid portion of the epiglottis and aryepiglottic folds) behave more like hypopharyngeal lesions, with higher tendency to spread to the base of tongue and adjacent pyriform sinuses and to metastasize more readily than tumors arising in the rest of the supraglottic larynx. On the other hand, they are less likely to spread to the preepilgottic space. Lesions of the *lingual surface* of the *epiglottis* behave like hypopharyngeal lesions and should be treated accordingly. *Management* of lesions of each of these three types by *partial* or *total laryngectomy* yields survival statistics as follows:[84] supraglottic, 76 percent, marginal, 53 percent, lingual surface of epiglottis, 48 percent.

2.   Choice of primary treatment. *Radiotherapy* alone offers survivals in the range of 30 to 50 percent overall, but does much better for early lesions (approximately 60 to 85 percent for T1 lesions).[4] Neck disease, on the other hand, is not well controlled by radiotherapy once clinically pal-

Table 13-6   Management of Supraglottic Carcinoma

T1	Partial laryngectomy (conventional or laser) *or* radiotherapy
T2,T3	High-dose planned (pre- or postoperative) radiotherapy *and* supraglottic laryngectomy
T3,T4	High-dose planned radiotherapy *and* total laryngectomy

Neck dissection is also performed where indicated

The major advantage of preoperative versus postoperative radiotherapy is in regard to completion of treatment. If surgery is carried out first and some complication or other change in the patient's condition ensues that does not permit timely delivery of radiation, completion of combined therapy may be delayed or even prevented. On the other hand, if radiotherapy is given preoperatively, treatment for the cancer will have been completed, even though there may be complications of healing from the surgery.—HMT

Bocca[88] has recommended so-called conservative neck dissection rather than classic radical neck dissection. In this technique, all soft tissues within fascial compartments (ostensibly including all lymph nodes) are removed, but all of the major muscles, the jugular vein, and all major nerves are spared. Besides its obvious cosmetic and functional advantages, this approach permits simultaneous, bilateral neck dissections to be carried out with much less probability of cerebral vascular complications.—HMT

pable nodes have appeared. Since total or even partial laryngectomy can be carried out for recurrences after radiotherapy (albeit with increased risk of surgical complications), irradiation may be a viable approach for early lesions, especially without cervical metastases. *Surgery* alone has a better survival rate than radiotherapy alone in every stage, with the possible exception of stage 1. Horizontal partial laryngectomy yields as good results as total laryngectomy for properly selected lesions.[85,86] *Planned combined radiotherapy* and *surgery* have generally offered the *best overall survival* statistics,[4,83] regardless of whether the radiotherapy is given preoperatively or postoperatively. *Complications* have essentially equal incidence and are of a similar nature by either approach, the only difference being the time during treatment at which they occur.◁

3. Nodal involvement. Incidence of lymph node metastasis in supraglottic carcinoma is reported as varying between 25 and 50 percent[47,49] depending on primary tumor site, stage, degree of differentiation, etc. Although there is some controversy[87] regarding sites to which laryngeal cancer metastasizes, nodes in the posterior triangle or along the spinal accessory nerve do not frequently become involved.[47] Although prophylactic radiotherapy is at least as effective as surgery for N0 disease,[81] it is generally agreed that therapeutic *radical neck dissection* is indicated *for palpable lymph node metastases.*◁ The more advanced the neck involvement at the time of initial treatment, the poorer the prognosis, with aggregate nodal involvement in excess of 6 cm in diameter or remaining fixed after preoperative radiotherapy, yielding essentially no long-term survivors.[89]

Subglottic Carcinoma

Primary lesions of the subglottic larynx are uncommon, except when they represent extension from above.[90] They comprise only about 5 percent of all laryngeal cancers. Because of location, *subglottic lesions* are often *silent* until they produce either *obstructive* symptoms or cervical *metastases.* Cartilage invasion is common. *Hoarseness* is usually seen only if the recurrent laryngeal nerve becomes involved by extralaryngeal extension. For all these reasons, prognosis is generally poor, even when subglottic cancer is correctly *treated* with *combined radiotherapy* and *total laryngectomy.* neck dissection is usually necessary, as well, and must often be carried out bilaterally. Subglottic extension from glottic lesions is treated similarly, although minimal subglottic involvement may be amenable to partial laryngectomy (see before).

In general, then, the *important steps in treatment* of *carcinoma of the larynx* are: (1) *early detection,* since cure rates and ability to preserve function are directly related to stage; (2) *accurate assessment* and *staging,* to permit selection of appropriate and most conservative approach to treatment, (3) *treatment planning,* including input from the surgeon, the radiotherapist, other appropriate medical personnel, *and* the patient, (4) *careful follow-up,* to permit prompt detection of persistent or recurrent disease while further treatment may still be effective for salvage. My *follow-up regimen* for any head and neck cancer is:

1. Monthly for the first 6 months after completion of definitive treatment
2. Bimonthly for the next 6 months
3. Every 3 months during the second year
4. Every 4 months for remaining 3 years of follow-up◁

Surgical Techniques for Carcinoma of the Larynx

Total Laryngectomy

This is the *baseline procedure* for attempted surgical cure of laryngeal carcinoma, against which the results of any *less conservative* technique must be measured.◁ *Indications* are: (1)Lesions too extensive for resection by subtotal procedures; (2) patients whose lesion is appropriate for conservation surgery, but whose medical status, age, or personal preference mitigate against accepting the risks of aspiration, higher complication rates and/or longer rehabilitation period of partial laryngetomy (see later); (3) salvage surgery after failed radiation (a relative indication, since some radiation failure cases are still amenable to partial laryngectomy); and (4) palliative local control of disease, wherein tracheotomy or diversionary feeding techniques are less satisfactory and where reasonably long-term survival can be expected. *Contraindications* include Lesions too extensive to permit complete resection of local disease, unacceptable medical risks, and patient refusal.

Technique

An apron flap is commonly used (although many other incisions will do) because it permits placement of the tracheostoma in the incision line, provides excellent exposure, and permits ready extension for uni- or bilateral neck dissection. (Fig. 13–2) The flap is elevated in the subplatysmal plane until the hyoid bone has been exposed. After completion of neck dissection, if one is being performed, the strap muscles are transected below the level of the anticipated stoma. The jugular vein and carotid artery are mobilized bilaterally and the omohyoid muscles are transected.

The thyroid isthmus is identified and transected. (Fig. 13–3) The thyroid lobe on the noninvolved side is preserved by mobilizing it from medial to lateral. On the involved side, the inferior thyroid vascular bundle is identified, transected, and suture ligated. The ipsilateral thyroid lobe is mobilized from lateral to medial and left attached to the trachea.

I prefer to transect the trachea at this point in the operation and to establish the anterior part of the tracheostoma. This can usually be done safely at a point below the second tracheal ring, unless there is significant subglottic extension. Rather than cutting the trachea on a bevel, I cut horizontally between two rings until the membranous posterior wall is reached. A tonguelike projection can be left at the membranous posterior portion of the trachea to increase the cross-sectional area of the stoma, without unecessary exposure of cartilage that occurs if the trachea is simply beveled (Fig. 13–4). At this point, the endotracheal tube may be removed from the mouth and replaced with a sterile one via the distal tracheal opening. The anterior wall of the distal trachea is anchored to the midline skin

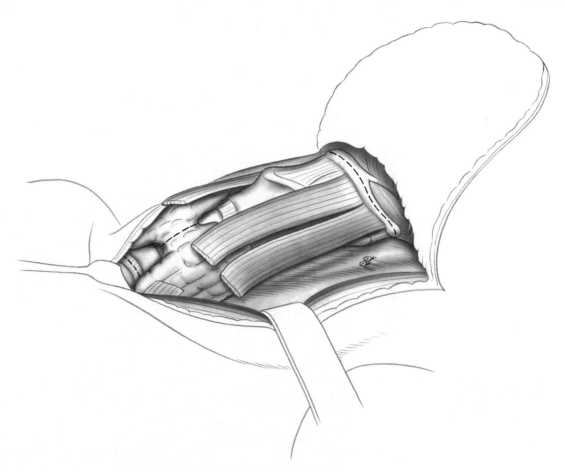

Figure 13–2. Apron flap incision for total laryngectomy. Strap muscles are transected low in the neck.

of the lower flap with interrupted sutures of 2–0 silk, placed as in the illustration, to draw the skin edge well within the tracheal opening. This technique allows eventual retraction of the skin-mucosa junction down into the neck after healing and thus minimizes exposure, crusting, and irritation of the mucosa.

The hyoid bone is separated from its upper muscular attachments by either sharp dissection or cutting cautery. The greater cornua are individually identified and dissected free of all attachments from their tips medially to the lesser cornu. the superior neurovascular bundle of the larynx is identified on the uninvolved side, doubly suture ligated, and divided. The same procedure can be carried out on the involved side, as well, unless there is disease in the vallecula or base of tongue, in which case the superior thyroid artery is identified and ligated at its point of origin as the first branch of the external carotid or as it arises from the bifurcation of the common carotid artery.

The thyroid cartilage is mobilized on the side of noninvolvement by placing a double hook retractor behind the lateral thyroid ala and entering the retropharyngeal space by sharp and blunt dissection. The inferior and middle constrictor muscle fibers are sharply dissected from the greater cornu, lateral margin, and lesser cornu of the thyroid cartilage. If tumor does not involve the pyriform sinus, the thyroid cartilage can be skeletonized on the ipsilateral side, as well.

The larynx can now be entered in any of several ways, depending on location of tumor and/or surgeon preference. I find the inferior approach to

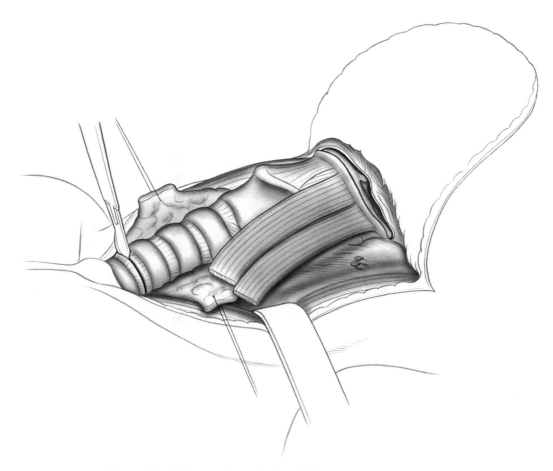

Figure 13–3. Transection of thyroid isthmus and incision to free supraglottic musculature from the hyoid bone.

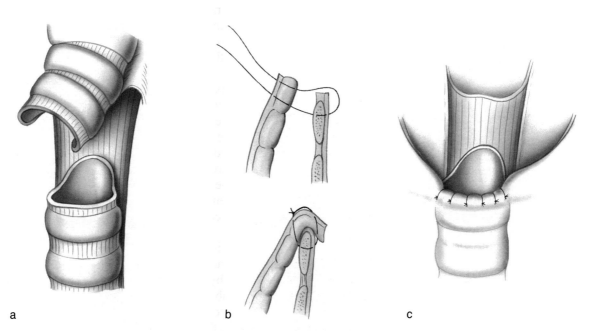

a   b   c

Figure 13–4. **a,** Beveled transection of the trachea produces a consistently wider laryngostoma. **b,** Placement of skin to tracheal sutures to draw skin inside the stoma and cover exposed cartilage. **c,** Anchoring stoma by closing anterior half. The posterior portion is closed when the apron flap is returned at the end of the procedure.

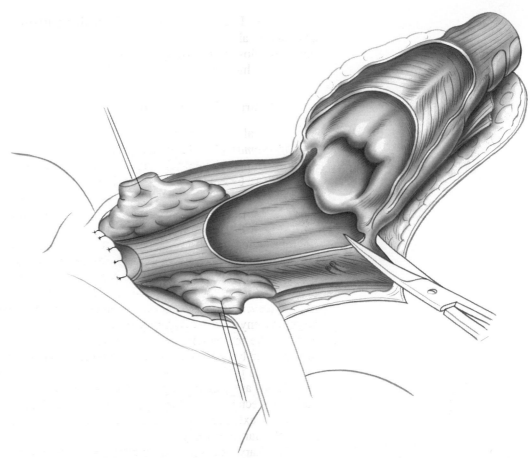

Figure 13–5. Removal of laryngectomy specimen. Approach from below allows maximal preservation of uninvolved hypopharyngeal mucosa.

The other two major approaches are via the uninvolved pyriform sinus and through the bed of the hyoid bone and valleculae. Either of these permits visualization of the extension along Broyles' ligament if the anterior commissure is involved. Once this has happened, spread to the Delphian node and, thereafter, metastasis to either midjugular chain of lymph nodes can occur.—HMT

Too tight a muscular ring has been incriminated in poor voice results after subsequent ''duck-bill'' prosthesis surgery.—HMT

be most useful, because there is rarely any disease in the postcricoid area and this technique allows maximal preservation of uninvolved hypopharyngeal mucosa.◁ The surgeon places an index finger or retractor into the transected laryngotrachea and carefully enters the loose areolar tissue in the party wall between it and the esophagus. Once this has been accomplished, it is possible bluntly to separate the esophagus from the trachea all the way up to the postcricoid area. The hypopharynx can then be entered by incising this mucosal reflection. Scissors are used to transect the remaining mucosal attachments on either side superiorly toward the base of the tongue and hyoid bone (Fig. 13–5). The line of transection desired in the vallecular area and across the base of the tongue is established under direct vision with the entire laryngotracheal specimen inverted, thus completing the resection.

Closure is begun after inspecting the specimen and obtaining frozen section margins when indicated. I prefer 3–0 chromic catgut in a running Connell-type suture to invert the mucosa, although almost any careful visceral suturing technique will do. If the defect permits, either horizontal or vertical straight line closure should be carried out, but it is almost always necessary to create a Y-shaped closure, beginning at each corner and joining at the midline. A second layer is desirable, providing it does not overly reduce the available lumen or reestablish continuity between the constrictor muscles.◁ If a radical neck dissection has been done, the exposed carotid artery should be covered against the risk of exposure if the wound breaks down later. I prefer a dermal graft for this purpose, although muscle-flap coverage is also satisfactory. Suction catheter drains are placed and the skin flaps are closed. Dressings are neither desirable nor necessary, provided continuous high wall suction is used.

Vertical Partial Laryngectomy

Vertical partial laryngeal procedures are most often employed in *glottic carcinomas* (T1, T2 where possible, T3 with subglottic extension not exceeding approximately 8 mm at the anterior commissure), although some success has been obtained with minimal transglottic disease. As with all conservation surgery, the onus of proper patient selection is on the surgeon, since properly done total laryngectomy should result in cure of virtually all of these lesions. Local recurrence is therefore a sign of less than optimal patient selection or inadequate extent of surgical resection.

Indications for vertical partial laryngectomy are for lesions that can be adequately resected *and* reconstructed by these techniques, and after radiation failures in which the lesion and patient's condition still permit partial surgery. *Contraindications* include lesions too extensive for subtotal laryngectomy (see individual procedures), and medical considerations that either make the patient a poor surgical risk in whom even minimal aspiration cannot be tolerated, or when preservation of voice is of little or no value to the patient (i.e., severe mental retardation or neurologic deficit).

There are four basic procedures that may be classified as vertical partial laryngectomies: (1)laryngofissure with cordectomy; (2) hemilaryngectomy, (3) extended or frontolateral vertical partial laryngectomy, and (4) near-total laryngectomy.

1. Laryngofissure with cordectomy. This procedure is suitable for T1 cancers limited to one membranous vocal fold and with no suggestion of deep invasion (Fig. 13–6). Most such lesions are treated successfully by radiotherapy with better voice results than are achieved with surgery (see next margin note). "A tracheotomy is performed in the usual location. Either a vertical midline incision or a small apron flap will give adequate exposure. The strap muscles are exposed and separated in the midline to give access to the thyroid cartilage. An incision is made in the anterior perichondrium of the thyroid cartilage at the midline and [it] is elevated laterally for 1 or 2 mm in each direction. Using a[n oscillating] saw, the thyroid cartilage is incised in the midline from the thyroid notch to the inferior margin. An incision is then made transversely in the thyrohyoid membrane just at the midline. A small hemostat is placed through this incision and . . . the operator looks from below upward to see the undersurface of the vocal cords. Using the spread hemostat to protect and separate the cords, a knife is inserted and the soft tissues of the larynx are incised from below upward directly through the anterior commissure to the petiole of the epiglottis (and for a short distance to one side of it). The separated halves of the thyroid ala may now be gently spread apart and held with small double hooks or retractors. This will give access under direct vision to the vocal cords on each side. The (involved) vocal cord and adjacent false cord can now be resected by elevating the inner perichondrium from the inner surface of the thyroid cartilage to separate all soft tissue from [it]. The necessary volume of tissue is excised under direct vision, and bleeding is controlled with cautery. . . . [N]o direct reconstruction is undertaken; . . . the raw surface thus produced is purposely left to granulate in and heal by second intention.◁ Closure is accomplished by . . . suturing the preserved edges of the anterior perichondrium to each other with fine absorb-

"Probably the major drawback to this procedure is . . . that the voice results are generally less satisfactory than those achieved by standard hemilaryngectomy. This is probably due to the rigid lateral thyroid cartilage left in place, which prevents collapse of the lateral soft tissues and the formation of a good band of scar tissue (pseudocord) in the area in which the cord was excised."—HMT[68]

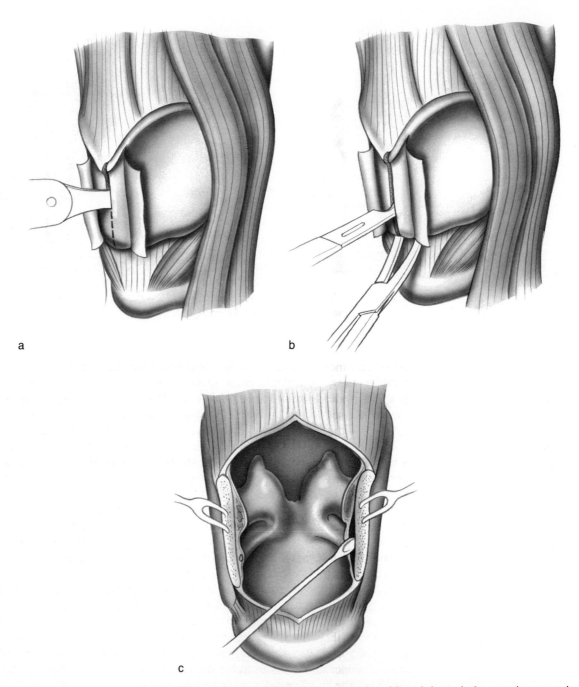

a

b

c

Figure 13–6. **a,** Midline thyrotomy is achieved through the anterior commissure of the thyroid cartilage with an oscillating saw. **b,** Broyles' ligament is bisected precisely at the anterior commissure under direct vision. **c,** Vocal fold to be resected is elevated from inner surface of thyroid cartilage in the subperichondrial plane.

able sutures. The strap muscles are then reapproximated and the neck incision closed in the usual fashion with placement of a (suction catheter) drain.''[68]

2. Hemilaryngectomy. This is the basic vertical partial laryngectomy and is appropriate to many glottic lesions. It is a good alternative to radiotherapy for cure in T1 lesions and may be applicable in T2 and even some T3 cancers of the glottis. At maximal extent, it permits resection of

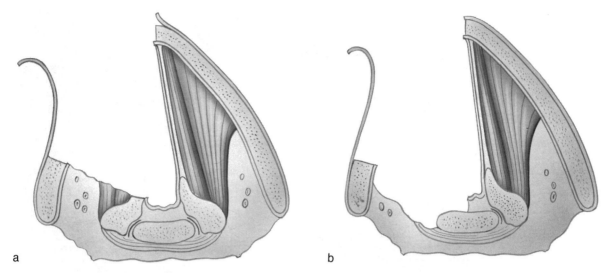

a   b

Figure 13–7. Vertical partial laryngectomy (hemilaryngectomy). **a,** Body of arytenoid cartilage preserved. **b,** Arytenoid cartilage removed.

See Chapter 6.

all of one membranous vocal fold and arytenoid cartilage (if necessary) as well as a few millimeters of the opposite vocal fold (Fig. 13–7). If more than approximately one-fourth of the less-involved membranous vocal fold must be resected to provide an adequate margin, consideration should be given to either frontolateral or near-total laryngectomy (see later).

Although there are many techniques advocated for this procedure[2]◁, I prefer the one used by Ogura and Biller.[91] Performance of tracheotomy, skin incision, anterior laryngeal exposure, and initial midline incision of the thyroid cartilage perichondrium are identical to the same steps as described for laryngofissure in the preceeding section (Fig. 13–8). Perichondrial cuts are extended at right angles to the vertical midline incision along the upper and lower borders of the thyroid alae, as far as the bases of the greater and lesser cornua on the involved side and for 2 to 3 mm on the uninvolved side. Perichondrial flaps are raised to these same landmarks bilaterally. An oscillating saw is used to make cartilage cuts as follows: (1) from the lower to upper border of the thyroid ala on the involved side, just anterior to the bases of the cornua and leaving a posterior cartilage strut connecting them; (2) at the midline, or, when necessary because of minimal anterior commissure involvement, 2 to 3 mm toward the uninvolved side. An incision is made along the lower border of the involved thyroid ala from the midline toward the lesser cornu. A small hemostat is introduced and is used to separate and protect the vocal cords while the operator inspects their undersurface and identifies the lesion from below. The larynx is entered by incising the soft tissues from below upward with a scalpel, either passing precisely through the midline, or, when the lesion demands, a few millimeters toward the uninvolved side. At least 1 to 2 mm of apparent clearance of the cordal lesion should be allowed when making this cut. The cut is continued with knife or scissors along the upper border of the involved thyroid ala, paralleling the lateral border of the epiglottis. The involved ala and its soft tissue contents can then be opened like a book to expose the laryngeal contents. The appropriate point for the posterior line of resection can then be determined under direct vision. This may be just at the tip of the vocal process, may transect the vocal process from the body of the arytenoid, or may remove the arytenoid cartilage entirely, depending on the extent of the lesion. In the course of this resec-

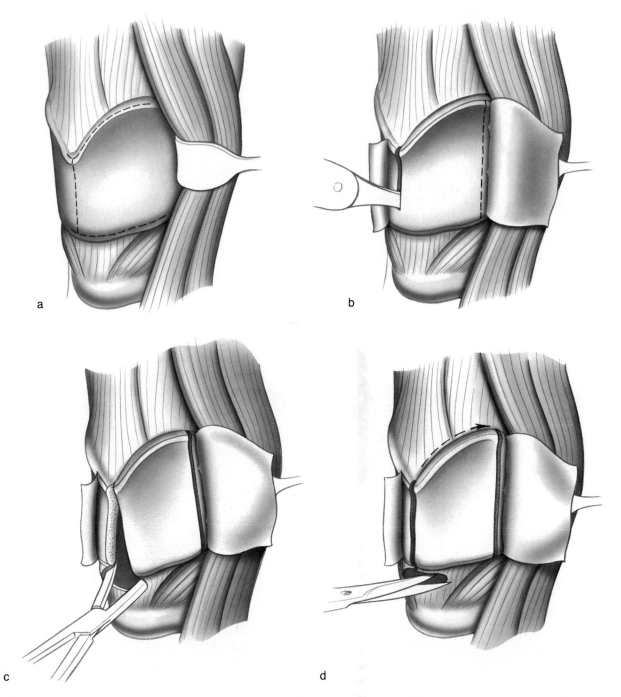

a

b

c

d

Figure 13–8. Vertical partial laryngectomy. **a,** Perichondrial cuts outlined. **b,** Perichondrium elevated, oscillating saw cut at midline. **c,** Midline cut completed under direct vision, aided by spread hemostat. **d,** Scissors cuts to complete hemilaryngectomy.

tion, one or two major bleeders will be encountered superolaterally. These must be identified and suture ligated. Other bleeding is usually minimal and can be controlled with judicious bipolar cautery. Frozen section margins can be obtained to be sure that adequate resection has been carried out before reconstruction is begun.

If the body of the arytenoid has been preserved, no real reconstruction is necessary. Indeed, the raw surface should not be covered with mucosal

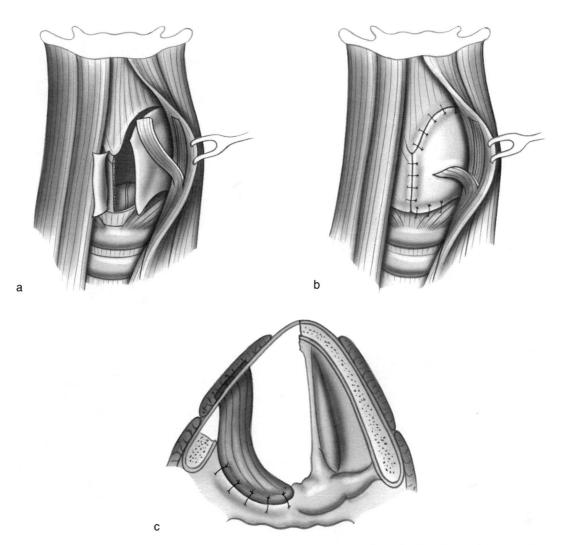

Figure 13–9. Muscle flap reconstruction after hemilaryngectomy with resection of entire arytenoid cartilage. **a,** Inferiorly based flap elevated from undersurface of strap muscle. **b,** Flap led through slit in perichondrium. **c,** Muscle flap sutured to bed of resected arytenoid cartilage.

The purpose of this flap is to provide bulk and to reestablish the buttress that separates the medial portion of the pyriform sinus from the glottis in order to help prevent spill-over and aspiration of liquids. It is not intended to reconstruct the vocal fold or to improve voice.
—HMT

flaps, since they will tend to prevent formation of a pseudocord and result in a less satisfactory voice. If the entire arytenoid cartilage has been removed, however, some bulk should be restored to the posterior part of the glottis in order to minimize chances for postoperative aspiration. Of the several techniques described to accomplish this,[92,93] I prefer the inferiorly based, single pedicle sternohyoid muscle flap[94] (Fig. 13–9). A short horizontal incision is made through the preserved thyroid perichondrial flap on the side of excision at the level of the remaining vocal cord. An inferiorly based partial thickness muscle flap is developed from the deep surface of the sternohyoid muscle, so situated that its point of attachment is at or slightly below the incision in the perichondrium. The free end of the flap is led through the perichondrial incision and sutured to the bed of the excised arytenoid cartilage. Adjacent pyriform sinus mucosa can be mobilized to cover the flap partially.◁ The perichondrial flaps are then approximated with interrupted 3–0 chromic sutures and the neck closed and drained with suction catheters.

3. Frontolateral hemilaryngectomy. Several techniques have been

Figure 13–10. Tantalum keel
used to prevent anterior
commissure webbing after
frontolateral laryngectomy.

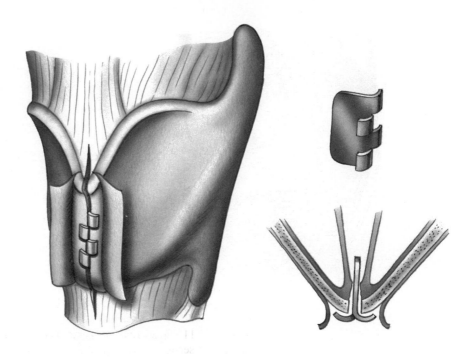

described to permit resection and reconstruction of defects that involve all or part of both membranous vocal folds.[2,95] All of these require either a two-stage procedure or prolonged stenting to prevent stenosis of the reconstructed glottis. Voice results are less satisfactory and risk of aspiration or inadequate airway are more common than after simple hemilaryngectomy.

Indications include lesions of the glottis that involve the anterior commissure, in which more than approximately one-third of the anterior aspects of both vocal folds must be removed. *Contraindications* are the same as for hemilaryngectomy and postradiation failure. A widely used procedure places a tantalum keel (Fig. 13–10) between the vocal cord remnants, which is left in place for 6 to 8 weeks. The patient is not decannulated until the airway has been deemed satisfactory after the second procedure.

4. Near-total laryngectomy with epiglottic reconstruction. A more recent technical improvement in extended and frontolateral partial laryngectomy has increased the surgeon's ability to resect most of the glottic larynx and still reconstruct a functioning and competent airway in a single stage procedure.[77,96] *Indications* are lesions that can be resected leaving the body of one arytenoid cartilage and a posterior strut of thyroid cartilage bilaterally. *Contraindications* are the same as for hemilaryngectomy and involvement or absence of the epiglottis. The procedure can be performed in patients who have had previous radiation, but with somewhat increased risk of complications of healing.

The procedure is performed as follows. Skin incision, tracheotomy, separation of strap muscles, and laryngeal exposure are carried out as for hemilaryngectomy. After exposure of the thyroid cartilage, an incision is made in the perichondrium at the midline, and then carried at right angles along the upper and lower borders of the thyroid alae, bilaterally (Fig. 13–11). Perichondrial flaps are elevated back to the bases of the greater and lesser cornua of the thyroid cartilage on both sides. Using an oscillating saw, a cut is made between the upper and lower borders of the cartilage, just anterior to the cornua on the side of greater involvement. This leaves a posterior cartilage strut between the cornua at the posterior thyroid ala. On the side of lesser involvement, the cartilage cut is made anywhere along the anteroposterior extent of the ala, depending on the degree of involve-

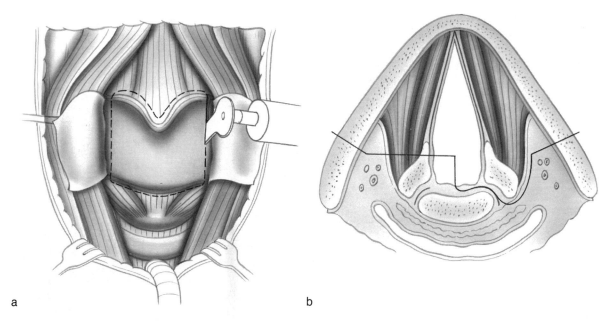

a   b

Figure 13–11. Near-total laryngectomy. **a,** Cartilage cuts. **b,** Possible maximal extent of resection leaves a posterior cartilage strut bilaterally and the body of at least one arytenoid cartilage.

ment, although it is usually at the same point as on the side of major involvement. An incision is made in the cricothyroid membrane connecting the cartilage cuts. A scissors is then used to transect the vocal cord and soft tissues on the side of lesser involvement to match the previously made cartilage cut, allowing sufficient margin of clearance from the lesion. This may be as far posterior as just anterior to the body of the arytenoid cartilage. The scissors are brought along the upper border of the thyroid alae, anterior to the epiglottis, toward the cartilage cut on the side of greater involvement. This maneuver severs the thyroepiglottic ligament in the middle and allows the larynx to be opened like a book to expose the side of greater involvement. The necessary posterior soft tissue cut on that side can then be made under direct vision. All of the vocal fold, including the entire arytenoid, may be resected on this side, if necessary.

Once margins have been checked by frozen section, reconstruction can begin. The petiole of the epiglottis is grasped with a tenaculum and the preepiglottic space is entered with sharp and blunt dissection (Fig. 13–12). The entire epiglottis is mobilized inferiorly as a composite flap supported on the reflection of vallecular mucosa. The median hyoepiglottic and lateral glossoepiglottic ligaments are encountered and transected in this process, care being taken not to penetrate the mucosal reflection at the base of the tongue. Moderate amounts of soft tissue are left with the epiglottis, since too meticulous dissection can interfere with its blood supply. Tension is relieved by grasping the cricoid cartilage and displacing it toward the epiglottis at the same time as the epiglottis is pulled downward. This relief of tension on the closure is maintained until the entire suture line has been completed. The epiglottis is sutured to the cut edges of the thyroid cartilage remnants bilaterally and to the cricothyroid membrane inferiorly, using interrupted, nonabsorbable sutures (I prefer 2–0 silk). No attempt is made to suture mucosa to mucosa. The preserved perichondrial leaflets are approximated with 3–0 chromic sutures, drains are placed, and the neck is closed as usual.

Postoperative management is essentially the same as for hemilaryn-

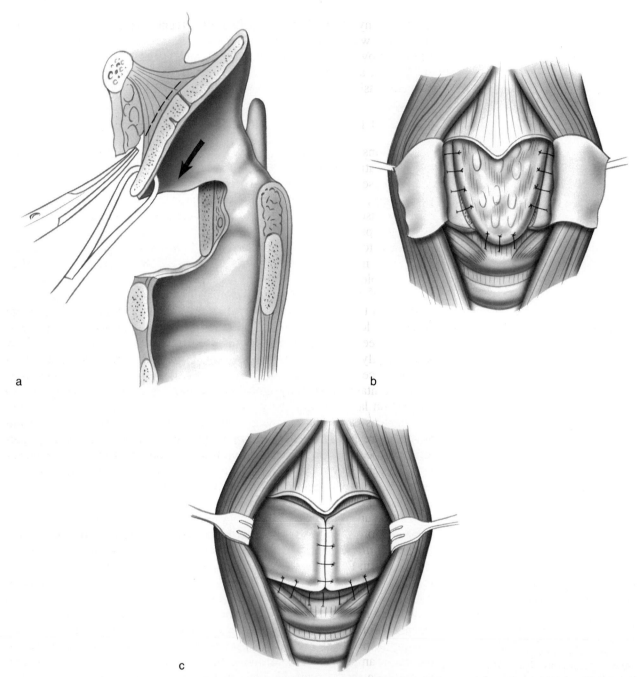

Figure 13–12. Epiglottic reconstruction after near-total laryngectomy. **a,** Mobilization of epiglottis. **b,** Epiglottis sutured to remaining cartilage struts and cricothyroid membrane. **c,** Perichondrial leaflets approximated.

gectomy, although there is usually somewhat more aspiration. Once the tracheotomy tube can be removed, however, swallowing without significant aspiration usually follows within a day or two. No patient in our series has failed of eventual decannulation with little or no aspiration, good airway, and a useful voice, even though half of the first 60 patients managed with this technique were radiation failures. In two of these the mobilized epiglottis sloughed, but ultimate healing and good function ensued in both of them without further surgical intervention. Three-year survivals have approximated results expected for comparable lesions treated with partial laryngectomy. There has been only a 50 percent 3-year nonrecurrence rate in patients with more than 6 mm subglottic extension at the anterior commissure, however. All recurrences have thus far been salvaged by total laryngectomy, although insufficient follow-up has as yet been possible to draw firm conclusions regarding this group of patients.

Horizontal Partial Laryngectomy

Lesions that are situated entirely above the plane of the ventricles can often be satisfactorily resected by variants of horizontal partial laryngectomy. These include supraglottic laryngectomy, extended supraglottic laryngectomy, and partial laryngopharyngectomy.

Because of the tendency for lesions in this area to remain "silent" for prolonged periods and to present with palpable neck nodes, it is frequently necessary to include neck dissection with these supraglottic procedures. Moreover, many of the cancers treated this way have been shown to offer best possible cure rates when planned, combined radiotherapy and surgery are used.[4,5] For these reasons, complications are higher after supraglottic procedures than after vertical partial laryngectomies, although still at quite acceptable levels around 10 to 20 percent. Although all patients aspirate to some degree after supraglottic laryngectomy, most eventually can swallow satisfactorily. Overall, about 6 percent of patients who have had supraglottic procedures are not able to swallow well enough to protect the lungs or to maintain satisfactory nutrition and must eventually be subjected to completion laryngectomy, even though the cancer may be cured.[97,98] Wound breakdowns, carotid blowout, fistula formation, and difficulties in decannulation are all encountered more frequently after supraglottic laryngectomy,[2] especially when radiotherapy has also played a part in the patient's management. Even though it has been shown that local disease control is the same for comparable lesions whether managed by supraglottic laryngectomy or total laryngectomy, the surgeon must select patients for conservation surgery with great care, weighing the increased risks against the potential for voice preservation and avoidance of long-term tracheotomy.

Indications are any lesion that can be resected by partial horizontal laryngectomy and that will allow margins of 1 to 2 cm in all areas except inferiorly. At the ventricular margin, 3 to 4 mm are adequate.[2] *Contraindications* are lesions that cannot be resected with adequate margins by this technique; radiation failures in lesions that were initially borderline or too extensive for partial laryngectomy, even though the persistent lesion is small enough to meet the criteria; vocal cord fixation, unless the immobility of the cord can be shown to be due to bulk of the lesion rather than invasion of cartilage, cricoarytenoid joint, or recurrent laryngeal nerve; cardiopulmonary compromise that makes it unlikely that the patient could tolerate the aspiration that follows all such procedures; patients in whom, because of mental or neurologic status, voice preservation is of no value and the ability to learn to swallow again is equivocal; and lack of informed consent. ◁

Technique of horizontal partial laryngectomy varies somewhat, depending on the extent of the procedure, although all techniques are based on supraglottic laryngectomy.

1. Supraglottic laryngectomy. This procedure seeks to remove the entire epiglottis, hyoid bone, preepiglottic space, false vocal folds, and the upper half of the thyroid cartilage. It usually spares the vocal folds and both arytenoid cartilages. The technique is as follows.[68] "An apron flap incision is used. If a radical neck dissection is to be performed simultaneously, it may be an asymmetric flap wherein the limb on the side of the

Chronologic age, per se, is not a contraindication to conservation surgery of the larynx.[99] Physiologic age, on the other hand, frequently makes it advisable to seek less risky approaches for management of supraglottic lesions. Since elderly patients do not generally tolerate radiotherapy as well as younger persons do, total laryngectomy is often the safest approach in this age group, even though the lesion itself might be amenable to supraglottic surgery.—HMT

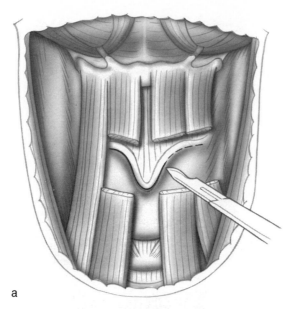

a

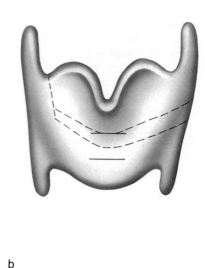

b

Figure 13–13. Supraglottic laryngectomy. **a,** Transection of strap muscles and incision of perichondrium of thyroid cartilage. **b,** Cartilage cuts: note that anterior commissure is traversed at the junction of the upper and lower halves in males and at the junction of the upper third and lower two-thirds in females.

neck dissection is carried along the posterior aspect of the sternocleido-mastoid muscle instead of the anterior border. . . . Tracheotomy may be performed at any time during the procedure that seems most appropriate to the surgeon. [T]he hyoid bone is grasped and, if the lesion is well away from it, preserved. If there is any question about involvement of the pre-epiglottic space or if the lesion comes close to the hyoid bone, it should be sacrificed. Using a cautery knife, the muscles are removed either from the lower border of the hyoid bone, or from the upper border if it is to be sacrificed. The greater cornu of the thyroid cartilage is exposed on the side of involvement, but usually not on the uninvolved side. This is done to protect the superior laryngeal artery, nerve, and vein in this area, which are so important to successful redevelopment of swallowing. The strap muscles are transected at approximately the upper border of the thyroid cartilage to expose it. An incision is then carried through the perichondrium along the upper border of the thyroid cartilage, beginning at the base of the greater cornu on the less involved side, and carrying it across to the lateral aspect of the thyroid cartilage on the more involved side. It is also extended down the lateral border of the thyroid cartilage on the involved side, in the process detaching some of the inferior constrictor fibers from the cartilage [Fig. 13–13a]. The perichondrium is then carefully elevated from above downward to expose sufficient cartilage to allow the appropriate cuts to be made. The anterior commissure of the vocal cords will be found approximately at the junction of the upper and lower halves of the thyroid cartilage in males and at the junction of the upper and middle thirds in females. [Fig. 13–13b] When the cartilage has been exposed, cuts are made from the base of the greater cornu, beginning at the upper border of the thyroid cartilage on the lesser involved side, and carried diagonally to the midline at the appropriate point. The cut continues transversely from this point to the base of the greater cornu on the lateral aspect of the thyroid cartilage on the involved side. With this skeletonization and mobilization of the structures to be removed, the surgeon may now decide where best to enter the larynx for exposure. If the lesion is close to the vallecula,

Figure 13–14. Supraglottic laryngectomy. Resection completed, including removal of most of the hyoid bone. Note that preservation of greater cornu of hyoid on the patient's right serves as a point of attachment of remaining suprahyoid muscles and as a protector of the superior laryngeal nerve on the same side.

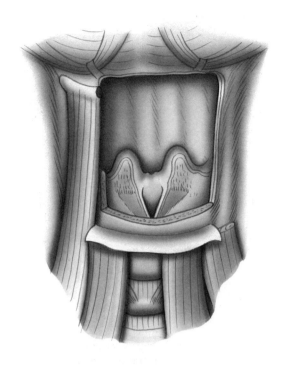

it is perhaps better to enter through the pyriform sinus on the involved side of the larynx, provided that the lesion does not enter this area as well. Once an entry has been achieved, the opening is gradually enlarged under direct vision towards the known location of the tumor. This is done a bit at a time to allow the surgeon to gradually gain exposure of the lesion without approaching it too closely. When it has been exposed, the resection can be carried out to allow adequate margins. In most cases, supraglottic laryngectomy will comprise removal of the entire false cord along the anterior face of the arytenoid on the uninvolved side down to and through the ventricle . . . ., along the the upper border of the true vocal cord to the anterior commissure, and from that point across the attachment of the petiole of the epiglottis, through the ventricle on the (involved) side, to the face of the arytenoid. If the lesion is such that the arytenoid on the involved side does not have to be removed, the dissection is then carried along its anterior surface to produce a mirror image of the dissection on the uninvolved side [Fig. 13–14]. . . . The upper margin of dissection will be carried either just below or just above the hyoid bone, depending on whether this structure can be preserved. When the specimen has been removed and bleeding controlled, a cricopharyngeal myotomy should be performed. This is done by placing a finger into the esophageal introitus from above, palpating the cricopharyngeus muscle, and rotating the larynx with the thumb so that the posterior pharyngeal wall is brought into view [Fig. 13–15]. A knife can then be used to carefully incise all of the transverse fibers of the cricopharyngeus muscle so that nothing is left at that point but mucosa. If this is done properly, the creases of the operator's finger can be seen through his glove and the (remaining) mucosa. Once the cricopharyngeal myotomy has been completed, . . . anesthesia should be lightened to the point where movement of the endotracheal tube will produce (motion) of the vocal cords as the patient coughs. This is necessary to be certain that both vocal cords are still innervated after the cricopharyngeal myotomy . . . (and so that if one is not moving it) can be fixed in the midline to prevent later aspiration.

"Closure of the supraglottic defect is then accomplished as follows: 2–0 . . . black silk is used throughout. Sutures are placed between the remaining musculature of the base of the tongue (or, if it has been pre-

Figure 13–15. Cricopharyngeal myotomy. Rotation of the laryngeal remanant facilitates transection of all fibers of the cricopharyngeus muscle.

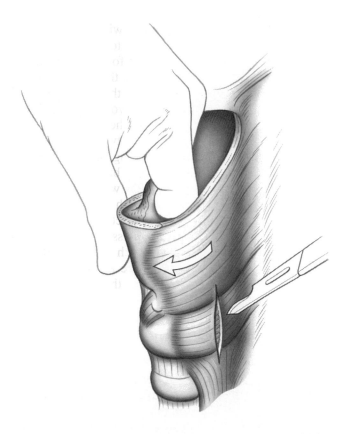

served, the hyoid bone) and the free margin of the preserved perichondrium of the larynx below. The sutures are carried through the muscle of the base of the tongue at a distance of approximately 4 or 5 mm from the free margin, deep into the muscle but not through the mucosa and out through the raw surface of the muscle (or around the hyoid bone). . . . [Fig. 13–16] Inferiorly, the stitch is carried through the free margin of the perichondrium. In this fashion, when the defect is closed the margin of the peri-

Figure 13–16. Closure of defect after supraglottic laryngectomy. Note "bunching" suture placed at the end of the defect on the side of greater resection.

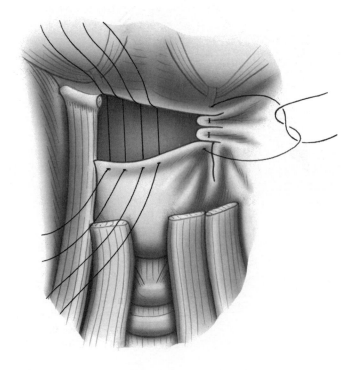

chondrium will be drawn up onto the raw surface of the cut edge of the base of the tongue, pulling the overhanging mucosa down inside the perichondrium for a short distance. . . . It is neither possible nor advisable to try to bring the mucosa of the cut edge of the base of the tongue down to the level of the true vocal cords. . . . The stitches are placed from the side of lesser involvement to the side of greater involvement, being sure to approximate the midline of the base of the tongue to the midline of the larynx. When two or three sutures remain as yet unplaced . . ., a single corner gathering suture . . . begins in the base of the tongue, exactly as with the others, but is then carried as an in-and-out stitch through the lateral pharyngeal wall until the free edge of the perichondrium is reached, and then through it as well. This will bunch and invert the tissue at the side of greater resection''[68] (Fig. 13–16). The sutures are then tied one at a time, while the assistant relieves tension by drawing the wound edges together. If any stitch breaks during tying, it can be replaced. The remaining strap muscles are approximated across the closure to relieve tension further and to buttress the suture line. The neck is closed in the usual fashion, after

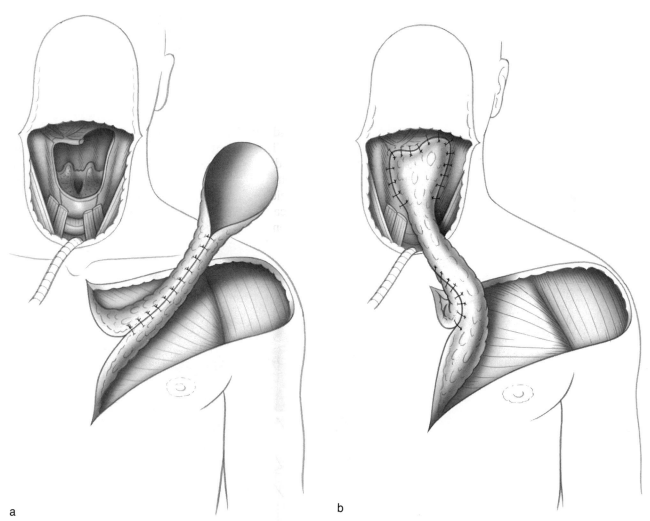

a   b

Figure 13–17. Closure of extended supraglottic laryngectomy or partial laryngopharyngectomy by undelayed deltopectoral flap. **a,** Note that flap is tubed skin side in. Use of a generous apron flap for exposure facilitates this reconstruction. **b,** Repair completed. Return of the apron flap covers most of the exposed portion of tubed deltopectoral flap, the rest of which is skin grafted.

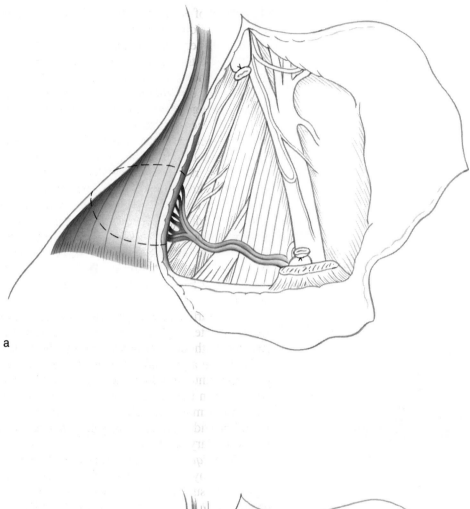

a

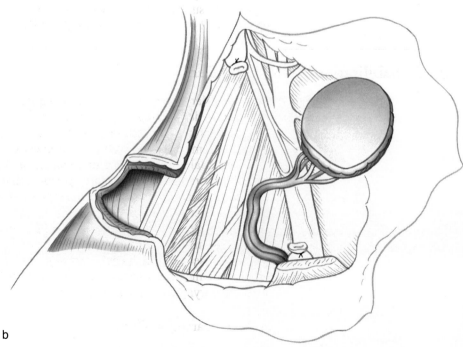

b

Figure 13–18. Transverse cervical trapezius myocutaneous island flap. **a,** Design of flap after isolation of transverse cervical artery and veins. **b,** Island of skin and underlying muscle raised, ready to be transposed into any cervical, oral cavity, or lower facial defect.

placement of suction catheter drains and a nasogastric tube. If a radical neck dissection has been done, carotid coverage is advisable.

2. Extended supraglottic laryngectomy. When lesions are limited to or extend to the base of the tongue, supraglottic laryngectomy may be extended to include resection up to the line of circumvallate papillae. The *indications, contraindications,* and *technique* are the same as for supraglottic laryngectomy, differing only in extent of resection and in certain aspects of reconstruction.

After completion of resection, reconstruction can sometimes be carried out as described for supraglottic laryngectomy. However, this approach can result in excess tension and, particularly in irradiated cases, wound breakdown and fistula formation are likely. A two-stage reconstruction, using an undelayed deltopectoral flap partially to replace the tissue removed, reduce tension, and to provide unirradiated tissue with good blood supply to one side of every suture line has been reported recently[100] (Fig. 13–17). The technique has the additional advantage that a dependent fistula is created that decompresses the suture line during healing. After approximately 5 weeks, the excess flap is returned and the planned fistula is closed.

3. Partial laryngopharyngectomy. Lesions that involve the pyriform sinus or lateral pharyngeal wall can sometimes be resected and reconstructed without total laryngectomy. *Indications* are lesions involving the body of the arytenoid cartilage, the medial wall, or the lateral wall of the pyriform sinus in which the apex is not involved, and lesions extending to or arising in the lateral pharyngeal wall, so that resection of the supraglottis and not more than 50 percent of the circumference of the hypopharynx would provide adequate margins. *Contraindications* are the same as for supraglottic laryngectomy.

Technique of partial pharyngolaryngectomy differs from supraglottic laryngectomy only in extent of resection. *Reconstruction* demands replacement of tissue. Undelayed deltopectoral flaps[100] or myocutaneous flaps[101] can be used for this purpose (Fig. 13–18).

Voice Rehabilitation After Total Laryngectomy*

Total laryngectomy results in complete loss of vocal function, which can have a devastating impact on the individual. The laryngectomized patient suffers many losses in personal, social, and occupational areas. Loss of selfesteem, poor motivation, dependency, and depression are common reactions. Salmon[103] showed that patients and spouses benefit significantly from both preoperative and early postoperative speech consultation to discuss various aspects of speech rehabilitation and associated personal, social, and occupational issues.

Three general means of alaryngeal communication are available to the laryngectomized patient: (1) artificial devices, (2) esophageal speech and, (3) tracheoesophageal speech. An objective discussion and willingness to apply each method is necessary to achieve greatest success and satisfaction with postlaryngectomy voice rehabilitation.

Artificial Laryngeal Devices

Artificial laryngeal devices can be activated electronically or pneumatically. The electronic device is battery operated and generates a me-

---

*This section written by Melinda Harrison, MA, CCC-SP.

chanical sound that is either introduced intraorally via a silastic tube or through the cervical soft tissues by application to the surface of the neck. For the pneumatic device, lung air via the stoma, sets a rubber diaphragm into vibration. The resultant sound is introduced intraorally. Previous theory suggested that use of artificial laryngeal devices early in rehabilitation would serve as a crutch and prevent development of esophageal speech; contemporary teaching, however, suggests that early use of an artificial device aids the patient's reentry into the speaking world, which allows for socialization and even return to work. Devices also provide a "back-up" in case of emergency, even after acquisition of esophageal or tracheoesophageal speech. Use of a device may even aid in the development of esophageal speech by eliminating the tendency for overly articulated, "whisper-like" speech and allowing time for the patient to firmly establish accurate technique.

The use of artificial laryngeal devices requires instruction for proper placement and activation as well as articulation and phrasing. Acquisition of intelligible speech is usually quite rapid. In the early postoperative period many patients can only use an intraoral-type device, due to cervical edema or fibrosis which precedes use of the transcervical type of prosthesis. In case of bilateral neck dissection or severe fibrosis following radiation therapy, long-term use of such an intraoral device may be necessary. While both types of devices require accurate articulation, the intraoral device is more sensitive to weakness of the tongue. If lingual weakness is significant, oral strengthening exercise may be necessary before any device can be used successfully.

Esophageal Speech

Esophageal speech is based upon the principle that when air is introduced into the esophagus and abruptly released, a vibratory event can occur.[104] The area responsible for vibration is called the pharyngoesophageal segment. It was once felt to consist primarily of the inferior constrictor and cricopharyngeus muscles.[105] However, more recent studies have suggested a much longer vibrating segment.[106,107]

Because the trachea and esophagus are separated following the removal of the larynx, lung air is not available to initiate speech; the esophagus and oral cavity must become the alternate air reservoir. Esophageal phonation is initiated when air is charged into the pharyngoesophagus, trapped, and released abruptly to be articulated in the oral cavity. Air charging is accomplished by either of two methods: (1) Injection method—involves compression of the lips or tongue tip against the alveolar ridge (glossopharyngeal press) to force air posteriorly. Syllables or words beginning with consonants which produce high intraoral air pressure (i.e., "p," "t," "k") are useful in establishing esophageal voice. (2) Inhalation method—during sharp inhalation with the mouth widely open, a differential in air pressure between the lungs and the outer walls of the esophagus causes air to be drawn into the esophagus.

Esophageal voice training requires intensive practice and emphasis on step-by-step progression from single sounds to words, phrases, and sentences. Often, useful esophageal speech does not occur for many months following initiation of therapy. Premature efforts to use esophageal voice in conversational speech can lead to faulty technique, prevent development of maximally fluent, refined speech, and may even inhibit intelligibility.

Overall quality of esophageal speech varies widely from patient to patient. Indeed, important acoustic limitations are noted even in superior esophageal speakers; these include low fundamental frequency, limited range of fundamental frequency for inflectional change, reduced intensity, and less than normal periodicity. In addition, restricted duration of phonation necessitates frequent air charge, which is associated with increased physical effort during speech.

Although widely varying results have been reported, it is apparent that esophageal speech has a rather high failure rate. The reasons for this failure have not been determined precisely although many have been postulated: (1) an excessively tight or loose pharyngoesophageal segment due to scarring or radiation changes; (2) anatomic narrowing of the pharyngoesophageal area; (3) lingual or palatal weakness; (4) hiatus hernia; (5) hearing loss; (6) poor patient motivation; (7) intellectional changes inhibiting learning potential, and (8) inadequate teaching.[107–110]

Tracheoesophageal Speech

Surgical-prosthetic methods for alaryngeal voice restoration date back to the early twentieth century. All such attempts have the common intention to establish lung air as the power supply for voice production. Earlier procedures were complicated by high morbidity with protracted recovery periods, potential compromise of surgical margins in an effort to expedite speech rehabilitation, aspiration, fistula stenosis, and the use of complicated, cumbersome prostheses.[111–112]

Singer and Blom introduced an uncomplicated endoscopic technique (Tracheo-esophageal Puncture, TEP) using a simple silicone prosthesis in 1979.[113] The surgical procedure establishes a midline puncture between the posterior wall of the trachea and upper esophagus. The tract is initially stented with a No. 14 Argyle catheter, which is replaced 48 hours or more after surgery with a one-way valved prosthesis which allows for air diversion into the esophagus while the stoma is occluded. The prosthesis maintains the integrity of the puncture tract and prevents aspiration.

When first introduced, it was recommended by Singer and Blom that TEP be performed as a secondary procedure, three to six months following total laryngectomy. However, recent modifications by Hamaker, Singer, and Blom[114] and Maves and Lingemann[115] have shown that TEP can be performed at the time of total laryngectomy.

Postoperative management includes accurate fitting and choice of the prosthesis, which needs to traverse the distance between the lumen of the esophagus and the outer edge of the tracheostoma. Choice of prostheses includes the traditional "duck-bill" type or the more recently introduced low pressure variation. Other variations have been reported in the literature, including the voice button developed by Panje,[116] the first voice prosthesis with an inner flange which allows selfretention of the prosthesis. Patients are instructed in insertion and removal as well as care and maintenance of the prosthesis.

Voice training consists of teaching patients to divert exhaled air efficiently under increased pressures to open the valve and allow tracheoesophageal airflow. Development of accurate digital stomal occlusion is necessary. Rapid acquisition of tracheoesophageal speech is typical.

In addition to prompt reacquisition of voice, acoustic studies have shown several advantages of tracheoesophageal speech over other means of voice rehabilitation, such as a higher fundamental frequency, greater intensity, longer duration, less pause time, and both greater periodicity and aperiodicity in tracheoesophageal as compared with esophageal speech. By every measure, tracheoesophageal patients perform more like laryngeal speakers.

Further advances in treatment have led to the development of a method to accomplish air diversion that does not require digital stomal occlusion.

Developed by Blom et al,[117] the tracheostomal valve closes the airway for phonation, but remains open for normal breathing by means of a flexible diaphragm. Individual respiratory needs during speech as well as during other activities are managed by differing thickness of the valve diaphragm.

Success rates for tracheoesophageal puncture rehabilitation of voice have ranged from 71% to 93%.[117-120] Success has been defined as the ability to communicate verbally better than preoperatively, as well as to manage the prosthesis. Failures have resulted from (1) inability to produce voice, (2) aspiration, (3) inability to care for the prosthesis or retain it in the puncture tract, and (4) patient dissatisfaction.

Failure to acquire voice may result from reflex hypertonicity of the pharyngoesophageal segment. This can be predicted by preoperative assessment with the *air insufflation test*. Failure to produce voice during the test indicates failure of the pharyngoesophageal transition zone to relax and allow passage of air. This phenomenon has been termed "pharyngoesophageal spasm." Patients with hypertonicity who show significant improvement in voice production following local anesthesia of the pharyngeal nerve plexus may be candidates for pharyngeal constrictor myotomy.

Persistent aspiration can occur because of (1) inadvertent dilation of the puncture tract, (2) misplacement of the puncture at or above the mucocutaneous puncture of the tracheostoma, or (3) stricture of the distal esophagus. Puncture dilatation is narrowed by cauterization, which may need to be applied repeatedly. Misplaced punctures are allowed to close either spontaneously or after surgical intervention, and repuncture is carried out thereafter. Suspected proximal esophageal stricture is confimred by barium swallow and may be improved by pharyngeal-superior esophageal myotomy.

With methods currently available for postlaryngectomy speech rehabilitation, prognosis for the patient's successful reentry into occupational, social, and personal areas is better than ever. Continued development of methods to aid restoration of effective communication of this population will further enhance their lives.

References

1. Alberti PW: The historical development of laryngectomy. II The evolution of laryngology and laryngectomy in the mid-nineteenth century. Laryngoscope, 85:288, 1975

2. Silver CE: Surgery for Cancer of the Larynx. New York, Churchill Livingstone, 1981

3. Stevenson RS: Morell Mackenzie, the Story of a Victorian Tragedy. London, William Heinemann, 1946

4. Fletcher GH, Goepfert H: Irradiation in management of squamous cell carcinoma of the larynx. In English GM (Ed): Otolaryngology, vol 5. Philadelphia, Harper & Row, 1984

5. Goldman JL, Silverstone SM: Combined preoperative irradiation and surgery for advanced carcinoma of the larynx and laryngopharynx. In English GM (Ed): Otolaryngology, vol 5. Philadelphia, Harper & Row, 1978

6. Conley JJ: Vocal rehabilitation by autogenous vein graft. Ann Otol Rhinol Laryngol, 68:990–995, 1959

7. Calcaterra TC, Jafek DW: Tracheoesophageal shunt for speech rehabilitation after total laryngectomy. Arch Otolaryngol, 94:124–128, 1971

8. Komorn RM: Vocal rehabilitation in the laryngectomized patient with a tracheoesophageal shunt. Ann Otol Rhinol Laryngol, 83:445–451, 1974

9. Sisson GA, et al: Voice rehabilitation after laryngectomy: Results with the use of a hypopharyngeal prosthesis. Arch Otolaryngol, 101:178–181, 1975

10. Taub S: Air bypass voice prosthesis for vocal rehabilitation of laryngectomees. Ann Otol Rhinol Laryngol, 84:45–48, 1975

11. Arslan M, Serafini I: Reconstructive laryngectomy: Report of the first 35 cases. Ann Otol Rhinol Laryngol, 81:479–486, 1972

12. Staffieri M, Serafini I: La riabilitazione chi-

rurgica della voce e della respirazione dopo laryngectomia totale. 29th National Congress of the Associazione Otologi Ospedalieri Italiana, Bologna, 1976

13. Singer MI, Blom ED: Tracheoesophageal puncture: A surgical prosthetic method for post laryngectomy speech restoration. Proceedings of the 3rd International Symposium on Plastic Reconstructive Surgery of the Head and Neck, New Orleans, 1979

14. Ogura JH, Kawasaki M, Takenouchi S, Yagi M: Replantation and transplantation of the canine larynx. Ann Otol Rhinol Laryngol, 75:295, 1966

15. Silver C, Liebert PS, Som ML: Autologous transplantation of the canine larynx. Arch Otolaryngol, 86:95, 1967

16. Tucker HM: Selective reinnervation of paralyzed musculature in the head and neck: Functioning autotransplantation of the canine larynx. Laryngoscope, 88:348–354, 1978

17. Kluyskens P, Ringoir S: Follow-up of a human larynx transplantation. Laryngoscope, 80:1244, 1970

18. Tucker, HM: Laryngeal transplantation: Current status 1974. Laryngoscope, 85:787–796, 1975

19. Young JL Jr, Percy CL, Asire AJ (Eds): Surveillance, epidemiology, and end results: incidence and mortality data, 1973–77. NCI Monograph 57, NIH, PHS, DHEW Publication #(NIH) 81-2330, 1981

20. Silverberg E: Cancer statistics, 1983. CA, 33:9–25, 1983

21. Jones GD, Gabriel CE: The incidence of carcinoma of the larynx in persons under twenty years of age. Laryngoscope, 79:251, 1969

22. Iwamoto H: An epidemiological study of laryngeal cancer in Japan (1960–1969). Laryngoscope, 85:1162, 1975

23. Kahn HA: The Dorn study of smoking and mortality among US veterans: Report on eight and one-half years of observation. NCI Monograph 19. Bethesda, MD, Public Health Service, 1966

24. Krajina Z, Kulcar Z, Konic-Carnelutti V: Epidemiology of laryngeal cancer. Laryngoscope, 85:1155, 1975

25. Bernfeld, P, Hamburger F, Soto E, Pai KJ: Cigarette smoke inhalation studies in in-bred Syrian golden hamsters, JNCI, 63:669–6675, 1979

26. Hiranandani LH: Panel on epidemiology and etiology of laryngeal carcinoma. Laryngoscope, 85:1197, 1975

27. Moore C: Cigarette smoking and cancer of the mouth, pharynx, and larynx: A continuous study. JAMA, 218:553–558, 1971

28. Vaughn CW, Strong MSS: Benign lesions of the larynx. In English GM (Ed): Otolaryngology, vol 5. Philadelphia, Harper & Row, 1983

29. Keller AZ: Cirrhosis of the liver, alcoholism and heavy smoking associated with cancer of the mouth and pharynx. Cancer, 20:1013–1022, 1967

30. Wynder EL, Covey LS, Mabuchi K, Mushinski M: Environmental factors in cancer of the larynx: A second look. Cancer, 38:1591–1601, 1976

31. Goolden AWG: Radiation cancer of the pharynx. Br Med J, 2:1110, 1951

32. Rabbett WF: Juvenile laryngeal papillomatosis: The relationship of irradiation to malignant degeneration in this disease. Ann Otol Rhinol Laryngol, 74:1149, 1965

33. Lawson, W, Som M: Second primary cancer after irradiation of laryngeal cancer. Ann Otol Rhinol Laryngol, 84:771, 1975

34. Stell PM, McGill T: Asbestos and laryngeal carcinoma. Lancet, 2:416, 1973

35. Morgan RW, Shettigara PT: Occupational asbestos exposure, smoking, and laryngeal carcinoma. Ann NY Acad Sci, 271:308, 1976

36. McGavran MH, Bauer WC, Ogura JH: Isolated laryngeal keratosis: Its relation to carcinoma of the larynx based on a clinicopathologic study of 87 consecutive cases with long term follow-up. Laryngoscope, 70:932–951, 1960

37. Hellquist H, Lundgren J, Olagsson V: Hyperplasia, keratosis, dysplasia, and carcinoma-in-situ of the vocal cords. A follow-up study. Clin Otolaryngol, 7:11–27, 1982

38. Norris CM, Peale AR: Keratosis of the larynx. J Laryngol Otol, 77:635, 1963

39. Putney FJ, O'Keefe JJ: The clinical significance of keratosis of the larynx as a premalignant lesion. Ann Otol Rhinol Laryngol, 62:348, 1953

40. Auerbach O, Hammond EC, Garfinkel L: Histologic changes in the larynx in relation to smoking habits. Cancer, 25:92, 1970

41. Batsakis JG: Tumors of the Head and Neck: Clinical and Pathological Considerations. Baltimore, Williams & Wilkins, 1974

42. Henry RC: The transformation of laryngeal leukoplakia to cancer. J Laryngol Otol, 93:447, 1979

43. Som ML: Surgery in premalignant lesions. In Alberti PW, Bryce DP (Eds): Workshops for the Centennial Conference on Cancer of the Larynx. New York, Appleton-Century-Crofts, 1976, p 145

44. McGavran MH, Stutsman MD, Ogura JH: In Alberti PW, Bryce DP (Eds): Workshops for the Centennial Conference on Cancer of the Larynx. New York, Appleton-Century-Crofts, 1976, p 151

45. Pressman JJ: Submucosal compartmentalization of the larynx. Ann Otol Rhinol Laryngol, 65:766, 1956

46. Tucker GF, Smith HR: A histological demonstration of the development of laryngeal connective tissue compartments. Trans Am Acad Opthalmol Otolaryngol, 66:308, 1962

47. McGavran M, Bauer W, Ogura JH: The incidence of cervical lymph node metastases from epidermoid carcinoma of the larynx and their relationship to certain characteristics of the primary tumor. Cancer, 14:55, 1961

48. Kirchner J, Som ML: Clinical and histological observations on supraglottic cancer. Ann Otol Rhinol Laryngol, 80:638, 1971

49. Shah JP, Tollefsen JR: Epidermoid carcinoma of the supraglottic larynx. Role of neck dissection in initial surgical treatment. Am J Surg, 128:494, 1974

50. Thawley, SE, Ogura, JH: Conservation laryngeal surgery and radical neck dissection. In English GE (Ed): Otolaryngology, vol 5. Philadelphia, Harper & Row, 1984

51. American Joint Committee for Cancer Staging and End Results Reporting: Manual for Staging of Cancer. 1977

52. Fisher, JR: Verrucous carcinoma of the larynx—A study of its pathological anatomy. In Alberti PW, Bryce DP (Eds): Workshops from the Centennial Conference on Laryngeal Cancer, New York, Appleton-Century-Crofts, 1976

53. Biller, HF, Bergman JA: Verrucous carcinoma of the larynx. Laryngoscope, 85:1698, 1975

54. Ackerman LV: Verrucous carcinoma of the oral cavity. Surgery, 23:670, 1948

55. Kraus F, Perez-Mesa C: Verrucous carcinoma: Clinical and pathological study of 105 cases involving oral cavity, larynx and genitalia. Cancer, 19:26, 1966

56. Van Nostrand AWP, Olofsson J: Verrucous carcinoma of the larynx. A clinical and pathologic study of 10 cases. Cancer, 30:691, 1972

57. Brodsky G: Carcino(pseudo)sarcoma of the larynx: The controversy continues. Otol Clin North Am, 17:185–197, 1984

58. Hyams VJ: Spindle cell carcinoma of the larynx. Can J Otolaryngol, 4:307–313, 1975

59. Sessions DG, Murray JP, BAuer WC, et al: Adenocarcinoma of the larynx. in Alberti PW, Bryce DP (Eds): Workshops from the Centennial Conference on Laryngeal Cancer. New York, Appleton-Century-Crofts, 1976

60. Fechner RE: Adenocarcinoma of the larynx. In Alberti PW, Bryce DP (Eds): Workshops from the Centennial Conference on Laryngeal Cancer. New York, Appleton-Century-Crofts, 1976

61. Hyams VJ, Rabuzzi DD: Cartilaginous tumors of the larynx. Laryngoscope, 80:755–767, 1970

62. Lavertu P, Tucker HM: Chondrosarcoma of the larynx: Case report and management philosophy. Ann Otol Rhinol Laryngol, 93:452–456, 1984

63. Hooley R, Levine HL, Flores TC, Wheeler T, Steiger E: Predicting postoperative head and neck complications utilizing nutritional assessment. (The prognostic nutritional index). Arch Otolaryngol, 109:83–85, 1983

64. Gluckman JL, Crissman JD: Survival rates in 548 patients with multiple neoplasms of the upper aerodigestive tract. Laryngoscope, 33:71, 1983

65. Strong MS: Laser management of premalignant lesions of the larynx. in Alberti PW, Bryce DP (Eds): Workshops from the Centennial Conference on Laryngeal Cancer. New York, Appleton-Century-Crofts, 1976

66. Stutsman AC, McGavran MH: Ultraconservative management of superficially invasive epidermoid carcinoma of the true vocal cord. Ann Otol Rhinol Laryngol, 80:507–512, 1971

67. DeSanto LW: Selection of treatment for in situ and early invasive carcinoma of the glottis. In Alberti PW, Bryce DP (Eds): Workshops from the Centennial Conference on Laryngeal Cancer. New York, Appleton-Century-Crofts, 1976

68. Tucker HM: Surgery for Phonatory Disorders. New York, Churchill Livingstone, 1981

69. Wang CC: Treatment of glottic carcinoma by megavoltage radiation therapy and results. Am J Roentgenol Rad Ther Nucl Med, 120:157, 1974

70. Constable WC, White RL, El-Mahdi AM, Fitz-Hugh GS: Radiotherapeutic management of cancer of the glottis, University of Virginia, 1956–1971. Laryngoscope, 85:1494, 1975

71. Fletcher GH, Lindberg RD, Hamberger A, Horiot JC: Reasons for irradiation failure in squamous cell carcinoma of the larynx. Laryngoscope, 85:987, 1975

72. Hawkins NV: The treatment of glottic carcinoma: An analysis of 800 cases. Laryngoscope, 85:1485, 1975

73. Lawson W, Biller HF: Cancer of the larynx. In Suen JY, Myers EN (Eds): Cancer of the Head and Neck. New York, Churchill Livingstone, 1981

74. Ballantyne AJ, Fletcher GH: Surgical management of radiation failures of non-fixed cancers of the glottic region. Am J Roentgenol Rad Ther Nucl Med, 120:164, 1974

75. Ogura JH, Sessions DG, Spector GJ: Analysis of surgical therapy for epidermoid

carcinoma of the laryngeal glottis. Laryngoscope, 85:1522, 1975

76. Hendrickson FR, Kline TC,Jr, Hibbs GG: Primary squamous cell carcinoma of the larynx. Laryngoscope, 85:1650, 1975

77. Tucker HM, Wood BG, Levine H, Katz R: Glottic reconstruction after near-total laryngectomy. Laryngoscope, 89:609, 1979

78. Kirchner JA, Som ML: Clinical significance of fixed vocal cord. Laryngoscope, 81:1029, 1971

79. Som ML: Cordal cancer with extension to vocal process. Laryngoscope, 85:1298, 1975

80. Jesse RH: I. The evaluation of treatment of patients with extensive squamous cell cancer of the vocal cords. Laryngoscope, 85:1424, 1975

81. Fletcher GH: Elective irradiation of subclinical disease in cancers of the head and neck. Cancer, 29:1450, 1972

82. Bryce DP, Hawkins NV: Primary radiotherapy for supraglottic laryngeal cancer. In Snow JB (Ed): Controversy in Otolaryngology, Philadelphia, WB Saunders 1980

83. Strong MS: The case for combined radiation therapy and surgery for supraglottic carcinoma. In Snow JB (Ed): Controversy in Otolaryngology. Philadelphia, WB Saunders, 1980

84. Sessions DG, Ogura JH: Classification of laryngeal cancer. In Alberti PW, Bryce DP (Eds): Workshops from the Centennial Conference on Laryngeal Cancer, Appleton-Century Crofts, New York, 1975

85. Coates HL, DeSanto LW, Devine KD, Elveback LA: Carcinoma of the supraglottic larynx. A review of 221 cases. Arch Otolaryngol, 102:686, 1976

86. Som ML: Conservation surgery for carcinoma of the supraglottis. J Laryngol Otol, 84:655, 1970

87. Schuller DE, Platz CE, Krause CJ: Spinal accessory lymph nodes: A prospective study of metastatic involvement. Laryngoscope, 88:439, 1978

88. Bocca E: Conservative neck dissection. Laryngoscope, 85:1511, 1975

89. Suen JY, Wetmore SJ: Cancer of the neck. In Suen JY, Wetmore SJ (Eds): Cancer of the Head and Neck. New York, Churchill Livingstone, 1981

90. Harrison DFN: The pathology and management of subglottic cancer. Ann Otol Rhinol Laryngol, 80:6, 1971

91. Ogura JH, Biller H: Conservation surgery in cancer of the head and neck. Otolaryngol Clin North Am, 2:641, 1969

92. Quinn JH: Free muscle transplant method of glottic reconstruction after hemilaryngectomy. Laryngoscope, 85:985, 1975

93. Bailey BJ: Glottic reconstruction after hemilaryngectomy: Bipedical muscle flap laryngoplasty. Laryngoscope, 85:960, 1975

94. Ogura JH, Biller H: Glottic reconstruction following extended frontolateral hemilaryngectomy. Laryngoscope, 79:2181, 1969

95. Som ML, Silver CE: The anterior commissure technique of partial laryngectomy. Arch Otolaryngol, 87:42, 1968

96. Schechter GL: Epiglottic reconstruction and subtotal laryngectomy. Laryngoscope, 93:729–734, 1983

97. Sessions DG, Ogura JH, Ciralsky RH: Late glottic insufficiency. Laryngoscope, 85:950, 1975

98. Flores TC, Levine HL, Wood BG, Tucker HM: Factors in successful deglutition following subtotal laryngeal surgery. Ann Otol Rhinol Laryngol, 91:579–583, 1982

99. Tucker HM: Conservation laryngeal surgery in the elderly patient. Laryngoscope, 87:1995, 1977

100. Wood BG, Tucker HM, Levine HL: Regional flap reconstruction during extended supraglottic laryngectomy/partial laryngopharyngectomy. Laryngoscope, 95: 1985

101. Tucker HM, Sobol SM, Levine HL, Wood BJ: Transverse cervical trapezius myocutaneous island flap. Arch Otolaryngol, 108:194–198, 1982

102. Schoenfeld DA: An estimate of the survival benefit of chemotherapy for advanced head and neck cancer and its implications to the design of clinical trials in Chretien, Betal P (Ed): Head and Neck Cancer, vol 1. Philadelphia, BC Decker, 1985, pp 78–83

103. Seeman M: Speech and voice without a larynx. Cus Lek Cesk, 41:369–373, 1922

104. Shipp T: Frequency, duration and perceptual measures in relation to judgments of alaryngeal speech acceptability. J Speech Hear Res, 10:417–427, 1967

105. Singer MI, Blom ED: Selective myotomy for voice restoration after total laryngectomy. Arch Otolaryngol, 107:670–673, 1981

106. Snidecor JC: Speech rehabilitation of the laryngectomized. Springfield, IL, Charles C. Thomas, 1962.

107. Diedrich WH, Youngstrom KA: Alaryngeal Speech. Springfield, IL, Charles C. Thomas, 1966

108. Gardner WH; Laryngectomy Speech and Rehabilitation. Springfield, IL, Charles C. Thomas, 1971

109. Dugeray MJ: Special problems of the alaryngeal speaker. In Keith RL, Darley FL (Eds): Laryngectomee Rehabilitation. Houston, TX, College-Hill Press, 1979

110. Dworkin JP, Sparker A: Surgical vocal rehabilitation following total laryngectomy: A state-of-the-art report. Clin Otolaryngol, 5:339–350, 1980

111. Singer MI: Tracheoesophageal speech: vocal rehabilitation after total laryngectomy. Laryngoscope, 93:1454–1464, 1983

112. Singer MI, Blom ED: An endoscopic technique for restoration of voice after laryngectomy. Ann Otolaryngol, 89(6):529–533, 1980

113. Hamaker RC, Singer MI, Blom ED, Daniels HA: Primary voice restoration at laryngectomy. Arch Otolaryngol, 111:182–187, 1985

114. Maves MD, Lingeman RE: Primary vocal rehabilitation using the Blom-Singer and Panje voice prostheses. Ann Otol Rhinol Laryngol, 91:458–460, 1982

115. Panje WR: Prosthetic vocal rehabilitation following laryngectomy: The voice button. Ann Otol Rhinol Laryngol, 90:116–119, 1981

116. Blom ED, Singer MI, Harkleroad BA: Self-activated pneumatic voicing system for ventilator dependent patients. Presented at the American Speech and Hearing Association Annual Convention, Toronto, 1982

117. Singer MI, et al: Further experience with voice restoration after total laryngectomy. Ann Otolaryngol, 90 (5):498–502, 1981

118. Wetmore SJ, et al: The Singer-Blom voice restoration procedure. Arch Otolaryngol, 107:674–678, 1981

119. Wetmore SJ, Krueger K, Wesson K: The Singer-Blom speech rehabilitation procedure. Laryngoscope, 91:101–117, 1981

120. Wood B, Rusnov M, Levine H, Tucker H: Tracheoesophageal puncture for alaryngeal voice restoration. Ann Otol Rhinol Laryngol, 90:492–494, 1981

Index